To Elizabeth Herrera

HOUSTON HEARTS

5/23/2014

For "Hearty" Reading

Wz Winters Jr.

HOUSTON HEARTS

A History Of Cardiovascular Surgery And Medicine

AND

The Methodist DeBakey Heart & Vascular Center

Houston Methodist Hospital

William L. Winters Jr., MD, MACC

With

Betsy Parish

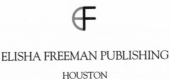

ELISHA FREEMAN PUBLISHING

HOUSTON

FIRST EDITION: MAY 2014.
Designed by Peter Layne.
Printed on acid-free paper.

Library of Congress Control Number: 2013946734

HOUSTON HEARTS ISBN: 978-0-9786200-8-0

ELISHA FREEMAN PUBLISHING

Unless otherwise noted, photographs are courtesy of William L. Winters Jr., MD, MACC.

The graphics on the cover of Houston Hearts and throughout the book were inspired by the design of the Houston Methodist Hospital George P. Noon, MD, Award.

Houston Hearts is dedicated to the genius of
Dr. Michael Ellis DeBakey.

CONTENTS

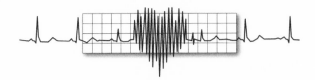

PREFACE

William L. Winters Jr., MD, MACC

The saga of cardiovascular surgery and medicine at The Methodist Hospital and Baylor College Of Medicine in Houston, Texas, began in 1944 with the arrival of Dr. Don W. Chapman, an Iowan trained in the specialty of cardiology. He joined the Department of Medicine at Baylor University College of Medicine as one of its first instructors.

Four years later, in 1948, Dr. Michael E. DeBakey was persuaded to leave Ochsner Clinic in New Orleans to become chairman of the fledgling Department of Surgery at Baylor University College of Medicine. For The Methodist Hospital, these two men formed the cornerstone of what was to become, over the next five decades, a highly respected and innovative cardiovascular surgical program with repercussions worldwide and, later, a premier cardiology department highly regarded for its clinical care, clinical training programs, basic science, and clinical research endeavors.

The story divides comfortably into three general periods. The first, from 1908 to the early 1940s, describes the formative period of The Methodist Hospital. The second, from the 1940s to the 1980s, is saturated with the surgical exploits of Dr. DeBakey and his surgical colleagues. Their counterparts, the cardiologists, played basically a necessary supporting role in those days for reasons that will become clear as this story of *Houston Hearts* unfolds.

In the third period, commencing in the 1970s with the arrival of Dr. Henry McIntosh to become chairman of the Department of Medicine at Baylor College of Medicine and The Methodist Hospital and later Drs. Antonio Gotto and Robert Roberts, the role of cardiology began to change rapidly and has continued to evolve for more than 40 years. Early on, the surgeons were the "doers," refining operations and techniques for circulatory support while repairing congenital heart defects, acquired valvular heart defects, and restoring coronary and other arterial circulations.

As drug therapy developed, imaging capabilities advanced, and catheter interventions evolved, cardiologists continued not only their supporting role but also became "doers" as well, particularly in the realm of coronary artery disease, valvular disease, and some forms of congenital heart disease. Their role has expanded from diagnostic procedures and medical therapy to that of therapeutic interventionalists.

Along the way, the distinction between cardiologists and cardiovascular surgeons started to blur. They now may work side by side in "hybrid rooms" that combine a catheterization laboratory and an operating room. One day not far away, I expect to see a single cardiovascular department replacing the traditional cardiology and cardiovascular surgery eponyms.

In essence, the evolution in the diagnosis and treatment of cardiovascular disease at The Methodist Hospital and Baylor College Of Medicine is a microcosm of the same scenario that has occurred on a national and international scale—the difference being that much of the innovation occurred right here in The Methodist Hospital, known as Houston Methodist Hospital since July 2013.

It has been an exciting time. I have had the pleasure and luxury of witnessing and working closely with all of the individuals described in this account. I hope you will absorb some of the excitement I have experienced along the way.

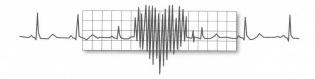

FOREWORD

William C. Roberts, MD, MACC

When Dr. William L. Winters Jr. calls and makes a request, it is very difficult to say "no." "Would you be willing to review my book?" "I would be honored," I replied, not realizing that in a few days a 607-page manuscript by he and Betsy Parish would be received. After reading only a few pages I realized that I had been given the privilege of reviewing a masterpiece. It was difficult to put down, and also for me difficult to review because the quantity of detailed information was enormous.

The book actually began in the early years of the 20th century when Dr. Winters began conducting video interviews, eventually numbering over 70, with long-standing members of The Methodist Hospital (TMH) staff to record the extraordinary changes that had taken place, particularly in cardiovascular disease, in the previous 60 years. Not long after starting the interviews Dr. Winters suggested to Ms. Betsy Parish, a longtime friend and patient of his, who had just finished writing *Legacy, 50 Years of Loving Care at Texas Children's Hospital 1954- 2004,* to collaborate with him on a history of cardiovascular medicine and surgery at TMH in Houston. She obviously agreed.

The product is a magnificent story. The book is divided into 20 chapters with an appropriate quote under each chapter title and what they call a "Blip"— mini-story—at the end of each chapter, followed by numerous "Endnotes" or references documenting their many sources –the interviews, Dr. Winters' inside 40-year recollections of the events, newspaper and magazine accounts, and medical publications. The book ends with an Epilogue by Dr. Winters in which he details the accomplishments of TMH since its tumultuous rupture in 2004 of its 50-year relationship with Baylor College of Medicine (BCM). And following the epilogue is "Reflections From Two Principals," personal recollections from Drs. Gotto and Noon, and a collection of poems penned seemingly effortlessly by Dr. Winters. This section is entitled "Addendum for Rhyme and Reason" and includes "Odes" to Antonio M. Gotto Jr., to William Zoghbi, to Don and Mary Louise Chapman, to Miguel Quiñones, to Jimmy Howell, to Richard Wainerdi, and to Michael E. DeBakey, plus one entitled "Healthcare Reform – A political plea." A detailed timeline of events effecting TMH also is included near the end of the book.

The star of the book and deservedly so is Michael E. DeBakey, who came to Houston in 1948, as chairman of the Department of Surgery of Baylor University College of Medicine (BUCM – later the "University" was dropped) which had moved from Dallas only 5 years earlier. On arrival, he had no hospital in which to operate but the visionary man from Lake Charles (initially) saw the potential. He was instrumental in rapidly setting up an affiliation of BUCM with the VA Hospital (years later to be named the Michael E. DeBakey VA Hospital), the Jefferson Davis Hospital, and beginning in1950, TMH, where he eventually limited his practice. In 1963, the Ben Taub General Hospital opened and also affiliated with BUCM. His surgical innovations and unique skills, his multiple publications (eventually totaling >1200) and presentations rapidly attracted patients from the world over and as the patients increased, Mr. Ted Bowen, TMH's dynamic president, increased the facilities accordingly – from 300 to eventually >1500 beds. It was not long before Dr. DeBakey attracted many talented associates including Oscar Creech Jr. (1949), Denton A. Cooley (1951), E. Stanley Crawford (1954), George C. Morris, Arthur C. Beall Jr., H. Edward Garrett, Jimmy F. Howell, Gerald Lawrie, George Noon, among others, and Dr. DeBakey gave them space to shine. For many years Dr. DeBakey daily averaged 100 patients on his hospital service and in 1965, an additional 100 other patients were waiting outside to get a bed. He would tell the cardiologists that he had gotten the patient out of the operating room and now it was their task to get the patient out of the hospital.

As his reputation grew, not only as an innovative and skilled surgeon but also as a major researcher, Dr. DeBakey expanded his national and international responsibilities. He became the US's top proponent for expanded cardiovascular research advising congressional committees, the National Heart Institute, and Mrs. Mary Lasker's initiatives among others. He traveled worldwide extensively giving presentations, receiving rewards (He eventually received 32 honorary degrees and the Congressional Gold Medal, the highest reward available to a US civilian), and consulting with prominent citizens and government leaders. Additionally, Dr. DeBakey was chairman of BCM's Department of Surgery for 40 years, and also either president or chancellor of BCM for 20 more years!

Although cardiovascular surgery drew the most attention at TMH in the 1950s and 1960s, the huge number of cardiovascular surgery patients at TMH led to a major expansion in the number of cardiologists, both fulltime at BUCM and also in the private realm (Volunteer faculty). Dr. Don Chapman, the first cardiologist in Houston and the first to perform a cardiac catheterization in Houston, started "The Chapman Group" in 1955 at TMH and Dr. Chapman became the "preeminent practicing cardiologist in Houston." At the same time, Dr. Edward W. Dennis, a cousin of mine by marriage, became the first full-time BUCM cardiologist at TMH and remained so until his untimely death in 1975 at age 52. At that time, his colleagues included Sam Kinard, Ben McCall, John Lancaster, and Manus O'Donnell.

The book describes in exquisite detail the development of cardiology at TMH and the town-gown relations that ensued. When coronary bypass became a successful procedure in the late 1960s, the number of patients further increased, the need for more cardiologists and cardiac catheterization laboratories expanded, and then when coronary angioplasty was introduced in the late 1970s further expansion was required. The hospital president Mr. Ted Bowen, also a visionary, did all he could to expand TMH facilities adequately to accommodate the additional onrush of patients.

Dr. DeBakey as BCM President and Chief Executive Officer beginning in 1969 worked among other endeavors to strengthen the non-surgical departments. Dr. Henry D. McIntosh in 1970, became chairman of the department of medicine and during his "tumultuous" 7-year reign a number of subsequently prominent cardiologists were recruited, including Dr. Antonio M. Gotto Jr., who later succeeded him as departmental chairman; Albert E. Raizner, who later headed the cardiac catheterization laboratories and was the instigator behind the Methodist DeBakey Heart Center, which unified all cardiovascular services; Miguel Quiñones, Mario S. Verani, Craig M. Pratt, James B. Young, William A. Zoghbi, Neal S. Kleiman and later Richard Miller, Douglas L. Morris, and Christie M. Ballantyne, to name a few. Simultaneously, The Chapman Group expanded to include H. Liston Beazley, Paul Peterson, Richard Cashion, William H. Spencer, and William L. Winters Jr., beginning in1968.

As each new "instrument of precision" was introduced—echocardiography, nuclear cardiology, computed tomography, magnetic resonance imaging, invasive procedures—the relations between the BCM faculty and the private practitioners at TMH had to be worked out. The different chairmen of the department of medicine had differing views on what constituted the best relationships between the town and gown cardiologists.

When coronary angioplasty entered the scene in the early 1980s at TMH the cardiac catheterization laboratories, as elsewhere, were converted from a purely diagnostic to a therapeutic laboratory as well, and this change altered for a spell the relations between the cardiovascular surgeons and the cardiologists. Interestingly, Dr. DeBakey was a strong supporter of percutaneous coronary intervention from the beginning.

During all the while, TMH kept growing through the efforts of its fine leaders – Ted Bowen, Larry Mathias, Peter Butler, and Ron Girotto. The damage ensued by Tropical Storm Allison in 2001 was a game changer in many ways. The major game changer, however, occurred in 2004 when the Baylor College of Medicine (BCM), and TMH ended their 50-year affiliation. Nearly all of the TMH cardiology staff stayed with the hospital and resigned from Baylor College of Medicine. Mr. Ron Girotto vowed to make TMH "an academic hospital" unassociated with a local medical school. Another wave of expansion occurred. By 2012, TMH was listed in the *U.S. News & World Report* as the number 1 hospital in Texas; as one of the best hospitals in 12 specialties, and named one of the top 15 major teaching hospitals in the USA. The TMH was listed as among the 100 best companies to work for 7 years in a row by *Fortune* Magazine, and one of the best places to work by *Forbes*. Mr. Girotto established ICARE (Integrity, Compassion, Accountability, Respect, and Excellence) to instill these values in every employee. As a consequence hospital turnover and vacancy rates dropped, and patient and employee/ physician satisfaction grew to the highest in its history.

And its physicians kept gaining prominence. Dr. Antonio Gotto served one year as president of the American Heart Association, and three other TMH physicians have each been president of the American College of Cardiology (Henry D. McIntosh, William L. Winters Jr., and William Zoghbi). As the years went by Drs. Chapman and Winters and many other TMH cardiologists received many local, national and international awards from many organizations.

This book presents a remarkable and inspiring story of how physicians and hospital administrators by working together can produce an awe inspiring institution.

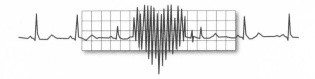

CHAPTER ONE

PERSEVERANCE
1948

"It does not matter how slowly you go, as long as you don't stop."
CONFUCIUS

Dedication ceremonies for the Methodist DeBakey Heart Center took place February 19, 2001, at The Methodist Hospital in Houston, Texas. It was to be renamed the Methodist DeBakey Heart & Vascular Center in 2008.

Established to honor medical pioneer and cardiovascular surgeon Dr. Michael Ellis DeBakey, the former heart surgery center at The Methodist Hospital comprised 10 operating rooms, eight catheterization labs, 154 acute care beds, and 30 beds for transplant candidates. More than 1,300 open-heart operations, 2,500 angioplasties, and 6,000 catheterizations were performed there each year. In its previous decade, more than 425 heart transplants were completed.

Although the Methodist DeBakey Heart Center was newly created in 2001, Dr. DeBakey's name and that of The Methodist Hospital had been inextricably linked for more than 52 years. It had been a symbiotic relationship, initially established shortly after the surgeon's 1948 arrival in Houston and nurtured for more than six decades. To many, their names became synonymous. This legendary pairing almost never had the opportunity to occur. Were it not for a set of extraordinary circumstances, which some even attribute to kismet, Dr. DeBakey's countless contributions to the field of cardiovascular surgery would not have taken place at The Methodist Hospital, or in Houston.

There was no certainty that Dr. DeBakey's career path would lead him to Houston. By the late 1940s, the Louisiana-born son of highly intelligent and successful Lebanese immigrants already had established himself as an exacting surgeon as well as a dedicated researcher and prolific writer. His was a career filled with accomplishments. He had authored or coauthored more than 100 articles in peer-reviewed journals; coauthored two books on surgery; served five years in the U.S. military as a surgical consultant in the U.S. Army Surgeon General's office in Washington, D.C.; and coauthored a detailed overview of the vascular injuries acquired during the fighting in World War II.[1,2] In 1948, at the age of 39, Dr. DeBakey was poised to continue his stellar career in New Orleans, where he was an associate professor of surgery at Tulane University School of Medicine.

The primary catalyst for inspiring Dr. DeBakey's coming to Houston was the relocation of Baylor University College of Medicine from Dallas. Invited by the M.D. Anderson Foundation to join the newly formed Texas Medical Center, the college opened in Houston on July 12, 1943, in a converted Sears, Roebuck & Co. building. Four years later, the college moved into its present site in the Roy and Lillie Cullen Building, the first building completed in the new Texas Medical Center.

It was in this new building that the college's dean, Dr. Walter H. Moursund, along with key members of the Houston Executive Committee of the Baylor University Board of Trustees, first began to contemplate the hiring of the college's first fulltime professor of surgery to serve as chairman of the Department of Surgery. Heretofore, the chairmanship was held by a Houston physician and volunteer faculty member, beginning with Dr. Judson L. Taylor in1943 and followed by Dr. H.F. Poyner, who assumed the position after Dr. Taylor's death in 1944.

While the particulars regarding the selection of Dr. DeBakey as the prime candidate for this position are not known, a participant at the April 1948 opening ceremonies for the Cullen Building in the Texas Medical Center no doubt played a major role in the preliminary process. It was guest speaker and Tulane University School of Medicine Professor of Surgery Dr. Alton J. Ochsner, who also served as a consultant to the Texas Medical Center.

In his presentation during the opening ceremonies, Dr. Ochsner addressed how "the increased incidence of the condition of primary bronchiogenic carcinoma parallels the increased frequency of smoking, and this probably is of etiologic importance," a finding he had published in a 1945 report.[3] One of the coauthors of that report was his protégé, Dr. DeBakey.

By 1948, their mentor-protégé collaboration at Tulane had spanned almost two decades. True to Dr. Ochsner's oft-repeated saying, "Early to bed, early to rise, work hard and publicize,"[4] together they had studied and published more than 71 reports on amebic hepatic abscess; subphrenic abscess; bezoars; venous thrombosis; and cancer of the lung, esophagus, and stomach, including the landmark publication that first linked smoking to lung cancer, "Primary Pulmonary Malignancy," in the February 1939 issue of *Surgery, Gynecology and Obstetrics*.[5]

In addition to these publishing efforts, Dr. Ochsner often invited Dr. DeBakey to accompany him to national medical association meetings where he introduced him to his peers, arguably the nation's most prominent physicians at that time. In addition to facilitating Dr. DeBakey's access to some of the most exclusive, established medical circles, Dr. Ochsner also included his young protégé in many of his new ventures. When the Society for Vascular Surgeons was founded in 1946, two of its nine founding members were Dr. Ochsner and Dr. DeBakey, who, at the age of 36, was the youngest of the group.

The two surgeons first met when Dr. DeBakey was a student at Tulane University School of Medicine. Dr. DeBakey attended Tulane University throughout his undergraduate and graduate education, receiving a bachelor's of science degree in 1930, followed by a medical degree in 1932, and a master's of science degree in 1935 from that university's school of medicine. From 1932 to 1933, he served as an intern at the Charity Hospital of New Orleans, where he also served for three additional years as a resident and instructor in surgery, all under the mentorship of Dr. Ochsner. "I became a surgeon because I had the greatest respect, admiration, and affection for Dr. Ochsner and because he invited me to enter the field and to work with him," Dr. DeBakey explained. "It was one of the greatest privileges of my life."[6]

The genesis of this mentor-protégé relationship took place during Dr. DeBakey's sophomore year in medical school when he worked as an assistant technician in the laboratory of another member of the medical faculty. "In my junior year, Dr. Ochsner sought me out, and in my senior year I worked in his lab," Dr. DeBakey recalled.[7] "As a medical student working in Dr. Ochsner's laboratory, I published my first professional article,[8] and thereafter we coauthored many publications on a variety of surgical subjects on which we were working. From him I learned the importance of bibliographic research, meticulous abstracting of publications, verification of data and references, and careful writing and documentation. It was a lesson that became a lifelong habit."[6]

Also attributed to Dr. Ochsner's inspiration were the two years, 1935 to 1937, Dr. DeBakey devoted to studying in Europe, then known as "the ultimate training ground" for many great U.S. surgeons including Dr. Ochsner.[7] At the suggestion of Dr. Rudolph Matas, the recognized American pioneer in vascular surgery and Dr. Ochsner's predecessor at Tulane, Dr. DeBakey studied in

Strasbourg, France, with Professor René Leriche, considered to be the world's most advanced surgeon in vascular surgery at the time. The next year, he studied with Professor Martin Kirschner, the renowned pioneer and gastroenterology surgeon who performed the first pulmonary embolectomy at the University of Heidelberg in Germany.[9] Already fluent in French, Dr. DeBakey had to learn German while in Heidelberg, becoming fluent within one year.

This ability to excel in conquering the unknown had been demonstrated during medical school. Before his European studies, while working as a technician in the research laboratory, Dr. DeBakey was asked by another faculty member to see if he could find a pump that could modify the pulse wave. Unable to find the kind of pump requested and realizing he knew nothing about pumps in general, Dr. DeBakey decided the only place to do research was at the Tulane School of Engineering Library, where he spent days reading about the history of pumps. It was an exercise that left him both fascinated and inspired. Upon learning about the initial uses of rubber tubing in the early 19th century, he got the idea that compressing a rubber tube to force fluid out might be the type of pump the faculty member needed. "After experimenting different ways to do this for several years, I developed the pump for him," Dr. DeBakey said. "If you roll that pump when you have fluid in it, the outlet tube will create a pressure. If you compress the tube, the pressure will go right up. So when you compress the tube and then release it, it will create a wave. Depending on how much pressure you create and how quickly you release it, the wave can be modified. That was what it was for."[7,10]

Or so he thought. It wasn't until he became a medical resident several years later that he realized his pump invention could also be used to expedite blood transfusions. Instead of placing the blood from the donor in a paraffin-coated glass, as before, the now-patented DeBakey Roller Pump could be used to transfer the blood directly from the donor to the patient. In response to physicians' requests, he would perform transfusions in several hospitals in New Orleans because he was the only one who had the device. "I must have used the roller pump on a couple of thousand patients for transfusions," he said. "This made me the 'expert.' I would go all around town giving blood transfusions with my pump. Of course, once we had blood banks, we no longer needed the pump, but it served its purpose."[7]

Although its original purpose was obsolesced by technological advances in the 1930s, the patented DeBakey Roller Pump was to become an integral component of a historic device that evolved two decades later. At the suggestion of Dr. DeBakey, Dr. John Gibbon incorporated the device into the heart-lung machine, the heralded invention that made possible the first successful open-heart operations in 1953.[10] In published reports, Dr. Gibbon credited Dr. DeBakey with his roller-pump contribution.[11] Reflecting on this accomplishment decades later, Dr. DeBakey said, "At the time I developed it, I had no idea that it would one day be used for that purpose."[12]

This admitted inability to foresee the future was also applicable to Dr. DeBakey's vision of his career path in 1937. Returning to New Orleans after his studies in Europe, Dr. DeBakey joined Dr. Ochsner on the faculty at Tulane University School of Medicine. He was "delighted to have the job as a full-time instructor in the Department of Surgery,"[7] as was his mentor, and both were anxious to continue their collaborative efforts indefinitely. "He loved to write and loved to do research," Dr. Ochsner said, recalling those years at Tulane together. "He didn't have much desire to operate except just to become proficient in doing an operation. After he had become proficient in doing an operation, he didn't have much desire in operating any more. But he was particularly desirous of doing research and writing."[13]

It was this dedication to research and writing that Dr. DeBakey credited as being instrumental in his successful American Board of Surgery Certification in 1938. When examiners Drs. Fred Rankin and Harvey B. Stone, both recognized as top leaders in American surgery, began to question him about subphrenic abscesses, Dr. Rankin suddenly interrupted the process. Instead of proceeding with the oral exam, Dr. Rankin told Dr. Stone the applicant knew more about the subject than they did, citing the recently published article "Subphrenic Abscess,"[14] written by Drs. Ochsner and DeBakey, in which they had reported on their own personal experience with 25 cases and presented a systematic review of 3,608 collected cases from world publications.[15] This experience culminated several months later in Dr. DeBakey's becoming the 172nd board-certified surgeon in the United States.

Reflecting on that memorable occasion six decades later, Dr. DeBakey said, "My own conviction is that critical bibliographic reviews, well-designed research, and participation in the preparation of manuscripts for publication during surgical training not only enhance professional maturation, but also contribute significantly to a rewarding and fulfilling career."[15]

The rewarding Tulane career Dr. DeBakey had envisioned in 1938 took an abrupt detour when World War II broke out in 1941. Like many of his colleagues, even though declared "essential" by Tulane University School of Medicine, he volunteered for the Army Medical Services. Learning of his enlistment, Dr. Rankin, who was then a colonel in the Army Medical Corps and chief consultant in surgery to the Army Surgeon General, requested Dr. DeBakey's transfer to the Surgical Consultants Division in the Office of the Surgeon General. During the next five war years, Lt. Col. DeBakey eventually rose to the level of colonel, becoming director of the Surgical Consultants Division in 1945.

Throughout his service in the U.S. Army, the conscientious surgeon capitalized on the traits with which he already had excelled in the field of medicine. Totally unfamiliar with military medicine, he first spent hours researching the subject in the archives of the Army Medical Museum and Library, a dilapidated building on the National Mall that he found to be in desperate need of repair. He authored numerous reports and papers based on both academic research at the library and firsthand knowledge in the field. His literary abilities were used to the fullest extent, not only as an author of "top secret" publications from the medical office of high command, but also as the medical editor of its classified publication, *Health*, distributed to all the theaters and commands. He also traveled throughout North Africa and Europe for observational visits with the surgeons and commanders of the First, Ninth, Seventh, and Third U.S. Armies.

His extensive travels included visits to battalion aid stations in action, various evacuation hospitals, convalescent hospitals, field hospitals, and collecting and clearing stations. After observing each area, Dr. DeBakey documented how the wounds of war were managed there. One of his observations about the delivery of surgical care in combat areas was a logistical problem he deemed solvable with staffing alterations. In his travels he found that "we did not have the most experienced surgeons assigned to the field or evacuation hospitals. The most experienced surgeons were in the general hospitals in the rear, doing almost nothing."[16]

His proposed solution to the surgeon general was to create mobile teams out of the well-trained personnel at the base hospitals and designate them "auxiliary surgical groups" (ASGs). This concept was approved and immediately implemented by the surgeon general during World War II in all the armies.

The opportunity for Dr. DeBakey to observe his concept in action came during the fall of 1943. The Second Auxiliary Surgical Group, comprising a chief surgeon, assistant surgeon, anesthesiologist, surgical nurse, and two enlisted technicians, was the first mobile surgical hospital and was activated in support of the Fifth Army in North Africa, Italy, and Sicily.[17-19] Dispatched by the surgeon general to join the Fifth Army in North Africa, Dr. DeBakey remained with them throughout the subsequent invasion of Italy and the allied forces' liberation of Rome in June 1944. During that period, Dr. DeBakey observed and documented the adaptability of the ASG and its ability to sustain surgical operations near the frontlines. The end result was a notable improvement because of the shorter evacuation times, earlier resuscitation of the wounded, and fewer casualty deaths.

After returning to the United States with this news, Dr. DeBakey and Army Surgeon General Norman T. Kirk addressed the District of Columbia Medical Society on October 7, 1944. In his presentation, the surgeon general stated that the record achieved by American army surgeons in care of the wounded is "unparalleled in the history of warfare and is little short of miraculous. The survival rate among our wounded at the present time is higher that it has ever been in any army in any war at any time."[20]

Throughout the remainder of World War II, statistical data confirmed that the additional ASGs implemented before the Allied invasion of Normandy, which included those to support the First, Third, Seventh, and Ninth Armies, 17 collectively reduced mortality from its previous high of 15 to 20 percent to 4 percent.[21] This proven concept eventually evolved into the even more effective Mobile Auxiliary Surgical Hospital (MASH) units during the Korean War, where mortality totaled less than 3 percent. For his contributions to its development, Dr. DeBakey received the Legion of Merit from the U.S. Army in 1945.

With the abrupt ending of the war after the surrender of Japan in September 1945 and thousands of casualties returning home for medical care and rehabilitation, the surgeon general asked Dr. DeBakey to remain as chief of the surgical consultants to oversee the transition. "Fortunately, we had had the foresight to establish specialized centers in vascular surgery, orthopedics, plastic surgery, and neurosurgery—all well-manned with civilians," Dr. DeBakey said, noting this was the genesis of the Veterans Affairs Medical Center System. "Had those centers not been organized, we would have been caught short, with no cohesive plan for this eventuality."[22]

Where the Army was caught short was with the potential void of surgical specialists, all of whom were planning an immediate return to civilian life after demobilization. With veterans who required further hospital, medical, and specialized surgical care returning stateside in droves, often numbering more than 3,000 a day, it was a looming crisis in need of a solution.

After acquiring the authority from the surgeon general and Tracy S. Voorhees, the assistant secretary of the Army, Dr. DeBakey began calling 100 enlisted specialists, most of whom he knew by name, to urge them to remain in the Army one more year. For their extended service of caring for the casualties and training of the military personnel, each would receive a promotion. Not a single one refused.

Even with that stopgap measure implemented, there remained an almost insurmountable problem in the postwar delivery of health care to veterans. "The Veterans Administration was not prepared to take over," DeBakey said. "It did not have facilities or personnel to be able to deal with the millions of veterans returning from the war."[16]

Beginning in early 1945, the Veterans Administration (VA) had been highly criticized in the press, beginning with a series of articles written by Albert Deutsch in the New York newspaper *PM*. After stating the VA was a "vast dehumanized bureaucracy, enmeshed in mountains of red tape, ingrown with entrenched mediocrity, undemocratically operated under autocratic control centered Washington, prescribing medieval medicine to its sick and disabled wards, highly susceptible to political pressures, rigidly resistant to proposed reforms," Mr. Deutsch garnered widespread publicity and inspired other journalists to address the problems at the VA.[23] Even Eleanor Roosevelt wrote in her syndicated column, "I imagine that most people are interested, as I am, in making sure that our returned veterans, if they need treatment at a veterans' hospital, receive the best medical care possible."[24] All of this eventually led to President Harry S. Truman's concession that the VA had to be "modernized" and his appointment of General Omar Bradley as the new administrator of the VA in June 1945.[23]

As chief of the surgical consultants in the surgeon general's office, Dr. DeBakey was placed on Gen. Bradley's newly formed committee to reorganize the VA. With fellow committee members and surgeons Dr. Paul R. Hawley and Dr. Paul B. Magnuson, Dr. DeBakey championed the idea of "making the VA a teaching hospital with medical school doctors in charge of patient care."[16] One integral aspect of the suggested plan directly attributable to Dr. DeBakey was the requirement of a dean's committee, composed of deans and senior faculty members from appropriate departments and divisions of the medical school, to supervise the VA education and training programs. Accepting and approving all of the committee's suggestions, Gen. Bradley issued a policy memorandum in January 1946 to establish a program of affiliation between the VA and the nation's medical schools.[25]

Another program instigated at the suggestion of Dr. DeBakey soon followed. Envisioning a joint undertaking of the U. S. Army, VA, and National Research Council, Dr. DeBakey submitted a memorandum to Surgeon General Norman Kirk on March 5, 1946, "pointing out the unprecedented amount of valuable clinical material available that should be turned to practical use by the establishment of a long-term follow-up clinical research program on Army material, to determine the natural and post treatment history of selected diseases and conditions."[22] Such a program, Dr. DeBakey advised, would provide a rational basis for the development of professional procedures and operational policies.

This proposal garnered praise from Dr. DeBakey's peers for his "ability to combine clinical practice and organizational vision in a way that rose above the immediate concerns of the military bureaucracy" and was approved by the surgeon general within two months of receipt.[26] Soon thereafter, a Committee on Veterans Medical Problems was appointed under the chairmanship of Dr. Edward D. Churchill; serving on that committee's staff was Dr. DeBakey, assigned by the surgeon general to temporary duty to work with Dr. Gilbert W. Beebe on this project at the National Academy of Sciences–National Research Council.

The initial report on the feasibility of a research program devoted to medical follow-up drafted by Drs. DeBakey and Beebe, along with Dr. DeBakey's original memo, became the two founding documents of the Medical Follow-up Agency, the first medical research undertaken by the VA. It marked the beginning of an entity that was to become the central repository of medical research data and analytical talent in the postwar period and indefinitely into the future.

This and other such programs instigated by Dr. DeBakey exemplified his newfound area of interest, one that was to remain prominent throughout his life. Reflecting on his experiences as a surgical consultant in the surgeon general's office, he said that the kind of work that he was involved in afforded him the opportunity to learn governmental medical services and "to become interested in what might be called the socioeconomic and administrative and organizational problems in medicine in the country."[27,28]

In 1947, Dr. DeBakey returned to civilian life to resume his career in New Orleans as an associate professor of surgery at Tulane University School of Medicine. His multiple noteworthy experiences during his five-year tenure in the Army deeply affected him, both at the time of service and throughout his life. At the age of 96, Dr. DeBakey recalled, "This assignment afforded me a most rewarding and maturing experience, which I shall always treasure."[15]

It was to this matured, accomplished Army veteran and noted Tulane surgeon that Dean Moursund addressed the letter with an offer to become the first chairman of the Department of Surgery at the fledgling Baylor University College of Medicine in Houston.

Upon reading it, Dr. DeBakey's initial thought was "to throw it away."[21] Regardless of his total disinterest, Dr. DeBakey nonetheless decided it was best to discuss such an opportunity with his mentor. "Dr. Ochsner, who was a consultant to the Texas Medical Center, told me, 'I think, Mike, you ought to look at it. They have got big plans and they don't have anybody there that knows what the Hell to do. You can help them,'" Dr. DeBakey recalled. "So, I went over to Houston for a visit and then I came back and wrote a three-page letter turning it down."[21]

The letter detailed what he encountered during his visit. First and foremost, the medical school had no university hospital and no affiliated teaching hospital. When told he would work at the Jefferson Davis Hospital, Houston's charity hospital, Dr. DeBakey questioned how he could do that without having an appointment there. The system at that hospital, he feared, was not only closed, but also politicized. He noted that even though the medical school students were already making rounds with the community doctors there, most of those physicians were general practitioners who also happened to perform surgery as opposed to being board-certified surgeons. He also found the existing Department of Surgery at the medical school to be lacking in expertise with no full-time professors. Because of all of these shortfalls, plus the pivotal lack of a clinical outlet, Dr. DeBakey concluded there was limited potential for him at Baylor University College of Medicine and he "turned down the job, telling them I couldn't have a residency program if I had no service."[29]

What did leave a favorable, lasting impression during Dr. DeBakey's first visit to Houston was the vast potential of the Texas Medical Center. "All that was out here was the Cullen Building," he said, recalling the expansive wooded acreage on the edge of Hermann Park. "In fact, I came out of that building one afternoon and there was a fellow out in the parking lot who said, 'If you had come out here 15 minutes ago you would have seen a man shooting a deer over there.'"[21]

Still in the hunt, however, was Dean Moursund. When Dr. DeBakey received an invitation from him to return to Houston shortly after his return to New Orleans, he was curious to learn what, if anything, had changed since his first visit. Not much, he quickly discovered.

Eager to provide a clinical outlet for Dr. DeBakey, Dean Moursund advised he was trying to arrange some type of affiliation with Hermann Hospital, the private hospital adjacent to the Texas Medical Center, but the arrangement was not secure. Unwilling to accept such tentative conditions, Dr. DeBakey once again told the persistent dean he would not come.

Convinced he had heard the last offer from Baylor, Dr. DeBakey devoted his efforts to his surgical service and continued research in his own laboratory at Tulane. In addition to his New Orleans duties, he made frequent trips to

Washington, D.C., where he remained a consultant to the surgeon general and continued to serve on the Armed Forces Medical Advisory Committee to the Secretary of Defense, also known as the Cooper Committee. When Assistant Secretary of Army Voorhees became chairman of the Task Force on Federal Medical Services of the Hoover Commission on Organization of the Executive Branch of the Government in 1948, he asked Dr. DeBakey to serve as a member of that task force and work closely with him as an executive assistant. This necessitated Dr. DeBakey's taking a leave of absence from Tulane to work virtually full time for more than nine months in Washington, D.C.

The Hoover Commission, authorized by Congress in 1947, was chaired by former President Herbert Hoover and comprised 24 task force committees, each delving into specific areas to examine ways to improve efficiency and effectiveness of the federal government.

Among the glaring deficiencies and examples of wastefulness discovered during his research of government agencies, Dr. DeBakey found a prime example to include in the medical services task force report. In the turn of events that would follow, his discovery was prescient.

Recalling his search of the archives and the resulting documentation, Dr. DeBakey said, "I unearthed a memorandum signed by President Roosevelt stating that at the end of the war the U.S. Naval Hospital in Houston would be turned over to the VA. It was already 1948 and the hospital still had not been turned over. The Navy wanted to retain the hospital even though they had no active Navy personnel as patients; they were all veterans. The Veterans Administration was going to build another hospital, right next door for 35 million dollars (a huge sum at the time!), and I stated that it was a complete waste of money."[7]

In the midst of his efforts to unearth other glaring examples of wastefulness to include in the task force's report, Dr. DeBakey received a phone call from Dean Moursund, who suggested they meet again, this time in New Orleans. He said the purpose of their reconvening was to discuss recent developments at Baylor University College of Medicine that might entice him to change his mind about becoming the chairman of the Department of Surgery.

When Dr. DeBakey returned to New Orleans for this meeting, he was skeptical about its outcome. Therefore, what the dean said caught him completely by surprise: "I think we have it settled. They have promised that you will have a 20-bed surgical service at the Hermann Hospital. I reread your letter with great care and you are absolutely correct, we don't have clinical facilities. And we can't get the facilities until you get here. What have we got to offer? We don't have a full time surgeon on the faculty. We can't offer any hospital much in the way of personnel and so that's why I need you."[7]

Tempted to change his mind after hearing what he thought was a reasoned approach, Dr. DeBakey still needed further convincing. When Dr. Ochsner told him, "You can leave and always come back here if you don't like it," he made his decision to join Baylor University College of Medicine as its chairman of the Department of Surgery. His sudden change of mind, he reiterated to Dean Moursund, was based predominantly on the promised 20-bed surgical service at Hermann Hospital.[7]

Due to his commitment to the Hoover Commission, Dr. DeBakey advised Dean Moursund that the medical services task force report he was compiling would not be finalized until December, and he would not arrive in Houston until after its completion. This delay did not deter the dean, who wasted no time in announcing Dr. DeBakey's appointment in the July 21, 1948, *Houston Chronicle*.

The front-page article, headlined "Baylor Names Chairman of Surgery Unit," gave a glowing review of Dr. DeBakey's education and previous accomplishments.[30] No doubt, this did not bode well with members of the Harris County Medical Society, the powerful and close-knit organization of Houston medical professionals who advocated and strictly enforced its no-personal-publicity regulations for Houston physicians. If this particular transgression were not a bone of contention at the time, Dr. DeBakey was to present ample opportunities for others.

A somewhat fractious history already existed between the society and Baylor University College of Medicine in 1948. Some members of that society previously had been at odds with the Texas Medical Center leaders in 1943 for having invited the medical college to move to Houston without the society's knowledge, or consultation.[31] After the Baylor move was a fait accompli, the society hastily organized a fact-finding committee to ascertain the worthiness of having a medical college in Houston. Upon receipt of the committee's positive report after a meeting with Dean Moursund, the society voted to cooperate with Baylor and issued a statement that welcomed the medical college as an asset to the city.[32]

The welcome extended to Dr. DeBakey by society members at Hermann Hospital was not the cordial one he expected. Upon his December 1948 arrival, the promised 20-bed surgical service at that hospital was nonexistent and remained so for more than a month. Growing restless about this stalemate, an exasperated Dr. DeBakey told Dean Moursund, "I can't get a residency program; I can't do anything. I have no service. Unless I get a service, I am wasting my time here, and I will go back to New Orleans or accept some other offer."[7]

It was a threat that prompted action, but not the desired results. At a hastily called meeting of society members on the hospital's surgical staff, the decision made was to appoint Dr. DeBakey "chief of teaching services" and not allow his establishment of a surgical service.

When told by the chief of staff his duties would be simply to teach the medical students and not care for the patients, who would remain the responsibility of society members on the staff, Dr. DeBakey deemed that arrangement incredulous. The conversation that ensued was to remain one of his vivid memories decades later: "I said, 'How can that work? Suppose I walk in there and say the operation that was done was wrong, or the patient shouldn't have been operated on.' The chief of staff said, 'That won't happen.' I said, 'From what I have seen around here, it will happen often.' I endeared myself right away, but I didn't care; I was displeased, and I had made up my mind to leave."[7]

Fed up and ready to resign, Dr. DeBakey requested and received a final meeting with both the dean and Earl C. Hankamer, the Houstonian who served as chairman of the Baylor University College of Medicine board of trustees. In their presence, he did not mince words, beginning with his voiced opinion that "the present medical school was third-rate" at best, and continuing with his personal assessment of the existing situation: "Do you realize that a student who graduates from Baylor University College of Medicine has to leave town to get any kind of specialty training, because he can't get any training here? There isn't an approved residency program in the whole city. This school is going to go nowhere; it's going to remain a third-rate medical school as long as it continues this way. You are not going to be able to get anybody worthwhile clinically to come here if he will not have a service"[7]

When the chairman of the board asked him to reconsider his resignation while he and the dean attempted to remedy the situation, Dr. DeBakey acquiesced. Doubtful that dramatic changes would take place, given his previous encounters with disgruntled members of the medical society at Hermann Hospital, he agreed to stay one more month and no longer, stating he was "wasting his time staying here under these circumstances."[7]

The thought of further protracting this uncharacteristic period of idleness only made Dr. DeBakey more anxious to return to his productive career at Tulane. Quite unexpectedly, an extraordinary change in circumstances took place within a matter of days of that meeting. "Fate intervened," Dr. DeBakey said, recalling a telephone call he received at home the following Sunday.[29]

The call was from his former colleague on Gen. Bradley's committee to reorganize the VA, Dr. Paul Magnuson, who had been named chief administrator of the VA in January 1948. His old friend had an enormous favor to ask of him. "Mike, we have just been ordered by President Truman to take over the Navy hospital," he said. "We don't have personnel to take care of it. Can you organize a faculty group and take it over?"[7]

It was a question that took Dr. DeBakey only moments to answer affirmatively, given his familiarity with the particulars. President Truman had ordered the takeover in response to the recommendations made in the Hoover Commission Federal Medical Services Task Force Report, the one compiled and written by Dr. DeBakey. First published in December 1948, the task force report's highlighting of the wastefulness found in the already-approved, future construction plans for future VA hospitals garnered nationwide publicity and a political uproar. In his January 10, 1949 Annual Budget Message to the Congress, President Truman announced that he had "directed that the program which I had previously authorized be curtailed by approximately 16,000 beds and asked the Administrator of Veterans Affairs to recommend specific adjustments in the program. I have approved his recommendations for the cancellation of 24 hospital projects, and the reduction in planned capacity of 14 additional hospitals."[33]

As for Dr. Magnuson, who originally was in favor of building a new 1,000-bed VA Hospital in Houston, he was horrified to learn the proposed location was "right across the street from a truly magnificent 1,000-bed wartime U.S. Naval Hospital which was now practically empty" and had "very strongly recommended that the Veterans Administration arrange to take over the U.S. Naval Hospital instead of building a new one, and I was so sure this had been settled long ago that I had completely forgotten about it."[34] After the Hoover Commission condemned this obviously overlooked project as a "wasteful and ridiculous duplication of the worst kind" in its December report, Dr. Magnuson soon received word from the White House that the Navy indeed was turning over the Houston hospital to the VA.[34]

The U.S. Naval Hospital in Houston had a capacity of 943 beds and was completed at an estimated cost of $11 million in 1946. Comprising 37 buildings built on 118 acres of property generously donated by the Houston Chamber of Commerce and the M.D. Anderson Foundation in 1944, it was a source of community pride, touted as one of the largest and most modern hospitals in the South. With its commanding location at the corner of what later became Alameda Road and Holcombe Boulevard, it was in close proximity to the Texas Medical Center and conveniently accessible for Baylor University College of Medicine faculty and students.[35]

When the January 21, 1949, official announcement stated the VA takeover of the U.S. Naval Hospital would take place April 15, 1949, there was little or no time to waste at Baylor University College of Medicine. Since the blueprint for the affiliation of a medical school and the VA was the product of a committee on which Dr. DeBakey previously served, he knew the exact building blocks required. First, he helped organize the prerequisite Dean's Committee composed of deans and senior faculty members at the medical school to supervise the education and training programs at the VA. Named to serve on the initial committee were Dr. Warren T. Brown, associate dean and professor of psychiatry as chairman; Dr. James A. Greene, professor of medicine; Dean Moursund, dean emeritus of Baylor University College of Medicine; and Dr. DeBakey, professor of surgery.[31]

The first step for the committee was to begin the process of arranging for resident training, as this was to be the first affiliated hospital for the Houston medical college. In the surgical area, this was a formidable challenge dictated by Dr. DeBakey's predicament. Without a surgical service, he had not received the required approval for residents from the American Board of Surgery, to which he belonged. To immediately remedy that situation, he began contacting fellow members of the board to explain his dilemma. In telephone call after telephone call, he requested temporary approval for a year, followed by an evaluation for permanent approval. To this reasonable approach, all agreed and granted permission for a resident surgical training program at the VA Hospital, the first of its kind in Houston.[8]

It was to be the first of many firsts in Dr. DeBakey's legendary Houston career, which, for all intents and purposes, officially did not begin until Dr. Magnuson's phone call. Throughout the hectic weeks and months that followed, he recruited new Department of Surgery faculty, began a nationwide search for possible residents, and organized the particulars of the surgical training program at the new Houston Veterans Administration Hospital.

To achieve these goals required Dr. DeBakey's spending an inordinate amount of time in the office, where fate once again intervened. Hired by Baylor University College of Medicine several months before his arrival was his secretary, June Clendenin Bowen, the newlywed wife of the assistant administrator of The Methodist Hospital, Ted Bowen. It was through this association that Dr. DeBakey first learned of that venerable, 100-bed hospital located midway between the Texas Medical Center and downtown Houston.

The serendipity of this chance encounter was not realized in 1948. The inevitability of this small organization's playing such a huge role in Dr. DeBakey's manifest destiny was to become foreseeable only in hindsight.

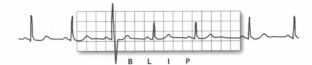

THE HANDS OF A SURGEON

*B*eginning in his youth, Dr. DeBakey concentrated on improving his dexterity. After learning as a child how to sew, knit, and crochet from observing his mother, he recognized his innate ability to work with his hands. He played the piano but was interested in joining the band at school, so he learned how to play a saxophone. At Tulane, when told he could not join the orchestra unless he played the clarinet, Dr. DeBakey taught himself how to play that instrument. Within six weeks he became a member of the Tulane orchestra. "I already knew how to read music and how to finger and how to play a reed instrument like the saxophone; I just needed to learn the fingering of a clarinet, which is a little different from a saxophone," Dr. DeBakey told an interviewer in 1998. "So it is that kind of neuromuscular coordination with your hands that you either have genetically, like a good athlete, or you don't. I think a surgeon needs that same quality, athletic coordination."[1]

---

1. Roberts WC. Michael Ellis DeBakey: a conversation with the editor. Interview with William C. Roberts. Am J Cardiol. 1997;79(7): 929-950.

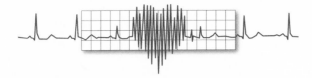

CHAPTER TWO

DELIBERATE DECISIONS BY STRONG WOMEN 1924 - 1929

"The most effective way to do it, is just to do it."
AMELIA EARHART

When The Methodist Hospital in Houston opened its doors to the public on June 12, 1924, it comprised two adjacent buildings with a total capacity of 90 beds and 10 bassinettes. Located at the corner of San Jacinto Street and Rosalie Avenue, in the residential district of downtown Houston, this "modern" hospital's opening garnered rave reviews from the citizenry and prompted one *Houston Post* reporter to exclaim, "Everything looked so comfortable and cozy that one was tempted to believe it would be a pleasure to be sick here."[1]

Such praise only served to enhance its already established reputation. Though chartered in 1919, The Methodist Hospital had more than a decade-long history of patient care when it opened. That was because the new hospital encompassed an old one, the four-story Norsworthy Hospital, originally built in 1908 by Dr. Oscar Laertius Norsworthy.

A general practitioner who developed a specialty in surgery, Dr. Norsworthy established the private, eponymous hospital for the care of his patients, most of whom were the city's most prominent citizens. What's more, he had been the attending physician at the Christmas Eve 1905 birth of a child who arguably was to become Houston's most famous son, Howard Robard Hughes Jr.[2]

Designating himself the hospital's surgeon-in-chief, Dr. Norsworthy installed an operating room on the top floor with all the accessories of a modern aseptic hospital, including Terrazzo floors, white enamel walls and ceiling, and excellent lighting for both day and night operations. Adjoining the operating room was a sterilizing room for instruments and dressings, a dressing and sterilizing room for surgeons, and an anesthesia room.

The hospital was built to accommodate 30 patients in ward beds, single rooms, or two connecting rooms, the latter two with or without private bathrooms. At the time, it was advertised as being "a new brick veneered building, three stories and an over-ground basement, built especially for hospital use...[that was] heated by hot water radiation, equipped with electric lights, call buzzers, private telephones, fans, elevators, dumb waiter and vacuum cleaners."[3]

From its beginning in 1908, the Norsworthy Hospital quickly became the best known of Houston's private hospitals.[4] Eleven years later, its future was in jeopardy when Dr. Norsworthy decided to devote all of his efforts to a new interest, radium research. To avoid closing the hospital, Dr. Norsworthy presented a unique plan to the Texas Conference of the Methodist Episcopal Church, South. His proposal included the sale of his hospital under generous terms, with one condition: that the church add a new hospital on the adjacent property, which he offered to sell to them at its appraised value. After suggesting the church raise funds for the purchase, he offered to continue operating the Norsworthy Hospital until the completion of the new building and to remain available as a consultant to the church on medical affairs. When the newly built hospital adjacent to the Norsworthy Hospital opened in 1924, the two structures were to become known as The Methodist Hospital.

The acceptance of the plan presented by Dr. Norsworthy in 1919 necessitated the creation of the first board of trustees of The Methodist Hospital. Dominated by Houstonians, the board also included members from Beaumont, Galveston, Huntsville, Jacksonville, Longview, Marlin, Nacogdoches, Pittsburg, Richmond, and Tyler, Texas. All were successful men, and most were self-made and self-educated; they included bankers, lawyers, and businessmen whose main areas of interest included cotton, timber, and oil. Individually and collectively, they personified the quintessential entrepreneurial spirit that permeated Houston in 1919.

The board's immediate decision to erect a 346-bed hospital was predicated on building the structure in four phases, with each phase projected to cost $200,000. To the trustees, this was not an overly ambitious plan. While they expected to solicit the funds from fellow church members in both Houston and the Conference in a timely manner, the board had not accomplished this goal by 1922. Instead of the amount necessary to begin phase one, the total pledged was less than $100,000, including a substantial contribution from each trustee. To appease Dr. Norsworthy, who served as a trustee and was anxious to hand over his hospital and devote time to radium research, the board scaled back their original plans and proceeded with a new one dictated by the limited budget.

Included in the architect's revised building plans was an additional structure, the Sarah Francelia Bell Home, to be erected on the south side of the Norsworthy Hospital on Rosalie Avenue. Since several trustees from the Bell Trust also served as trustees for The Methodist Hospital, the request to purchase a portion of Dr. Norsworthy's property to erect a three-story residence was approved in 1922. It was to be the residence stipulated in the July 1911 will of Sarah Francelia Bell, who bequeathed funds for "providing living assistance for indigent widows of Methodist ministers in Houston."[5] Although the same architect simultaneously designed the new hospital and the Bell Home with a similar brick-veneer appearance, the Bell Home was not intended to be a part of The Methodist Hospital. It eventually, however, became just that.

During the construction of these facilities in 1923, The Methodist Hospital board of trustees hired Sam R. Hay Jr., the son and namesake of Methodist Bishop Sam R. Hay, to be the superintendent of The Methodist Hospital. In turn, the new superintendent hired Josie Mooring Roberts, a young widow who worked as a troubleshooter and personnel trainer for the Texas telephone company, to serve as business manager. Neither had hospital experience, but each was willing to learn. "It was something new, sounded challenging," Mrs. Roberts said, recalling their initial conversations. " Hay built it up where it was just something we would have a good time doing and I never regretted it for one minute."[6]

The one who did have regrets was Mr. Hay, who resigned on December 31, 1925, after just two years on the job. Explaining to the board his desire to pursue other business opportunities, he later would admit another reason for leaving: "Every time a patient died, I couldn't sleep that night, thinking there might have been something we didn't do right. I lost 20 pounds in one year and gained it back within six months after I left."[7]

Also offering to resign when the new superintendent, the Reverend D. H. Hotchkiss, arrived, Mrs. Roberts said, "I told him I didn't want him to feel that he had to keep me in any way. He threw up his hands and said, 'Oh, I'm depending on you. I'm depending on you.' And I said, 'I don't want to leave, but I do want it understood that you could bring in someone if you had a preference.'"[6]

For the following five years, the Reverend Hotchkiss devoted the majority of his time to public relations in the community and left the managing of the hospital in Mrs. Roberts' very capable hands. "He was quite elderly," Mrs. Rogers explained. "And he didn't know anything about hospitals." He knew even less about managing budgets. During the Depression years, when The Methodist Hospital was going deeper and deeper in debt, Mrs. Roberts found that the Reverend Hotchkiss was "afraid to do anything about it. So we just got to owing more and more and more. As the old saying goes, I took the bull by the horn, and believe me, I got 'em out of debt." [6]

In recognition of her valiant efforts, resourcefulness, and ingenuity, Mrs. Roberts was named administrator of The Methodist Hospital in 1931. Throughout the Depression and the next 17 years, she presided over the ever-evolving hospital with a keen eye for details and her finger on the pulse of the community. When the infantile paralysis outbreaks in the 1920s and 1930s resulted in an overflow in the hospital's children's ward, Mrs. Roberts seized the opportunity to fulfill a need and contacted Methodist Bishop A. Frank Smith with her idea. In turn, Bishop Smith advised the Blue Bird Circle, a unique organization of women volunteers who had banded together to promote the well-being of humanity through the betterment of the community. Eager to be involved with a permanent project such as this, the Blue Bird Circle funded the erection of the 30-bed Children's Building, also referred to as the "little hospital," on the grounds of The Methodist Hospital, establishing what was to become known as The Blue Bird Clinic.

Working closely with both her hospital staff of 30 and a growing medical staff, Mrs. Roberts responded to the needs of both in a timely and efficient manner. With an ever-mindful eye on the budget and cutting costs wherever she could, she was able to add new equipment when needed, but always judiciously and often purchased by the Women's Auxiliary. In 1938, when the patient population began to exceed the number of beds available, she joined the Sarah Francelia Bell Home to the original hospital to provide 18 more beds. Over the years, Mrs. Roberts transformed wasted spaces into usable ones; from cubbyholes to closets to reception areas, every available square foot was repurposed to the best advantage. When she exhausted all the possibilities, only then did she turn to the board of trustees for a solution. The only answer, she reasoned, was expansion.

The board of trustees for obvious reasons had tabled all thoughts of possible expansion during the Depression years. It was not until the unexpected January 5, 1935, death of Dr. Norsworthy that the subject was raised again, and this time it was out of necessity. The trustees learned Dr. Norsworthy had bequeathed his entire estate to the hospital on the condition that the hospital expand to 200 beds within five years or 300 beds within 10 years. The Methodist Hospital trustees agreed the biggest question was whether this expansion would take place at the current site, or elsewhere. One thing was certain: Should The Methodist Hospital not meet Dr. Norsworthy's posthumous terms, the entire estate would go to Hermann Hospital.

A secret plan to solve this dilemma was devised by trustee Walter W. Fondren, one of the founders of Humble Oil. He and his wife, Ella Cochrum Fondren, had kept in close contact with Mrs. Roberts ever since her 1924 arrival at The Methodist Hospital. It was said, although never documented, that during the first few years of the hospital's existence, Mr. Fondren, one of the original trustees, worked closely with Mrs. Roberts on all expenses incurred and quietly picked up the deficits.[8]

Again working in secret without the knowledge of the board, Mr. and Mrs. Fondren authorized Mrs. Roberts to purchase a block of land on San Jacinto Street across from the hospital in 1938. They then asked Mrs. Roberts to announce to the trustees that an anonymous benefactor was willing to donate the land and a 75-bed children's hospital thereon as well as underwrite 15 percent of the cost of building another new hospital to meet Dr. Norsworthy's requirements, provided it did not exceed $500,000. At the annual October 1938 board meeting, that's exactly what she announced, and the trustees' reaction was memorable. "Well, you can imagine telling a bunch of men something and their not knowing who it was," Mrs. Roberts recalled decades later, still amused at the thought. "There was an awful lot of discussion. Fondren finally got up and told them that he and his wife were the ones that were making the proposal."[6]

The Fondrens' generosity was celebrated by the board and formally announced to Bishops Smith and Hay, as well as influential local pastors, in a hastily called meeting the following day. Theirs was a welcomed solution by all, but one destined to become a victim of extenuating circumstances. Shortly after the announcement, Mr. Fondren died unexpectedly during a January 1939 visit to San Antonio. "Nothing was done then for quite a while," Mrs. Roberts said. "Then the war came and we couldn't build. But as soon as World War II was over, we started working on plans."[6]

To prepare for the eventuality of expansion, Mrs. Roberts embarked on a mission to expand her knowledge of hospitals throughout the country. A member of the American Hospital Association since 1931 and the American College of Hospital Administrators since 1935, she became president of the Texas Hospital Association in 1938 and became the first woman elected to serve on the board of directors of the American Hospital Association in

1943. She also served on the boards of the Texas Hospital Association, the Group Hospital Service of Texas, and the American Protestant Hospital Association.

Accompanying Mrs. Roberts to various conferences and workshops sponsored by these associations was Mrs. Fondren, the newly instated trustee of The Methodist Hospital after the death of her husband. "I had nothing to do and I paid my own way and went everywhere, went with her around St. Louis, Chicago, San Francisco, well, all the places there. Wherever I went, I was always inquiring about their hospital work. I wanted to know what other people were doing," Mrs. Fondren said, recalling her learning experiences as Mrs. Roberts's travel companion. "I knew so little about it myself, but I listened to her."[6]

When Mrs. Fondren accepted the board's invitation to assume her late husband's vacancy, she viewed the role as her obligation to "take up some of the steps he had been taking."[6] Although disappointed in 1939 to learn of the board's inability to meet the financial requirements set forth by the Fondrens for the new hospital building, she completed the purchase of the land on San Jacinto Street and maintained her hopes of building a children's hospital there. She was present at the May 27, 1942, board meeting when the trustees discussed the M.D. Anderson Foundation's reported plans to build a medical center on land near the Hermann Hospital and concurred with its decision to inquire about a possible site there for The Methodist Hospital.

Two years later, when the M.D. Anderson Foundation made a definite offer of land to The Methodist Hospital, the board of trustees was indecisive as to whether to accept it or build on the Fondren property across the street. The final decision, trustee Robert A. Shepherd recalled, "depended to some extent on how Mrs. Fondren felt about it."[9]

What convincingly persuaded Mrs. Fondren and the other trustees to abandon any previous planned sites and concentrate on a new one occurred quite unexpectedly in 1945. For the board of trustees, that year had not begun well. Because the Depression and World War II years had taken their toll on both the hospital and fund-raising efforts, the inability to raise the necessary funds for expansion had a measurable consequence. It resulted in the board's reluctantly advising the Norsworthy estate administrators that the stipulated requirements of the bequest could not be fulfilled. To the board's dismay, the entire estate went to Hermann Hospital, as specified.

Disappointed but determined to reinvigorate its efforts to expand The Methodist Hospital, the trustees and pillars of the church community planned to embark on a new fund-raising campaign after the war. Exactly how to begin again was the question. The answer came from William N. Blanton, executive vice-president of the Houston Chamber of Commerce and a member of St. Luke's Methodist Church, who recognized and seized upon an extraordinary opportunity.

One of the first to learn the news about the million-dollar checks contributed by "King of the Wildcatters" Hugh Roy Cullen and his wife Lillie to both the Baptist Memorial Hospital and Hermann Hospital on Friday, March 2, Mr. Blanton made an appointment with Mr. Cullen that afternoon to discuss the needs of The Methodist Hospital. "He must have told a very good tale," Mr. Cullen recalled during the 1950 laying of the cornerstone for The Methodist Hospital in the Texas Medical Center. "I couldn't get it off my mind. So one evening I phoned him that we would give The Methodist Hospital $1 million."[10]

Cullen actually decided on the spot, telling Blanton to have Bishop Smith to call him for confirmation the following day. Unlike Dr. Norsworthy's donations, there were no strings attached to the Cullens' gift, with the use of the money left to the discretion of the board of trustees. For Bishop Smith, their generosity was "a God-given opportunity to do what we have wanted to do through the years. We would be lacking in our duty not to make the most of it."[11]

Without their planning it, the trustees realized the new building campaign officially began with the announcement of the Cullens' gift on the front pages of the Houston newspapers on Sunday, March 4, 1945. Reporting that this gift "to The Methodist Hospital will be used for the construction of a new hospital plant," *The Houston Post* also pointed out the fact that a location of the plant is yet to be announced.[12] It was a conundrum that was to be solved within a matter of weeks, courtesy of another unexpected gift.

At the end of March 1945, the trustees of the M.D. Anderson Foundation sweetened their previous offer to The Methodist Hospital. In addition to giving land in the Texas Medical Center at no cost for the new hospital, the trustees tendered an offer of a challenge grant, promising to give The Methodist Hospital one-half dollar for every dollar raised up to a total of $500,000. Such a grant was precisely the impetus needed to persuade Mrs. Fondren and all the other trustees to abandon plans to build on the Fondren property and unanimously accept the Texas Medical Center site. The proposed size of the new hospital remained to be determined.

The existing hospital was unable to meet the demands for patient care in 1945. Having only 125 beds while sometimes accommodating more than

150 patients, the hospital was turning away an average of 15 to 20 patients daily. With all the cost-cutting measures taken during the lean years of the Depression and war, Mrs. Roberts had expertly used every nook and cranny but was woefully short on securing new equipment and updated amenities. Although tempted to spend some of the newly acquired funds on updating the old equipment, she instead concentrated her efforts on the new. "We started working on the new plans," said Mrs. Roberts, who continued to visit hospitals across the country "to see if I could get any ideas that I wanted to incorporate in the new hospital."[6]

By 1947, the building campaign was progressing at a healthy pace, and the board of trustees began to address future staff needs. Its decision to recruit an assistant administrator inspired trustee E. Moore Decker to suggest Ted Bowen from his hometown of Alto, Texas, as a likely candidate. A graduate of Stephen F. Austin State University with a major in accounting, Mr. Bowen had enlisted in the Army and spent three and one-half years during the war as a master sergeant assigned to the medical corps at the 2,100-bed hospital at Camp Gruber, Oklahoma. After returning to civilian life in 1946, he had entered the newly created graduate program in hospital administration at Washington University School of Medicine in St. Louis, a one-year academic program followed by a year of residency at Barnes Hospital, a 900-bed general hospital run by the Methodist Church and affiliated with Washington University. One of only seven graduate students in the program, Mr. Bowen excelled and his performance became the standard against which other students were measured—so much so that he was the only one asked to serve under the preceptorship of Dr. F. R. Bradley, the originator of the graduate program.

The opportunity to interview Mr. Bowen presented itself in an unusual way in the fall of 1947. Since Mrs. Roberts and Mrs. Fondren were traveling together by train to a conference in Chicago, they called him to arrange a brief meeting when the train stopped in St. Louis. "I went down to the train station and met Mrs. Fondren and Mrs. Roberts. I had never met either of them before, so I was rather in the dark about the people in Houston," Mr. Bowen said. "After we three had talked, Mrs. Roberts and I had an opportunity to sit and have a cup of coffee and talk for thirty or forty minutes."[13]

As a result of Mrs. Roberts' favorable recommendation, Mr. Bowen traveled to Houston the following spring for his second interview, which turned out to be his last. In the plush office surroundings of trustee Hines Baker, an executive vice president of Humble Oil and Refining Company,

Mr. Bowen received and accepted the offer to become Mrs. Roberts' administrative assistant. "He was careful to keep me from seeing the buildings until after I had agreed to take the position," Mr. Bowen recalled decades later. "I thought, really, when I first saw the hospital that I made a bad mistake. The hospital was operating under adverse conditions. However, I found a wonderful, remarkable esprit de corps in the board of trustees, in the medical staff, and among the employees. Looking back now, I find it astounding that we could have such fine people in such an antiquated building."[14]

The apparent deterioration of the facilities, coupled with the hospital's fragile financial structure, was to remain a challenge for the new assistant administrator after his July 1948 arrival. As the board of trustees continued to debate the parameters of the proposed new hospital, unable to concur on the exact size or precise location within the medical center, Mr. Bowen and Mrs. Roberts immersed themselves with the detailed, day-to-day management of the existing one. Exactly how they would share those responsibilities was never a question.

From the time of his arrival in July, it was agreed that Mr. Bowen was to assume a role similar to that of a chief operating officer to Mrs. Roberts' chief executive officer. His priorities were clearly defined by existing circumstances. Twenty-four years into its existence, The Methodist Hospital had maintained its reputation for excellent health care, albeit delivered in less-than-ideal facilities. Nonetheless, with new and modern equipment added as needed in the laboratories, X-ray department, and surgery, the hospital remained totally up-to-date and its popularity in the community was reflected in its operational statistics. For the 12-month period ending September 30, 1948, year-end records indicated 5,925 patients admitted for treatment; 2,839 individuals treated as outpatients; 841 babies born; 72,500 laboratory examinations performed; 10,996 X-ray examinations made; 333,144 meals prepared and served; and 2,863 surgical procedures performed.[15]

In 1948, the hospital had an average occupancy of 116 patients per day and a medical staff comprised of 131 active and 35 consulting physicians in the community. According to Mr. Bowen, the formation of this excellent medical staff and its sound organizational structure represented Mrs. Roberts's "most outstanding accomplishment."[14] Another was her 1946 selection of Dr. Hatch Cummings as chief of the medicine service. A member of the medical staff since 1932 and one of the first board-certified internists in Houston, Dr. Cummings shared Mrs. Roberts' interest in establishing a medical-service teaching program for interns and residents. Their mutual goal resulted in the 1947 establishment of a comprehensive training program approved by the American College of Surgeons and the American Medical Association. By the time of Mr. Bowen's arrival in 1948, this program comprised three interns and 14 residents in internal medicine, surgery, obstetrics, neurosurgery, pediatrics, and radiology.

A learning experience for the entire medical staff existed in pathology, which was under the direction of Dr. Stewart A. Wallace, chairman of the department of pathology at Baylor University College of Medicine. Dr. Wallace had been asked by the board of trustees in 1945 to serve temporarily in this capacity when pathologist Dr. Martha Wood became ill and took a leave of absence. When Dr. Wood did not recover, Dr. Wallace remained permanently, thereby establishing one of the first formal affiliations enacted between the fledgling medical college and a Houston hospital. After bringing in his college associates to manage the laboratories and creating sections of biochemistry and bacteriology, he and associate Dr. Paul Wheeler would conduct Friday afternoon teaching sessions in which specimens were presented for microscopic inspection and discussion. Often, the audience comprised more than 50 members of the medical staff, indicative of the perceived value of such informative lessons.

While The Methodist Hospital had many positive aspects in 1948, the only detrimental one obvious to Mr. Bowen was the lack of air-conditioning in the aging facilities. During the hot, humid summer months, it was a shortcoming that caused immeasurable discomfort for both patients and staff. Heretofore, this was not unusual for a hospital in Houston, or any other structure for that matter. During the Depression and war years, the only "cooled summer air" in town was available in one bank, one hotel, and several downtown movie theaters, but the upcoming post-war construction boom was to enable Houston to become known as "the world's most air-conditioned city."[16] Instrumental in laying the foundation for that boastful claim in 1948 was the construction of the country's "first fully air-conditioned hospital," the seven-story, 300-bed addition to Houston's Hermann Hospital set to open in 1949.[17] Other Houston hospitals had also announced expansion projects, most of which included air-conditioned facilities.

Although apprehensive about the projected, steady decline in patient population as a result of such modernized competition and shackled with the constraints of a limited budget, both Mrs. Roberts and Mr. Bowen remained characteristically optimistic about the future survival of The

Methodist Hospital. Theirs was a sentiment instilled in and shared by the entire administrative and medical staff, which served to further inspire Mr. Bowen. Decades later, he was to recall his warranted optimism: "It was obvious that we couldn't fail in the long run." [13]

Also destined for success was Mrs. Roberts, whose alleviated workload permitted her total immersion in developing plans for the new hospital. When she and Mrs. Fondren received their 1948 appointment by Chairman of the Board Walter L. Goldston to serve on the board's building committee, they continued their travels and enhanced their close working relationship. Both were horrified to learn of fellow committee member Baker's selection of the proposed new hospital's site in the medical center. Next to Hermann Hospital, the selected site was not only directly across from the Hermann Park Zoo but also was limited in size to preclude any possible future expansion.

Together, the two women voiced their objections to this site because of its inaccessibility and confining restrictions as well as the zoo's odoriferous implications. Unable to dissuade Mr. Baker, they took it upon themselves to ameliorate the situation. In a subsequent meeting with Dr. Ernst W. Bertner, the newly appointed president of the Texas Medical Center, the women selected and a signed a contract for the parcel of land they wanted—acreage between Bertner Avenue and Fannin Street. When Mr. Baker took offense at the temerity of their actions, he tendered his resignation, but the board firmly declined to accept it.

What the board did not reject or even question was the women's selection of a new location in the Texas Medical Center, a testament to the formidable power rarely wielded by Mrs. Fondren. As the only woman on the board of trustees, for more than a decade she traditionally had agreed with the men's decisions, never voicing a contrarian's view. But an opportunity to do exactly that presented itself during the board's meeting to finalize the proposed building plans on February 22, 1949. Following a lengthy discussion about the economic realities of downsizing the oft-debated, original 300-bed plan to a more manageable 220-bed facility, Mrs. Fondren unequivocally stated, "Gentlemen, I have only one vote, but let's have one thing clear. I for one refuse to support a building of less than 300 beds. Not one penny of my money will go into a hospital of less than 300 beds." The resounding silence that followed her pronouncement inspired one of the trustees to recall later, "We just sat there, kind of stunned, blinking like bullfrogs in a hailstorm." [18]

Such an adamant statement from Mrs. Fondren gave the trustees pause, but they remained undecided for months afterward. Dependent on her financial support for the new building, board members nonetheless argued that a 300-bed facility was unfeasible in the current economy, particularly since the existing hospital already was experiencing dire financial difficulties. Unperturbed by that fact, Mrs. Fondren prevailed and the plans for 300-bed facility finally were approved. "I wouldn't have put my okay behind it if it hadn't," Mrs. Fondren recalled, believing her rigid stance was in keeping with the original vision she shared with her late husband for The Methodist Hospital.[19] To further achieve their mutual desire to improve education, health, and human services in Houston and to manage the resources of her late husband's estate, valued at more than $33 million at the time of his death in 1939, Mrs. Fondren established the Fondren Foundation in 1948.[20]

With a sizable donation from the Fondren Foundation secured, the future plans for The Methodist Hospital in the Texas Medical Center finally were solidified in 1949, but the hospital on Rosalie Avenue continued to deteriorate. When the patient population dwindled to less than half-capacity, the continuing existence of The Methodist Hospital in its original location was jeopardized. "For a while it appeared that the practical approach would be to suspend the hospital's operations until completion of the new building in the Texas Medical Center," Mr. Bowen said. "However, this would have been a drastic step. As usual, Mrs. Fondren and Mr. Goldston, the chairman of the board, stepped to the forefront and underwrote the deficit for about a year and a half in order that we would have a nucleus of staff and employees to open our new building."[14]

In addition to the financial uncertainty at The Methodist Hospital in the late 1940s, the decline in patient population continued as many Houston physicians began to admit their patients elsewhere. One of the more popular alternatives was to be the newly opened air-conditioned pavilion at Hermann Hospital in early 1949. When the influx of new patients at that hospital began to impede its previous arrangement with Baylor University College of Medicine, The Methodist Hospital reaped incalculable benefits at the time. The existing, teaching-only program with the medical college at the Hermann Hospital did not allow any hands-on interaction with the hospital's patients. Instead, the hospital had committed 40 beds for the exclusive use by the private patients of the full-time faculty. When this insufficient allotment did not meet the growing needs of faculty members, they began to admit their patients to other Houston hospitals,[21] one of which was The Methodist Hospital.

With the exception of those in the pathology department who had established an exemplary working arrangement at The Methodist Hospital, and Dr. DeBakey, the new chairman of the Department of Surgery whose secretary was Mr. Bowen's wife, many faculty members previously had been unaware of that small downtown hospital. Recalling his first visit, Dr. DeBakey explained why he began to admit his private patients there, "It was a ramshackle building, but it was a very warm place and they took an interest in their patients. I liked The Methodist Hospital, even though it was not as nice a building as Hermann. They had a very nice woman administrator, who was very kind to me."[22]

The first of Mrs. Roberts' gestures of kindness to Dr. DeBakey occurred during his initial visit to the hospital, and stories about this incident were to gain legendary proportions when recounted in future decades. According to onlookers, upon seeing the antiquated floor fans utilized in the operating room, Dr. DeBakey demanded their replacement with air-conditioning units. Instead of denying this oft-heard request, as she had so many times in the past, Mrs. Roberts immediately turned to her staffers and said, "Give him anything he wants."[23]

According to legend, it was that precise moment that marked the beginning of Dr. DeBakey's six-decade relationship with The Methodist Hospital, one that led to the 2001 establishment of the Methodist DeBakey Heart & Vascular Center.

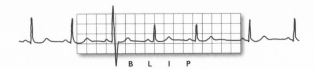

B   L   I   P

NOSE FOR OIL

Miss Ella Florence Cochrum was working at her family's boardinghouse in Corsicana, Texas, in the late 1890s when she first met Walter W. Fondren, a driller in the nearby oilfields. Following their wedding on February 14, 1904, Mr. Fondren was to become one of the major stockholders in Humble Oil, now ExxonMobil, and amass a sizable fortune by concentrating his drilling in the Humble oilfields. He and his wife would devote hours to smelling the samples of sand and mud he would bring home from the oilfields. Often crediting Mrs. Fondren with determining some of his most successful oil acquisitions, Mr. Fondren said, "She's got the best nose for oil I've ever seen."[1]

---

1. Kirkland Innis V. Walter and Ella Fondren: benefactors and builders. *The Flyleaf: Friends of the Fondren Library*. Winter-Spring 1982.

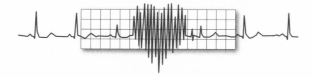

CHAPTER THREE

ASSEMBLING THE TEAM
1943 - 1950

"The strength of the team is each individual member. The strength of each member is the team."
COACH PHIL JACKSON

D r. DeBakey's ability to succeed where others had failed was to become
his trademark not only at The Methodist Hospital but also at Jefferson
Davis Hospital, the city-county charity hospital in Houston.

Originally built in 1924 at the urging of the Harris County Medical Society, the publicly owned hospital named for the president of the Confederate
States of America was located northwest of downtown Houston on Elder
Street and comprised 240 beds for indigent patients. When the Houston
population doubled to 292,352 in 1930, making the need for a larger public
hospital evident, city officials devoted the next eight years to the development and construction of a new 500-bed facility in Houston's Fourth Ward.
Completed in 1938 and located south of the bayou on Buffalo Drive, later
to be named Allen Parkway, the 11-story art deco structure was the largest
Depression-era construction project in Houston.

Five years later, when the Baylor University College of Medicine opened
in its temporary headquarters in the former Sears, Roebuck and Co. building on Buffalo Drive, the location was in close proximity to the new hospital. Capitalizing on the availability of such a convenient setting for the
medical college's education program, Dean Walter H. Moursund met with
the medical staff to request its cooperation and received approval in 1943
from both the staff and the board of managers. Their resulting agreement,
much like the one arranged by the dean with Hermann Hospital medical
staff, allowed only "clinical teaching" privileges for the medical school but
no other hands-on patient care.

These limitations were unacceptable to Dr. DeBakey, and in 1949 he decided a change was needed. Having voiced his displeasure with the similar parameters of the Hermann Hospital arrangement, he already had established his maverick status with the Harris County Medical Society. To avert the possibility of further fruitless altercations with the society and to achieve what he desired at Jefferson Davis Hospital, he chose to communicate his needs directly with the hospital's Chairman of the Board Ben Taub.

One of Houston's largest and most successful real estate developers, Mr. Taub also owned lumber companies, a molding company, and a concrete manufacturing concern. Well known in the community, he was a native Houstonian whose lifelong, behind-the-scenes philanthropic efforts focused on the indigent, ill, elderly, and children in his hometown. He served as chairman of the board of DePelchin Children's Center, a children's home, and two homes for widows, the Flake Home and the Wolfe Home. While taking impromptu walks through the hallways of the charity hospital, he often interacted with patients, displaying compassionate concern for each.[1]

Aware of Mr. Taub's sterling reputation in the community, Dr. DeBakey did not hesitate to contact him, an experience he vividly recalled: "It was the month following our taking over the VA Hospital in 1949 and I had called him on the phone; I had never met him before. I said, 'Mr. Taub, I am Mike DeBakey and I am new here and have recently been named chairman of the Department of Surgery at Baylor. I know you are interested in your patients' welfare at the Jefferson Davis Hospital. I want to talk with you. I only want 15 minutes of your time.' And he said, 'All right, come on.'"[2]

During their initial meeting, Dr. DeBakey presented his affiliation proposal within the allotted time requested, but when he announced, "I have used up my time," Mr. Taub replied, "I have plenty of time, and if you don't have to go I have some questions."[2] Their conversation continued for more than two hours, during which Mr. Taub displayed great interest in having the physicians, surgeons, and specialists at Baylor University College of Medicine assume the responsibility for the proper care of the sick patients at Jefferson Davis Hospital, the outpatient clinics, and emergency services.

In order to implement this mutually desired goal, the businessman suggested a plan, one that the surgeon deemed to be both ingenious and infallible. Since the Jefferson Davis Hospital had what was called a "closed staff" strictly comprised of members of the Harris County Medical Society and no one else, the mere suggestion of the hospital's possible affiliation with the medical college was certain to generate organized opposition. "To show you how crafty he was, Mr. Taub thought it would be a good idea to call in a consultant to look at it and make the recommendation," Dr. DeBakey said. "It would be a very strong point because these doctors would have a horrible time objecting. So, that's what we did." [2]

Another result of their initial meeting was that each considered the other to be an individual worth knowing better, a mutual admiration that marked the beginning of what would become a lifelong friendship. Believing the two were kindred spirits except in one specific area, Mr. Taub said, "He didn't care about money. I know very many men who don't care about money—and I'm not one of them because I care very much about money."[3] In the coming years, the two men were to spend a great deal of time together. During their traditional Sunday mornings together, not only at Jefferson Davis Hospital but also at Mr. Taub's home, as well as impromptu visits when time allowed, the two men found themselves to be deep in conversation. "We'd sit and talk and he would tell me about his projects and his dreams," Mr. Taub recalled. "He's always had more things going than you could believe. I knew there would be no stopping that fellow."[4]

Nor was there any impediment to the two men's plan to engender support for the affiliation of Jefferson Davis Hospital with Baylor University College of Medicine. Having worked closely at Tulane with a highly respected consultant, Dr. Basil C. McLean in Rochester, New York, during World War II, Dr. DeBakey knew him well. "He was a very close friend," Dr. DeBakey said. "So I called him on the phone and told him the background and told him Mr. Taub thought it would be a good idea to call a consultant to look at it and make the recommendation. I told him, 'If you would recommend it, it would be a very strong point because these doctors would have a very difficult time objecting.' He had the report written before he even came here!"[2]

After meeting with the consultant, the co-conspirators decided to further boost the chances for their proposal by taking him to meet one of the most influential members of the board of managers, Mr. Cullen. It was to be Dr. DeBakey's first meeting with the philanthropist, an opportunity for which he felt indebted to Mr. Taub. "He was a tremendous help to me, in so many ways," Dr. DeBakey often said in praise of his friend. "He had such tremendous influence and he could get friends to support ideas."[2]

The subsequent delivery of the consultant's report to the medical staff and board of managers at Jefferson Davis Hospital resulted in tumultuous conferences held by each group. As expected, there were multiple physicians who voiced strong opposition, but Mr. Taub remained confident that all eventually would accept the consultant's proposed affiliation. When he ascertained the majority of the board was in agreement, he called for a final, unanimous vote, saying, "If anything was worth doing halfway, it should be worth doing 100 percent."[5]

With the contractual agreement signed by the governing bodies of the two institutions, the affiliation became effective August 1, 1949. As previously offered by the college, each member of the hospital's active staff was to be given appointment to the faculty, if so desired. As a member of the volunteer faculty, each was to play an integral role in the college's clinical teaching program. Since the agreement stated only faculty members acceptable to the hospital's board of managers "shall serve on the staff of the Jefferson Davis Hospital,"[6] many of the most disgruntled members of the Harris County Medical Society begrudgingly complied. Their resulting sentiments were evident, especially to Dr. DeBakey, who later confessed, "I was not very popular."[7]

The opposite reaction was received from Dr. DeBakey's associates at the college, who shared an enthusiastic view of the affiliation. "This was a welcomed step in the growth of the Baylor University College of Medicine, as now there were two hospitals in which to make teaching rounds," said Dr. Don W. Chapman, an Iowan who had arrived at the college in July 1944 as one of its first full-time instructors.[8] The Chapman family had a strong medical tradition evidenced by every male in the Chapman family since The Civil War having become a physician, a total of 14.

Trained in medicine and cardiology at the University of Iowa, Dr. Chapman was destined to play a pivotal role in the developing field of cardiology in the decades to follow. He was enthusiastic about expanding the availability of cardiology services at Jefferson Davis Hospital in the late 1940s and early 1950s and also of all the other planned new services, recalling, "The volunteer faculty was eager to cover these commitments, and gradually the full time staff increased."[8]

As a faculty member who was keenly aware of the prevalence of hypertensive vascular disease among the indigent population, Dr. Chapman established a hypertension clinic at the hospital to address those patients' medical and surgical needs. In addition, specific clinics for valvular heart disease, congenital heart disease, coronary artery disease, and peripheral vascular disease were to come into existence in the months following the affiliation. To capitalize on the increased diagnostic capabilities made possible by right heart catheterization, a new technology,[9,10] a catheterization laboratory was established by converting a windowless, un-air-conditioned, inside room at the hospital. On Houston's hot summer days, Dr. Chapman admitted, "We may have measured the effect of heat on ourselves as much as we measured the patients' heart problems. Despite this, we continued to make progress in our catheterization research."[8]

Regardless of the obvious limitations of the new catheterization laboratory at Jefferson Davis Hospital, it was a notable improvement over the makeshift locale made available to Dr. Chapman at Hermann Hospital, where he had performed Houston's first cardiac catheterization in 1946. Having learned what he called the "new-fangled" diagnostic procedure while studying with one of its pioneers, Dr. Lewis Dexter at the Peter Bent Brigham Hospital in Boston, Dr. Chapman seized the opportunity to use Dr. Dexter's technique of wedging a small, elongated, plastic tube with a lumen (catheter) into a pulmonary artery as far as it would go to record the height of pulmonary capillary pressure.[11] The principal piece of equipment needed for this procedure was an X-ray unit, and the only one available at Hermann Hospital was devoted to gastrointestinal studies. When told by the head of the X-ray department there was no time available for catheterization procedures during normal working hours, Dr. Chapman had to improvise.

The resulting workable arrangement was to inspire a nickname for both Dr. Chapman and the group of residents involved in this pioneering endeavor: the "Dawn Patrol." Beginning at 5:00 A.M., residents Dr. Lynn Bernard, Dr. Rugeley Livesay, Dr. Ray Skaggs, Dr. Robert McConn, Dr. Robert Morse, and Dr. Lloyd J. Gugle joined Dr. Chapman on a rotating basis each weekday in the X-ray department at the Hermann Hospital. "Ultimately, we found that if we started at 6:00 A.M. in the morning, we could catheterize as long as we got everything out of there by 7:30 A.M.," Dr. Chapman recalled. "We could catheterize at least one patient per day."[12]

At the beginning, the Dawn Patrol was an enigma to the staff at Hermann Hospital, with few physicians able to appreciate the benefits of such heretofore untried procedures. This was to be expected in such a new field, one only recently introduced in the United States in 1941 by Dr. André Cournand and Dr. Dickinson Richards. With the surgical advances made during the late 1930s and early 1940s for the alteration or correction of certain congenital defects of the heart, the Dawn Patrol initially concentrated its efforts on developing techniques to provide a more accurate diagnosis of these lesions. Appropriate to the group's nickname, it was the dawning of the heart surgery era, and four congenital heart defects—patent ductus arteriosus,[13] coarctation of the aorta,[14] pulmonary stenosis, and tetralogy of Fallot[15]—became operable for the first time.

By the late 1940s, there were several practicing cardiologists in Houston. In addition to Dr. Chapman at The Methodist Hospital, Dr. Sydney Schnur practiced at St. Joseph Hospital downtown and brothers Dr. Paul V. Ledbetter and Dr. Abbe A. Ledbetter practiced at Baptist Memorial Hospital, also downtown.[16] Following in Dr. Abbe A. Ledbetter's footsteps was his son, Dr. Abbe A. Ledbetter Jr., who received his cardiology training in the early 1960s at Temple University Hospital in Philadelphia under Dr. William L. Winters Jr.

The Houston contingent of cardiologists in 1948 was aware that intravenous catheterization of the heart had been performed by Dr. Chapman and the residents at Hermann Hospital on more than 58 patients suspected of having congenital defects of the hearts or great vessels. "The results illustrate its value to ascertain whether or not the patient has a defect, to indicate operability when defects are discovered, and to suggest the prognosis," Dr. Chapman reported to the hospital's medical staff, which, in turn, immediately endorsed the new procedures.[17] Although this was welcomed by Dr. Chapman, he nonetheless found himself to be in a conundrum: "We were making accurate diagnoses from the heart catheterization lab, but no one was doing anything about it regarding the necessary surgery."[18,19]

At the time, while incremental advances in cardiac surgery were taking place elsewhere in the United States and Europe, Dr. DeBakey primarily performed general surgery in Houston, including a limited amount of vascular surgery for ulcers, varicose veins, and sympathectomies, a comparatively new surgical technique for treating diminished blood flow to the legs caused by arteriosclerosis. Speaking at a meeting of the American College of Surgeons held in Houston in 1949, Dr. DeBakey referenced a study he had completed at Tulane in which 80 patients underwent this procedure to sever certain sympathetic nerves. Stating that this surgery "saved over half of these from a major amputation," he went on to explain, "By severing the nerve leading to the auxiliary arteries, the vessels are allowed to dilate, thus increasing the flow of blood within the arm or leg."[20,21]

Another area of surgical interest to Dr. DeBakey at that time was the emergency room at Jefferson Davis Hospital. In a city destined to be named "Murder Capital of the United States"[22] in 1981, there was an unending emergency room parade of citizens who suffered from shotgun and handgun wounds, razor or knife lacerations, and ice-pick wounds, all remarkably similar to the penetrating vascular injuries experienced by soldiers in World War II. After being awarded a special U.S. Army grant to study these injuries,[23] Dr. DeBakey established the country's first civilian trauma center at Jefferson Davis Hospital in 1949.[24] The predominance of surgical procedures for vascular injuries there was recalled by one former resident, who said, "I would say 90 percent of what we did was trauma, because we didn't have time for elective surgery."[25]

To meet these and other escalating demands presented by the two newly affiliated hospitals in 1949, Dr. DeBakey began to expand the Department of Surgery at Baylor University College of Medicine. The first to join the full-time faculty was Dr. Oscar Creech Jr., a vascular surgeon who had just completed his surgical residency at Tulane University. As one of his mentors there, Dr. DeBakey had been "very impressed" with his work, a high opinion that was not to waiver throughout his protégé's career.[7] In Houston for the following seven years, Dr. Creech was to devote his efforts to basic experimental and clinical work on arteriosclerotic lesions, on the clinical approach to vascular disease, and on a better understanding of the use of arterial homografts and synthetic grafts.[26]

Within one year of Dr. Creech's 1949 arrival in Houston, Dr. DeBakey began to escalate his expansion plans for the Department of Surgery after the announcement of another hospital affiliation for Baylor University College of Medicine. An agreement signed October 3, 1951, by the board of trustees at The Methodist Hospital and the Houston executive committee of the board of trustees of Baylor University was effective for 30 years, with the provision that it could be terminated at any time by mutual consent or by either party's giving the other party 18 months written notice of termination.[27]

Similar to the affiliation agreement enacted at the Jefferson Davis Hospital, there was a requirement that all members of the medical staff at The Methodist Hospital were eligible to receive clinical appointments on the faculty of Baylor University College of Medicine. As was the case with Jefferson Davis Hospital, the existing medical staff members were invited to join the faculty as members of the volunteer clinical faculty, if so desired. It was a stipulation fully embraced by Dr. Hatch Cummings, chief of the hospital's medicine department, who believed this was the only way to avoid the problems exhibited at Hermann Hospital, where he said the staff believed they were in charge of the patients and the Baylor faculty "could make rounds on them and talk about them and teach off of them, but wouldn't have control of their care."[28]

Because the affiliation also was to improve the education programs that Dr. Cummings previously had instigated and championed at The Methodist Hospital, he was an avid supporter of the agreement and of the boards' mutually shared goals stated therein. In writing, both parties agreed in good faith to carry out a program for the advancement of medical service through professional care of the sick; training of medical and ancillary personnel;

promotion of personal and community health; and advancement of medical knowledge through investigation.[29]

The inclusion of The Methodist Hospital in the medical college's affiliation program presented the opportunity to create one of the nation's first inclusive, multihospital teaching programs, one that was to be greatly enhanced by the volunteer faculty's participation.[30] The new program's first surgical resident in general and thoracic surgery was Dr. George Cooper Morris Jr., who received his medical degree at the University of Pennsylvania. After completing his internship and residency in surgical pathology there, he came to Baylor University College of Medicine in 1950 as a resident and was to remain there for more than 46 years, holding many academic appointments, including professor of surgery. In retrospect, Dr. DeBakey was to say that because Dr. Morris possessed and demonstrated "all the qualities essential to surgery—technical ability, absolute integrity, a good basic foundation in anatomy, pathology, and physiology, and a compassionate concern for the patient," he was one of the best surgeons he ever trained.[31]

In addition to the arrival of his first resident in 1950, Dr. DeBakey also was expecting to welcome the first surgeon he had appointed to the faculty for the expressed purpose of organizing a cardiovascular program, Dr. Denton A. Cooley.[32] However, after completing his surgical residency at Johns Hopkins with Dr. Alfred Blalock, Dr. Cooley had been invited by the renowned surgeon Dr. Russell Brock to train for an additional year at the Brompton Hospital in London. When he had asked permission to arrive in Houston one year later than planned, Dr. DeBakey not only agreed but also encouraged his seizing the opportunity to receive advanced training from one of the world's recognized pioneers in cardiac surgery.

At that time, Dr. Brock, later to become Lord Brock of Wimbledon, was one of the first surgeons to perfect mitral valve surgery. He had produced three successful results in 1948 by using a self-designed mechanical dilator to better separate the commissures of the valve. His keen interest in congenital heart disease and Dr. Blalock's breakthrough "blue baby" operation resulted in his developing another mechanical dilator, a pulmonary valvulotome, to directly attack pulmonary stenosis.[33] During an exchange-program visit to Johns Hopkins in 1948, Lord Brock, with an assist from Dr. Cooley, performed demonstrative operations using this instrument with a retractable, spade-shaped blade to open the pulmonary valves of children suffering from tetralogy of Fallot.[34]

Because of these procedures and Dr. Cooley's other recognized accomplishments at Johns Hopkins, Dr. DeBakey already knew him to be "well trained and a damn good surgeon."[2] A native Houstonian, Dr. Cooley had attended the University of Texas Medical Branch in Galveston before switching to Johns Hopkins University School of Medicine, where he earned his medical degree. As a first-year surgical intern at Johns Hopkins Hospital in 1944, he had worked with the legendary cardiologist Dr. Helen Taussig and assisted Dr. Blalock when he performed the first Blalock-Taussig shunt for treating tetralogy of Fallot, known as "the blue baby" operation.[15] "The striking results from this procedure, which increased the circulation through the pulmonary arterial system, caused much excitement in the surgical community," Dr. Cooley said, noting the personal impact of being a part of that first "blue baby" operation. "I witnessed the dawn of heart surgery."[35]

He also experienced Johns Hopkins Hospital's becoming the epicenter for congenital heart case referrals in the country. While training with Dr. Blalock, he assisted or independently performed more than 200 Blalock-Taussig shunts as well as countless other surgical procedures, including two successful outcomes in surgical repair of aortic aneurysms.[36] A member of the Army Specialty Training Program, Dr. Cooley was called to active duty in 1946 and spent two years as a general surgeon and chief of surgery at the 124th Station Hospital in Linz, Austria. Returning to Johns Hopkins in 1948, he was appointed chief resident, one of the most coveted and prestigious postgraduate surgical positions in the United States.[37]

When belated news of Dr. Cooley's accepting Dr. DeBakey's appointment finally reached Dr. Chapman, the heretofore frustrated cardiologist thought his conundrum of making accurate diagnoses without having experienced surgeons to operate was soon to be solved. Without knowing him, Dr. Chapman wrote Dr. Cooley a letter at Johns Hopkins to express his delight about his imminent arrival in 1950, stating that there already were quite a few patients in need of his expertise. Dr. Cooley's reply advised that his arrival would be delayed until after his training in London and included advice about Dr. Chapman's patients: "I will be back in a year. Keep 'em on ice."[18]

While in London in 1950 for his training with Lord Brock as a senior surgical registrar, the equivalent of senior resident in the United States, Dr. Cooley learned fundamental diagnostics and other techniques usually performed by cardiology specialists in the United States. Because of his interest in learning more about his mentor's pioneering techniques with internal heart surgery, like opening the pulmonary valves of children suffering from tetralogy of Fallot, and his genius in lung surgery and mitral stenosis, Dr. Cooley preferred to be with him in the operating room and soon grew restless with his inability to do so more often. He was known to be swift and skillful at Johns Hopkins and found the deliberately slow and methodical diagnostic process practiced at the Brompton Hospital to be a waste of time. Labeling it the "Sherlock Holmes" approach,[38] he felt it caused patients to wait needlessly for surgery, which he was anxious to do expeditiously for as many as possible on any given day. Convinced that the opportunity to do exactly that awaited him at Baylor University College of Medicine, Dr. Cooley became anxious to return to the United States.

This anxiety was obvious to Lord Brock, who offered this perspective of his protégé's year at Brompton Hospital: "Denton Cooley was eager to return home for two reasons: there was the Korean War—which may have been an excuse, though he was liable to military duty—and then it admittedly was the restlessness of his nature. He believed he had gotten as much in nine months here as the average man would have gotten in a year—which was probably true. It stands to reason that the world will not produce a second Denton Cooley; and, frankly, I have my doubts if the world could handle another one. He spun in and out of here like a whirlwind, though not without leaving his mark—indeed, several marks."[39]

The indelible marks Dr. Cooley was to leave at Baylor University College of Medicine became obvious immediately following his arrival on June 11, 1951. Within the first few weeks of his joining the full-time faculty as an associate professor, the highly anticipated beginning of Dr. DeBakey's cardiovascular program occurred unexpectedly at Jefferson Davis Hospital. While making one of their first rounds together, the two surgeons encountered a patient with a syphilitic aneurysm of the aortic arch, an abnormal bulge on the wall of the body's largest artery. It was diagnosed as a saccular aneurysm, an asymmetrical blister on the weakened artery wall that could rupture, causing life-threatening bleeding, but the proper surgical treatment of such aneurysms was debatable at that time.

"Aneurysms of the aorta were always the big challenge," Dr. DeBakey said, pointing out that only incremental advances had been made in the diagnosis and treatment of an aneurysm since it was first identified in the 2nd century.[2] One advance made in 1903 by Dr. Matas at Tulane was the introduction of his concept of endoaneurysmorrhaphy, the obliteration of the aneurismal sac and suturing it to preserve blood flow. Before publishing *The Principles and Practice of Medicine* textbook in 1892, Dr. William Osler had performed more than 1,000 autopsies to develop his clinical acumen and professional expertise and knowledge of aneurysms. A decade later, the highly regarded internist and first physician-in-chief at Johns Hopkins Hospital remained perplexed about the diagnostic aspects and surgical treatment of aneurysms in 1910, stating, "There is no disease more conducive to clinical humility than aneurysm of the aorta."[40]

In the early decades of the 20th century, physicians had found that aortic diseases were common among those afflicted with syphilis, with most aneurysms occurring predominantly in the thoracic area. Though the patient at Jefferson Davis Hospital was receiving 12 million units of penicillin, whether such treatment would be adequate to alter a syphilitic aneurysm causing pain in his lower left chest was not known in 1951.[41] As most patients with syphilitic aneurysms died within a year after onset of symptoms, his prognosis was poor.[42] "Even specific medicinal measures in syphilitic and mycotic aneurysms have usually proved ineffectual in controlling the fatal consequences once the aneurysm is well developed," Dr. DeBakey explained. "The surgical treatment of intrathoracic aneurysms of the aorta and its major tributaries remains a difficult problem and, for the most part, unsatisfactory despite the remarkable advances in vascular surgery that have been made in recent years."[43]

In addition to Dr. Matas's endoaneurysmorrhaphy, existing procedures for the surgical treatment of saccular aneurysms in 1951 were the use of fibrogenic material, such as cellophane, to wrap the aneurysm to promote blood clotting and the introduction of a foreign material, such as wiring, to promote coagulation of the blood. When Dr. DeBakey asked which of these procedures Dr. Cooley recommended for this particular patient, he replied his preference was for none of them. Instead, he suggested excision, a rarely utilized aneurysm procedure that he had previously performed, with two successful outcomes, at Johns Hopkins. "I think if you put a clamp across the base of it, you could take the thing off and the man would recover," Dr. Cooley said. "He sure doesn't have a chance lying there in bed."[44]

Several days later, Dr. Cooley operated on the patient at Jefferson Davis Hospital, successfully performing the proposed aneurysmectomy that later was to be termed "a tangential excision and lateral aortorrhaphy."[36] Subsequently, following a succession of procedures performed on three additional patients who presented with aortic aneurysms, he and Dr. DeBakey presented a report of their pioneering efforts to the Southern Surgical Association in Hot Springs, Arkansas, on December 4, 1951. Advocating the excision of aortic aneurysms as the method of choice when possible, the two surgeons received an enthusiastic response from a majority of their peers and effectively established themselves as aortic aneurysm experts, even among those who said their new technique soon was to become outdated. "Five of the first six patients had syphilitic aneurysms," said Dr. Cooley. "I can readily recall the comment of the renowned Dr. Evarts Graham of Barnes Hospital. He said that the technique, unfortunately, was untimely because the advent of penicillin would make aortic syphilitic aneurysms rare. That was true, but atherosclerosis and trauma soon provided an abundance of pathologic material for clinical trials."[45]

Another certainty in the future was more critical acclaim for the two Baylor University College of Medicine cardiovascular surgeons, as this was only the first of many innovative surgical procedures to be introduced. Also to gain a reputation for its impressive volume of surgical treatments performed, "The Houston Group," as it was to become known among its peers around the world, wasted no time in laying the foundation for that accolade. With the evaluation services rendered by the cardiac catheterizations performed by Dr. Chapman and his "Dawn Patrol," the two surgeons were able to begin a series of 50 consecutive cases of surgical treatment of mitral stenosis by commissurotomy in 1951 at both Jefferson Davis and the VA hospitals. Included in a 1953 published report authored by Drs. Cooley, Chapman, and DeBakey was an additional 13 patients who underwent the procedure, bringing the consecutive total to 63.[46] Since such a large number was in stark contrast to Lord Brock's published 1948 report about his first three surgical treatments of mitral stenosis, the medical community began to take notice of the "Houston Group," soon discovering their volume of cardiovascular surgical treatments was to increase exponentially during the coming years.[47]

One area of that growth was to be in the surgical treatment of aortic diseases. Inspired by the initial successes resulting from their direct approach to the treatment of saccular aneurysms, Dr. DeBakey set his sights on a plan "to work my way around the aorta," a seldom taken path for surgeons in 1951.[2] The impetus for this ambitious plan was the advances made in the surgical corrections of congenital heart defects during the 1940s, in particular the procedures for vascular anomalies such as patent ductus and coarctation of the aorta, which was introduced in 1938 by Bostonian Dr. Robert E. Gross. Also of great interest to Dr. DeBakey was the continuing research of aortic repairs at Georgetown University by Dr. Charles Hufnagel, who began experimenting with artificial valves in 1946. But the predominant motivation to focus on aortic disease stemmed from the fact that cardiovascular disease remained the underlying cause of more than 75 percent of U.S. deaths in the 1950s. "One of the fatal aortic diseases was dissection of the aorta," Dr. DeBakey said. "All studies that were done on the national history of aortic dissection showed that 50 percent died within 48 hours after occurrence, 90 percent in three months, and rarely did anyone live a year."[7]

Determined to devise surgical procedures to improve the prognosis for aortic dissection and all other fatal aortic diseases, Dr. DeBakey embarked on his ambitious plan in 1951. "The only aortic disease that was treatable was coarctation of the aorta and there was no effective treatment for fusiform aneurysms," he said, referring to the symmetrical ballooning on the weakened artery wall. "Treatment of coarctation actually gave me the idea that other problems with the aorta might be treatable. Gross and Hufnagel presented some experimental work showing that in animals they could bridge an aortic defect with a homograft. That gave me the idea: why not use a homograft for an aneurysm?"[7]

A homograft, now known as an allograft, was a homologous arterial graft transplanted between genetically nonidentical individuals of the same species. Since the primary source for such blood vessels was cadavers, Dr. DeBakey conceived a plan not only to harvest his own supply but also to establish a viable source for future procedures in a tissue bank. "I was in the fortunate position at the time of having access to all the autopsies that the coroner had to do at Jefferson Davis Hospital," Dr. DeBakey said. "The coroner at that time was a very nice fellow, but lazy as hell. He didn't like to get up in the middle of [the] night to do an autopsy."[2] Seizing the opportunity, Dr. DeBakey told him that "my residents and I would do all his autopsies, because I wanted to train them by this means; he readily agreed. At Charity Hospital in New Orleans, when a patient died, we went to the autopsy room. I considered it a great teaching experience. By doing the autopsies, we had a ready opportunity to obtain homografts."[7]

The next step in Dr. DeBakey's formulated plan for the surgical treatment of aortic diseases would be taken within a matter of months, but not at Jefferson Davis Hospital. It was to occur in a newly opened 300-bed facility located in the Texas Medical Center, The Methodist Hospital, which, in tandem with the pioneering advances in cardiovascular surgery made therein, was to be propelled into the national spotlight thereafter.

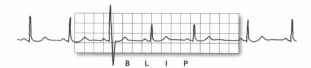

THE FAST LANE

*F*rom the onset of the collaborative efforts of Drs. DeBakey and Cooley, the pair became the fodder for urban legends. One example of Texas Medical Center lore from the 1950s and 60s, according to Dr. S. Ward Casscells, was this story: "As he often did, Dr. DeBakey was racing his sports car to the medical center, in green scrubs ready to round and operate, residents at attention to park the car and hold the elevators, teams lined up nervously, secretly hoping he would not come, just as the patients yearned to see him. The policeman who stopped him for speeding was unfazed when the driver said, 'Surely you know who I am, and how important it is that I get to the hospital immediately!' Not realizing he was speaking to the mentor and not the rising star, the officer said, 'Sir, I would have to give you this ticket even if you were Dr. Denton Cooley himself.'"[1]

1. S. Ward Casscells, MD, *Remembering A Legend, Dr. Michael DeBakey*, U.S. Department of Defense Military Health System, July 12, 2008. Military Health System web site: http://www.health.mil/News_And_Multimedia/News/detail/08-07-12/Remembering_a_Legend_-_Dr._Michael_DeBakey.aspx. Accessed May 18, 2013.

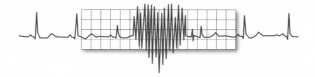

CHAPTER FOUR

INSIDE THE BEATING HEART
1949 - 1956

"It is the feet that you move, but it is with your heart that you dance."
AALAYNAH THOMPSON

In the two years following the December 1949 groundbreaking ceremonies for The Methodist Hospital at the Texas Medical Center, there were growing doubts among the board of trustees about its decision to build a 300-bed facility. Even those who originally supported Mrs. Fondren's ultimatum to build such a large facility began to express apprehensions about whether there would be enough patients to fill the beds.

The fear of low occupancy was legitimate at the time, since it was an existing problem at The Methodist Hospital on Rosalie Avenue in 1951. This fact strongly influenced the board's decision to limit the number of beds for the November 1951 opening of The Methodist Hospital in the Texas Medical Center. Instead of the full 300-bed occupancy, there were to be only 193 beds available for immediate occupancy.[1] Fearful that even this number of beds would go unoccupied, one board member, O'Banion Williams, decided to drum up business by imploring the medical staff to strongly encourage other doctors in the community to admit their patients to the new hospital.

Such concern reflected the past, when the steadily diminishing number of patients on Rosalie Avenue caused the board to implement many cost-saving measures during Mr. Bowen's first few years as assistant administrator. With a constrained operating budget, he often found himself improvising solutions to the problems presented by a limited income. By his side to help accomplish many of those extracurricular tasks was his wife, who viewed their collaborative efforts during the early years as necessary under the circumstances. "At that time, you did anything that needed to be done," she said, recalling how the hospital was "working on a shoestring."[2]

An example of the Bowens' ingenuity followed the board's futile search for the architectural plans for Dr. Norsworthy's original structure, as well as all subsequent additions to the structure, to present to possible buyers of the Rosalie Avenue facilities. Since the expense of hiring an architect to document the floor plans was declared prohibitive by the board, the Bowens took matters into their own hands. "We went down and I've forgotten how long it took us to do it, but with a ruler and a tape measure he would measure and I would draw," Mrs. Bowen said. "They were amateurish, of course, but we did draw an acceptable set of plans so they could use them."[2]

Another artistic endeavor created by the Bowens in 1949 was in response to an expense deemed unnecessary by the board of trustees, a sign to mark "The Site of The New Methodist Hospital" in the Texas Medical Center. "They said we'd have to do without a sign, but we wanted a sign, so we painted one and it was very adequate and it stood up through the whole building process," they said decades later, still proud of the two pieces of board cobbled together by the hospital's carpenters.[2]

What also remained during the entire construction process of the new facility was the operating deficit at the Rosalie Avenue site. In order to keep the hospital open, Mrs. Fondren and Mr. Goldston continued to anonymously contribute the necessary funds to cover the monthly shortages. With the expectations that the new hospital also would lose money during its opening period, the board turned to the bank to borrow $80,000 for startup purposes.[1] "It was an exciting time and interesting time and a time that you really develop a whole lot with some adversity here and there," Mr. Bowen said. "I think all of us developed with that challenge that we had, not only me, but the other members of the staff and the doctors."[2]

Singularly saddled with the challenge of designing and creating the new hospital was Mrs. Roberts, who had delegated most of her administrative duties to Mr. Bowen. "She worked day and night almost 24 hours a day to supervise its construction," said Robert A. Shepherd, chairman of the board of trustees.[3] Although he and the board had offered to hire a consultant to help design the new hospital, Mrs. Roberts was confident she could deliver the desired results without incurring the additional expense of a consultant.

During the previous 28 years, Mrs. Roberts had traveled extensively in search of ideas to incorporate into a new hospital, taking copious notes about each innovation she encountered along the way. Her resulting design plans were meticulous, and as construction progressed on the new hospital, she and Mr. Shepherd would periodically inspect every nook and cranny to ensure all of her specifications had been met. "I think everybody has a fond-ness and respect for her for what she did," Mr. Bowen said. "She spent lit-erally thousands of hours designing that building. There are very few things wrong with the first main building, from an operating standpoint as well as the structural, architectural and so forth standpoint. She devoted her latter years to practically that and that alone and did a marvelous job." [2]

The fruits of Mrs. Roberts' labor were clearly evident not only to the dignitaries gathered at the formal dedication of The Methodist Hospital on November 10, 1951, but also to members of the media given a "peek-a-boo preview" beforehand. [4] Serving as the tour guide for this group of reporters and photographers, Mrs. Roberts emphasized the technical advances in-corporated for efficiency, the design nuances introduced especially for the patients' comfort, and both the beauty and maintenance practicalities of the washable wallpaper, fiberglass drapes, and plastic blinds. Reported one newsman in the group, "When she talks about the new $4,500,000 medical wonderland she helped create, her blue eyes dance with excitement, and her voice vibrates as she describes the many innovations that make the hospital one of the most modern in the nation." [5]

Among the innovative features enthusiastically described to the media by Mrs. Roberts were those found in the second-floor operating suite. Com-prising 11 separate operating rooms, the suite included two designated for urology procedures, one for orthopedic procedures, and eight for major sur-gery, one of which was specifically designed for neurosurgery, a specialty pi-oneered at the Rosalie Avenue location by Houston's first neurosurgeon, Dr. James A. Greenwood. Four of the major surgery operating rooms were con-structed with observation booths, and all 11 operating rooms were wired for televised viewing in the nearby doctors' staff suite, an area constructed with finances donated by the medical staff. Adjacent to the operating rooms was an eight-bed recovery unit for the observation of patients immediately after surgery, the first of its kind in Houston and a modernism championed by Dr. Presley H. Chalmers, the hospital's newly named chief of anesthesiology.

Following Mrs. Roberts' informative tour and the formal dedication cere-monies, both the local and national media published glowing reviews about the opening of The Methodist Hospital in the Texas Medical Center. *The New York Times* noted its "incorporating many advances in hospital con-struction" and praised the "many installations for saving time and energy." Echoing the praise given in 1924 to Dr. Norsworthy's hospital on Rosalie Avenue was one Houston reporter's observation that "being a patient in the new 315-bed hospital will be a virtual pleasure" [4]

Newspapers across the country heralded the "most modern hospital in the South,"[6] and though most published reports included information about the availability of Dr. Greenwood's diagnostic and treatment center for neurological and brain-disease patients, there was no mention of a diagnostic and treatment center for vascular- and heart-disease patients nor the pioneering surgical efforts of Dr. DeBakey. This was not an oversight; his was a yet-to-be-established specialty at The Methodist Hospital, and its resulting dramatic impact on that new facility, as well as the field of vascular surgery, was unimaginable in 1951.

What was unthinkable to the hospital's board of trustees at that time was the immediate demand for more available beds. In less than one week after transferring 63 patients from Rosalie Avenue to the new hospital, Mrs. Roberts reported occupancy had more than doubled to 143 patients, necessitating her arranging for more available beds within a matter of weeks. Seven months after opening, she reported the average occupancy was 220.8 patients. At the conclusion of the hospital's first full year of operation in 1952, she announced an average of 86 percent occupancy for all 300 beds and an upcoming vacancy in the administration office.[6]

In celebration of her accomplishments and to commemorate her 29 years of service, Mrs. Roberts informed the board of her decision to retire on the upcoming anniversary date of employment in February 1953. "When I came to Houston, to The Methodist Hospital, I said I had three purposes in life that I hoped to fulfill," she said. "One was to raise a good, Christian daughter. The other was to see her educated and happily married. The third was to build a hospital. I accomplished those three things."[7]

Named by the board to succeed Mrs. Roberts was the candidate she had not only groomed for the position but also had recommended to the search committee, Ted Bowen, her 32-year-old assistant. Initially given the title of acting administrator in February 1953, Mr. Bowen was named administrator several months later, becoming the youngest head of a major hospital in Texas.[8] Confident in his new role, he stressed that the key ingredient necessary to managing a successful hospital was an equally balanced triad comprised of medical staff, board of trustees, and administration. In his role as administrator, he was "dedicated to increasing our research capabilities and our educational capabilities, along with our clinical excellence" and strived to establish "a comprehensive institution with quality care, education, and all sorts of research going on in every part."[2] To accomplish this mission, his working seven days a week, often more than 18 hours a day, soon became the norm as The Methodist Hospital rapidly evolved from its presupposed role in the community to its unexpected debut and continuing presence on the world stage.

This evolution was propelled by Dr. DeBakey's succession of pioneering accomplishments in the field of vascular surgery at The Methodist Hospital. Progressing in his stated goal to work his way around the aorta, he and Dr. Cooley continued to make noteworthy strides, eventually establishing themselves as the recognized experts in the field of aortic aneurysms. As envisioned, Dr. DeBakey began to use homografts successfully during arterial repair procedures shortly after the new hospital opened in 1951.[9-10]

These innovative operations generated newspaper headlines that ranged from "Dead Man's Arteries Save Life"[11] in a Connecticut patient's hometown paper to "Rare Operation Patches Aorta With Accident Victim's Artery,"[12] a nationally syndicated Associated Press story about another patient's homograft surgery. More often than not, unlike the articles published elsewhere in the country, the Houston newspapers deferred to the Harris County Medical Society's ban on personal publicity and omitted the surgeons' names when reporting these surgical advances.

Impossible to ignore by the local media or the medical society was the worldwide recognition given to Dr. DeBakey in March 1952 for his invaluable contribution to a history making surgical operation in Philadelphia. It was the first use of Dr. John H. Gibbon Jr.'s "mechanical heart," an apparatus introduced to keep a patient's blood flowing for the duration of the surgical procedure.[13] Described by a spokesman as "an improved version of the pump developed in 1932 by Dr. Michael DeBakey,"[11-15] this new invention was to be perfected by Dr. Gibbon in the coming year. On May 6, 1953, it officially became known as the "heart-lung machine" when it was used to approximate those organs' functions in the first open-heart operation successfully performed in Philadelphia, one of the most important advances in the history of cardiac diseases.[16]

Also destined for the history books was a first-of-its-kind procedure performed in January 1953 by Drs. DeBakey and Cooley at The Methodist Hospital. Credited by name in the June 29, 1953, issue of Time magazine for successfully performing "an operation which was unthinkable until a few years ago," the two surgeons described the four-and-one-half hour successful resection of a syphilitic fusiform aneurysm of the descending thoracic aorta that was successfully resected with restoration of normal blood flow by means of an aortic homograft.[17]

Public reaction to that Time article, coupled with the medical community's response to the surgeons' published report in the June 20, 1953, issue of the *Journal of the American Medical Association*, [18] was measurable at The Methodist Hospital. "No one else was performing this operation, so physicians were referring their patients to me," Dr. DeBakey said. "As my service began to increase, I was using more and more beds; at one time I had a service of about 100 beds."[19]

Among the growing number of referrals were patients of physicians who had had the occasion to hear Dr. DeBakey speak, an extracurricular activity in which he excelled. Invited to address medical organizations throughout the world, he rarely declined an opportunity to express his opinion or demonstrate his expertise. His travels were extensive, and the origins of his referred patient population often reflected the cities, states, and countries in which he spoke. One such patient from Georgia, who underwent surgery for an aortic aneurysm in 1953, told the *Houston Chronicle*, "Our doctor was in Florida and heard a paper delivered at a medical meeting by the Baylor surgeon who fixed me up. That's what brought me here. I'm anxious to get home, but I sure hate to leave this hospital. I'll admit they do things right in Texas."[20]

As the surgeons' reputation continued to grow, the hospital began to admit referred patients who had been diagnosed with arterial diseases for which proven surgical treatments did not exist. "In 1953, I saw a patient with symptoms of circulatory insufficiency in the left carotid arterial bed and left side of his brain, which, on the basis of the clinical manifestations, I believed to be due to arteriosclerotic occlusion of the left carotid artery," Dr. DeBakey recalled. Because of the "considerable favorable results" from the surgical removal of plaque from a blocked artery, a procedure known as endarterectomy, and graft replacement for segmental lesions causing insufficient circulation in other arteries, particularly those in the legs, Dr. DeBakey "believed that the same procedure would restore normal circulation in the left carotid artery in this patient." Upon learning the surgical risk was slight, the patient expressed his confidence in the surgeon and agreed to the experimental surgery. On August 7, 1953, Dr. DeBakey performed the first successful carotid endarterectomy, thereby establishing the field of surgery for strokes.[21]

Another first at The Methodist Hospital in August 1953 was the Walter L. Goldston Cardiac Clinic, a cardiac catheterization laboratory for private patients. Its advent was hailed from afar by Dr. Chapman, who had been called to service in the U.S. Army Medical Corps and was assigned to the 5th General Hospital in Stuttgart Bad-Cannstatt during the Korean War.[22]

The new cardiac clinic and catheterization laboratory, located on the hospital's ninth floor, was named in tribute to one of the hospital's most generous benefactors, Mr. Goldston. Under the direction of Dr. Ray K. Skaggs of the medical department, the clinic began to average one catheterization per week, mostly "congenital abnormalities of the heart, but a few with acquired heart disease," mostly of rheumatic origins.[23-25] Patients with congenital abnormalities of the heart were those who predominantly had been referred to Dr. Cooley, the surgeon with the recognized expertise in that field in 1953. Recalling those early days of congenital heart surgery, Dr. Cooley said, "Our methods of diagnosis were extremely crude by today's standards, because most were made on physical findings rather than using the more sophisticated diagnostic techniques available today."[26]

Equally antiquated in retrospect was the diagnostic tool known as roentgenograms, the medical terminology for X-ray pictures that were used to confirm aortic aneurysms in the early 1950s. By 1954, Drs. DeBakey and Cooley had experience with the excision of aortic aneurysms and replacement with homografts in more than 29 cases.[27-30] Although there were six deaths, the surgeons were gratified with the early results and other clinical observations on the use of aortic homografts "encourage us to believe that this method of therapy constitutes the most effective surgical approach to the problem of the aneurysms of the aorta."[31]

Because of these pioneering successes with homografts for vascular replacement, Dr. DeBakey quickly realized that an increasing demand for homografts soon would far surpass the quantity available. To prepare for that inevitability and to address the need to establish an inventory of the various sizes needed to perform vascular replacements, he began his research to develop a suitable arterial substitute. After reading in 1952 about the experimental use of Vinyon "N"— the synthetic cloth used to make spinnaker sails—to create such arterial grafts at Columbia University School of Physicians and Surgeons, he went to a Houston department store in search of the same material.

Disappointed to learn Vinyon "N" was not available for purchase at the store, Dr. DeBakey asked whether a similar synthetic fabric might be available. "They said, 'We are fresh out of nylon, but we do have a new material called Dacron.' I felt it, and it looked good to me, so I bought a yard of it," he explained. "You have to remember that my mother was kind of a sewing instructor. In those days when you were growing up as a boy, girls were supposed to sew. So, after school, she would always have about six or seven young girls come to the house, and she would spend an hour with them teaching them how to sew. She saw I was interested, so she taught me how to sew. In fact, I taught my wife how to sew. So I had this sense of what you could do with a sewing machine."[32]

With that exact thought in his mind, Dr. DeBakey took the Dacron fabric home to work on his wife's sewing machine. "I cut two sheets in the width I wanted, sewed the edges on both sides, and made a tube out of it," he said. Later, in the laboratory with Dr. Creech, "we made our own crimping. We put the graft on a stent, wrapped nylon thread around it, pushed it together, and baked it. That would change the 'memory' in the fiber, and it would crimp. We did that all ourselves in the laboratory. After about two or three years of laboratory work, on my own, I decided that it was time to put the graft in a human being."[32-33]

The opportunity to utilize this laboratory-tested Dacron arterial substitute in a patient came during an abdominal aortic aneurysm resection in 1954. In the four years following the success of that operation, Dr. DeBakey's team of surgeons, which included Drs. Cooley, Creech, Morris, and a new member, Dr. E. Stanley Crawford, performed more than 654 procedures to replace or bypass aortic and peripheral arterial lesions at The Methodist Hospital. In the first 317 patients, they implanted a variety of synthetic tubes, but in the last consecutive 237 cases, he and his team exclusively implanted the new, flexible, knitted Dacron tube as a vascular replacement. Subsequently in 1958, these surgeons reported their collective belief that the Dacron tube was the most satisfactory available vascular replacement.[34] This pioneering work by Dr. DeBakey was to popularize both woven and knitted grafts all over the world and serve as a catalyst for the rapid development of the field of reconstructive arterial surgery.[35]

Also destined to gain international attention in the years to come was Dr. Crawford, an Alabama native educated at The University of Alabama and Harvard Medical School. His arrival in the Department of Surgery at Baylor University College of Medicine in 1954, following the completion of his surgical residency as chief resident at Massachusetts General Hospital, marked the beginning of his 38-year career in Houston. A master surgeon, he was to become known for his innovative surgical techniques in the treatment of complex aortic diseases, particularly Marfan syndrome and aortic dissection. While in Houston, be was to become a prodigious scholar and teacher and the author of more than 300 peer-reviewed publications and book chapters. His book, *Diseases of the Aorta*, published in 1984 with his surgeon son, Dr. John Lloyd Crawford II, was to be considered as one of the standard reference texts on aortic surgery.[36]

Already recognized in 1954 by their peers for their pioneering surgical treatments of aortic aneurysms, Drs. DeBakey, Cooley, and Creech became known to a large segment of the general public by making their national television debut together on December 5, 1954. Filmed while performing an aortic aneurysm operation at The Methodist Hospital, the surgeons appeared before an estimated audience of 10 million viewers who had tuned in to watch the *March of Medicine* program on NBC. Afterward, newspapers around the country documented this "life and death drama staged in an operating room," noting that "it was the first time in medical history that such an operation had been televised for the public."[37]

Such a precedent was to generate a measurable increase in the number of referred patients from across the country to The Methodist Hospital and the surgical services available therein. What's more, Dr. DeBakey also was receiving media attention for his participation in former President Hoover's second Commission on Organization of the Executive Branch of the Government. Appointed one of the 15 members of the task force on the medical services in 1953, Dr. DeBakey gained nationwide recognition for his efforts to transfer the Army Medical Library to the National Institutes of Health.

Ever since he spent hours of research time in the dilapidated Army Medical Library during the war, Dr. DeBakey actively had participated in the ongoing fruitless efforts to create national awareness for the need to construct a new facility to house its treasure trove of medical information. "I was therefore convinced that the problem of the library could not be resolved without adequate legislation to define its responsibilities and establish it clearly as the National Library of Medicine," he said, recalling not only how this conviction was included in the task force's report but also how he personally emphasized "the direness of the needs" to President Hoover.[38] As a result, Dr. DeBakey said, "That became one of the most important medical recommendations in the Hoover Commission Report."[19]

After the commission's report was submitted to the U.S. Congress, Dr. DeBakey and "a number of us who had been working on the recommendation encouraged Senators Lister Hill and John F. Kennedy to prepare legislation for its implementation."[38] On March 13, 1956, those two senators introduced Bill S 3430, later amended to include a provision for the Public Health Service's operation of the new library to be "erected in or near the District of Columbia," which was passed by the Senate on June 11, 1956.[39] Instead of being presented to the House of Representatives, eleven representatives and one senator from Illinois introduced a June 19 bill that was identical to the Hill-Kennedy bill except for the specification that the new library was to be built in Chicago. Staunch opposition to this change of location resulted in a bottleneck and a vote of no action for this bill.

Because the Democratic National Convention was to be held in Chicago that year, the influential speaker of the house, the legendary Texas Democrat, Sam Rayburn, decided it was not an opportune time to call for a vote on the Hill-Kennedy bill because its provision for locating the new library elsewhere was likely to create a political problem. When a stalemate became obvious, Senator Hill called Dr. DeBakey to see if anyone in Houston had any influence with Congressman Rayburn. Such an individual did not come to mind, but, "it suddenly dawned on me that I had performed an aneurysmal resection on the husband of the secretary of the National Democratic Party, Dorothy Vredenberg," Dr. DeBakey said, recalling how he befriended her at that time. Receptive to his telephoned request for assistance, Mrs. Vredenberg contacted Speaker Rayburn and called Dr. DeBakey back the next day with the news of her successful mission. "Right after she called me, Senator Hill called me and said, 'Mike, I don't know what you did, but we are going to get the library through,'" he said. "That's how we got the library."[19]

It also took some clever maneuvering by the politicians to avoid the aforementioned political brouhaha in the House of Representatives. In the final bill presented for vote in the House on July 23, 1956, the specified location for the library was omitted, allowing instead for the proposed library's board of regents to have the responsibility for site selection. After the Senate agreed to the House amendments, President Dwight David Eisenhower approved the bill on August 3. Named a member of the founding board of regents, Dr. DeBakey was the one who "suggested a lovely spot adjacent to the NIH (National Institutes of Health)—an old golf course—which I thought would be an ideal site," where it ultimately was built. On the 125th anniversary of the original library's founding, the newly named National Library of Medicine was dedicated on December 14, 1961, and formally opened in early 1962.[38] The efforts expended by Dr. DeBakey toward its creation marked the beginning of his career as a medical statesman and was, in his opinion, one of his major accomplishments.

It was during his multiple visits to Washington, D.C. in the mid-1950s that Dr. DeBakey first met the individual whom he later would credit with providing the multidimensional trajectory of his career as a medical statesman. Her name was Mary Woodard Lasker, the recent widow of advertising genius Albert Lasker, who died in 1952. With her husband, she had established the Albert and Mary Lasker Foundation to further medical education and research in 1942, and the couple successfully had used their money, administrative talents, and influence in 1943 to transform the American Cancer Society into a successful lobbying and research organization. With the National Cancer Institute Act of 1937 as the inspiration, she convinced lawmakers in 1948 to create the legislation that established the National Heart Institute. Appointed one of the first nonmedical members on the National Advisory Heart Council in 1948, she was to become fully aware of Dr. DeBakey's pioneering achievements in surgery long before she had the opportunity to meet him in person.

Exactly how and where the philanthropist met the surgeon was not documented, but reports of their many collaborative efforts in the following decades would capture the essence of what was to become known as the perfect mentor-protégé relationship. Beginning in 1955, Mrs. Lasker devoted her time and efforts to lobbying Congress, in particular Senator Hill's appropriation committee, for increased government funding for medical research at the National Institutes of Health (NIH). It was an objective in which Dr. DeBakey was to excel as one of her "citizen witnesses," joining the likes of Harvard's Dr. Sidney Farber and New York University's Dr. Howard Rusk. All of these recognized leaders from the medical scientific community were to gain the nicknames of "Mary's little lambs" and "noble conspirators."[40] A member of the Lasker Foundation observed many of this group's testimonies to Congress and commented: "DeBakey is unique; he has the aura of the surgeon, he's articulate, enthusiastic. Most doctors are not enthusiastic, not used to the verbal give and take. The Rusks, Farbers, DeBakeys had evangelistic pizzazz. Put a tambourine in their hands and they go to work."[41]

Within the first year of Mrs. Lasker's concentrated, sophisticated lobbying tactics to increase research funding, the NIH budget jumped from $98.5 million in 1956 to $213 million in the next fiscal year. By 1961 the NIH budget topped $450 million and was to reach $1 billion by the late 1960s.[42] She was to become a ubiquitous figure in the hallways of Congress, and though her goal in Washington, D.C. was to fundraise for research, Mrs. Lasker would say she was there to "friend raise."[43] As far as Dr. DeBakey was concerned, she excelled in both and was a living institution unto herself. "The NIH has flowered because in many ways she gave birth to it and nursed it," he said. "It was in existence, but it was she who got funding for it."[44]

For many of her upcoming efforts to increase community awareness of medical research as well as funds, Mrs. Lasker was to rely heavily on the expertise provided by her newly inducted fellow conspirator in Houston.

"Whenever Mrs. Lasker would call me to ask me to do certain things, I would drop what I was doing to do it," Dr. DeBakey said.[45] "Mary called on me because she knew I was interested in these activities, and I became in a sense one of her coworkers. Whenever she needed help in going to Congress, she would call on me and say, 'I want you to come with me.' So we would walk the halls of Congress lobbying."[46]

There were to be many such occasions in the future, all of which scheduled so as not to impede Dr. DeBakey's rapidly increasing number of surgical procedures performed at The Methodist Hospital. In addition to impromptu Washington trips were his travels in July 1955 to medical meetings across the country where he reported the successes experienced in his and Dr. Cooley's 245 aneurysm repairs to date. Together, the two surgeons also worked their way throughout Europe in August 1956 to lecture and demonstrate aneurysm surgery, effectively introducing their unique procedures to a worldwide audience.

A more geographically convenient opportunity for Dr. Cooley to expand his patient population came into existence with the February 1954 opening of Texas Children's Hospital in the Texas Medical Center. Also affiliated with Baylor University College of Medicine, the 106-bed hospital offered specialized care of infants and children, including surgical care in operating suite facilities shared with St. Luke's Episcopal Hospital. Having established himself as an expert in infant heart surgery at Johns Hopkins, where he relied on the diagnostic capabilities of renowned pediatric cardiologist Dr. Helen Taussig, he was thrilled to learn one of her trainees had joined the new hospital's staff. "When Dr. Dan McNamara arrived at Texas Children's Hospital in 1959, he was to me the real ray of hope which I had, to have a trained pediatric cardiologist in the Texas Medical Center," Dr. Cooley said.[26]

Since Texas Children's Hospital was located in close proximity to The Methodist Hospital, Dr. Cooley soon was performing operations at both hospitals. The surgeries he performed in the newly opened hospital were predominantly on children diagnosed with congenital heart defects. At that time, these surgical procedures were palliative, not curative, and performed on the closed heart. Though Dr. Taussig and other experts believed that surgical intervention for congenital heart defects was not warranted in the first year of life, Drs. McNamara and Cooley thought otherwise, a conviction based on the fact that 64 percent of children with congenital heart defects died within a year of birth. In the mid- to late-1950s, while other congenital heart surgeons around the world reported a limited number of such cases, Dr. Cooley had operated on 120 infants younger than one year old, including 13 younger than 1 month old. In a peer-reviewed journal Cooley reported, "Although many had been in severe cardiac failure at the time of their operation, more than 70 percent survived."[47]

Reflecting decades later on those early experiences with extracardiac procedures, Dr. Cooley said that the closed heart techniques employed "proved that circulation could be diverted and that the heart could be manipulated for brief periods without damage. With the success of these procedures, however, the need to perform operations in the heart, under direct vision, became increasingly obvious."[48]

By early 1955 there had been limited progress in the new field of open-heart surgery heralded by the 1953 successful procedure performed with Dr. Gibbon's heart lung machine with the modified DeBakey pump. The utilization of Dr. Gibbon's cardiopulmonary apparatus in four procedures performed inside the hearts of children with congenital heart defects resulted in dismal results. When only one patient survived this series of operations, Dr. Gibbon called a personal halt to the clinical use of his invention. Though he also ceased all plans to further perfect his apparatus, his successful efforts to temporarily interrupt circulation by bypassing the heart and lungs was an inspiration to other physician scientists, particularly Dr. DeBakey, who began to research additional methods to achieve a bloodless field for direct-vision operations of the heart.

One such innovative technique was the brainchild of Dr. C. Walton Lillehei at the University of Minnesota in 1954. As an alternative to a mechanical apparatus to replicate the heart's contracting function and the lungs' oxygenating function, he researched the possibility of utilizing extracorporeal cross-circulation between two animals. Though considered by his peers to be a departure from established procedures and a radical concept, the concept previously had been used elsewhere for the treatment of human beings who suffered from end-stage uremia and toxemia. "The thought of taking a normal human being to the operating room to provide a donor circulation (with potential risks, however small), even temporarily, was considered unacceptable, even 'immoral' by some critics," Dr. Lillehei explained.[49] To prove otherwise and to illustrate that the utilization of his concept of total-body perfusion was "to permit successful operations otherwise impossible,"[50] between March 1954 and February 1955 Dr. Lillehei and his associates used cross-circulation from parent to child in 32 successful open-heart operations on children with major cardiac malformations not previously correctable.

The specifics of these procedures were detailed in a paper presented by Dr. Lillehei to the Society of University Surgeons during its February 1955 meeting at Baylor University College of Medicine. At the conclusion of his presentation, which also included a film demonstrating controlled cross-circulation during an operation, the audience was encouraged to participate in a discussion about it. It was at this point that Dr. DeBakey stood up to stay, "I rise not to discuss this paper, but to express tribute to Dr. Lillehei and his associates for this superb piece of work. I think it is perfectly wonderful and I think they deserve a great deal of credit for their imagination, for their boldness, and for their demonstration of this technique as a practical and successful procedure. I am sure every member of this audience shares my feeling that this is really and truly inspiring work."[51]

Equally awestruck in the audience was Dr. Cooley, who later vividly recalled his reaction to viewing Dr. Lillehei's filmed operation: "My first view inside the beating heart was indeed a moving experience—almost like looking into the gates of heaven."[50] Impatiently waiting for the opportunity to perform open-heart surgeries on children with congenital heart malformations, Dr. Cooley conceived a plan. Though he expected the long awaited extracorporeal circulation apparatus designed by Dr. DeBakey to be available soon, he was anxious to begin open-heart surgeries immediately. With that thought in mind, he and Dr. McNamara scheduled a trip to observe Dr. Lillehei as he performed controlled cross-circulation surgery at the University of Minnesota in Minneapolis, the only place in the world where open-heart surgeries were being performed.

Before the Houston doctors' June 1955 visit to Minneapolis, an event at the Mayo Clinic in Rochester, Minnesota, necessitated its addition to their itinerary.[52] In March 1955, Dr. John Kirklin performed successful open-heart surgery using the Mayo-Gibbon heart-lung machine, a pump oxygenator similar to the original Gibbon machine but modified by Mayo Clinic engineers. This newsworthy procedure was to be the first in a series of eight consecutive patients, four of whom would survive, and the beginning of an intracardiac surgery program. Suddenly, the only two cities in the world where open-heart surgeries were being performed successfully were not only in the same state but also only 90 miles from each other.

As close as the two Minnesota surgeons were geographically, their methods of alternative extracorporeal circulation could not have been further apart. For Drs. Cooley and McNamara, the opportunity to observe both possibilities of achieving their desired goal of direct-vision, open-heart surgeries in Houston came in June 1955. After observing the cross-circulation procedure, the Houston doctors deemed it to be too risky for the patient and the donor, but to their surprise, they also learned of another method, one that Dr. Cooley immediately embraced. It was a new apparatus, a disposable bubble oxygenator, which had been devised by Dr. Lillehei and his resident Dr. Richard A. DeWall and first utilized in May 1955.[53] Revolutionary for its efficient simplicity and built by Dr. DeWall, it had no moving parts and comprised a couple of metal stands, some beer hose, a cork, needles, and two filters. As simple as it appeared to be, when connected to a Sigma-motor pump, it nonetheless performed the complicated replication of the heart's contracting function as a pump and the lung's oxygenating function. What's more, the total sum of its parts was $15, a mere pittance when compared to the estimated $25,000 cost of Dr. Kirklin's Mayo-Gibbon heart-lung machine.

Also noted by the two Houston doctors during their visit was another dramatic contrast between the two institutions and the two surgeons in Minnesota. During Dr. Lillehei's cross-circulation operation, his surgical team was composed mostly of house staff while Dr. Kirklin's team comprised physiologists, biochemists, cardiologists, and others necessary to perform operations using the Mayo-Gibbon apparatus. "Such a device was beyond my organizational capacity and financial reach," Dr. Cooley said. "Thus I was deeply disappointed on our return to Houston when Dr. McNamara stated that he would not permit me to operate on his patients unless I had a Mayo-Gibbons apparatus."[54]

Not deterred by Dr. McNamara's ultimatum, Dr. Cooley set out to convince him that a simplified method of extracorporeal circulation was more than adequate. Upon returning to Houston, he enlisted the assistance of several Houston associates—Dr. Benjamin Belmonte, Dr. Joseph R. Latson, and Dr. Robert D. Leachman—who previously had been in the process of designing a heart-lung machine of their own. Within a matter of months, these physicians helped Dr. Cooley develop a disposable bubble oxygenator similar to the DeWall-Lillehei apparatus. "We were able to secure most of our materials from hardware stores; what wasn't available there, we had made in metal shops," Dr. Cooley said. "Commercial Kitchens did most of the major custom work; for that reason, I guess, they called it the 'Cooley Coffee Pot.'"[55]

The debut of this eponymous bubble oxygenator occurred at The Methodist Hospital on April 5, 1956. The successful use of the apparatus during the emergency repair of a usually fatal injury to the heart, a hole the size of a half-dollar in the septum between the ventricles, of an adult patient by Dr. Cooley was of historic importance: it marked the beginning of the era of open-heart surgery in Houston. Reported in the April 30, 1956, issue of Time magazine, the "daring" operation took five hours and was described by one of the surgeon's colleagues as "the ultimate" in heart surgery, "the achievement we have been waiting for. It is now possible to lay open the fine muscles of the heart—the wires, so to speak—control circulation, patch a blowout and then repair the muscles and restore circulation. We can now repair some of the most serious damage there can be to the adult human heart."[56]

One Houston cardiologist who immediately responded to this breakthrough was Dr. Chapman, who had returned from the service in 1955, established a private practice, and joined the clinical staff at Baylor University College of Medicine. During the six weeks following the first open-heart surgery at The Methodist Hospital, he was to refer five other patients with congenital septal defects to Dr. Cooley for total correction, all of whom survived the procedure.[57]

In the subsequent seven months of 1956, Dr. Cooley was to perform 95 open-heart procedures on both adults and children at The Methodist Hospital, Texas Children's Hospital, and St. Luke's Episcopal Hospital. Decades later, when reflecting on the sudden exponential growth of the open-heart surgery program in Houston during its first year of existence, Dr. Cooley was to credit the courageous steps first taken by Dr. Lillehei to establish the field, praising him as the innovator who "provided the can opener for the largest picnic thoracic surgeons will ever know."[51]

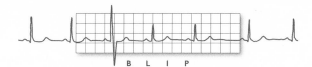

B L I P

AORTIC DISSECTION LESSON

More than five decades after devising the surgical repair of torn aortas, Dr. DeBakey self-diagnosed his own aortic dissection and underwent the operation at the age of 97: "The pain came like a bullet out of the blue. I was alone when it started. My wife and my daughter had gone out. The pain is often described as the worst pain you can have. The pain was so severe that I would have welcomed anything to relieve it—including death. I wasn't going to fight it. I look upon death as a part of living, just as some trees lose all their leaves in the winter and have them replaced in the spring. But at the same time, part of me was thinking, 'What caused this pain?' Part of me was doing a diagnosis on myself—which, as it turned out, was correct. Aortic dissection. I'd written more articles about the condition than anybody in the world, and I resigned myself to having a heart stoppage. The pain didn't teach me anything about the heart. It simply emphasized what I had already learned. I was a little surprised to find myself recovering after the surgery. Then gratified to have been given a second life. The doctor who operated on me only a few years ago was one that I trained. I was lucky to have somebody like that." [1]

---

1. Fussman C. What I've Learned: Michael DeBakey. Esquire website. http://www.esquire. com/features/what-ive-learned/michael-debakey-0308. Created July 14, 2008. Accessed October 1, 2013.

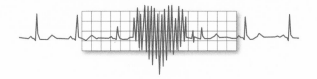

CHAPTER FIVE

THE POWER OF PERSUASION
1956 - 1960

"Persuasion is often more effectual than force."

AESOP

The 1956 advent of the open-heart surgery era, in tandem with the pioneering surgical advances in cardiovascular surgery performed by Drs. DeBakey, Cooley, Creech, and Crawford in the early 1950s, was to impact The Methodist Hospital in the Texas Medical Center in ways that previously had been unimaginable to its board of trustees.

Instead of being consumed with worry about the hospital's inability to fill the 300 beds mandated by Mrs. Fondren, the trustees found themselves challenged with precisely the opposite scenario—an escalating demand for additional beds. Such needs had been foreseeable by the trustees as only a possibility in the distant future during the original planning of the hospital, but they became increasingly inevitable during the hospital's first four years in the Texas Medical Center. In 1955, having successfully generated the income necessary to economically operate satisfactorily, the hospital no longer was operating at a deficit, an accomplishment that was to be replicated in all subsequent years.

As the hospital's reputation for excellent medical and surgical care continued to grow, and the patient population began to multiply at an even more rapid pace in 1956, the resulting repercussions created problems that, if not addressed immediately, were destined to become insurmountable. To the beleaguered hospital administrator, the obvious solution was one he heartily recommended to the board of trustees. "We had waiting lists all over the place, doctors mad, and patients mad," Mr. Bowen said. "It was getting to be critical, so we knew we had to expand."[1]

An inescapable fact was that the patient population comprised an inordinate number of cardiovascular patients. When Dr. Creech returned to New Orleans to become the chairman of the Department of Surgery at Tulane University School of Medicine in 1956, Dr. Crawford had assumed his vacated position as director of the peripheral vascular laboratory at The Methodist Hospital, attracting a steadily growing number of patients. In addition, as first established as the norm in the mid-1950s, the daily total of Dr. DeBakey's patients more often than not exceeded 100 beds. "I was actually creating a problem with some of the doctors here," Dr. DeBakey recalled. "They couldn't get their patients admitted here because there wasn't any room. They said, 'DeBakey's got all the beds.'"[2]

It was an overcrowded predicament that Dr. Cooley was able to accommodate, but not easily. With numerous patients and insufficient space to accommodate them, he became a master of improvisation. Already established as an expeditious surgeon, he was also to become known for a dizzying pace of multiple procedures performed on a daily basis in three different hospitals. To fulfill the growing demand for open-heart surgery for congenital malformations, he continued to operate at The Methodist Hospital but began to more frequently utilize the surgical facilities available to him at St. Luke's Episcopal Hospital and Texas Children's Hospital. "In those days, I would schedule operations in all three on the same day," Cooley later recalled. "I had to race across the parking lot between operations. And it would seem that just about the time I would get over to Texas Children's Hospital to do an operation, they would call me from Methodist to say there was some complication that needed immediate attention."[3]

Accompanying Dr. Cooley on what were to become known as "legendary" sprints between hospitals in 1956 and 1957 was his usual entourage of surgical assistants and nurses as well as someone to transport the "Cooley Coffee Pot" bubble oxygenator, the only one available at the time. On many occasions, the individual charged with that responsibility was his wife, Louise Cooley, who later recalled moving the invaluable apparatus in the back of her car from hospital to hospital.[4] Though the exact number of times this occurred was not documented, Dr. Cooley had operated on more than 200 patients with the bubble oxygenator in all three hospitals by the end of 1957, a total that was approximately three times the combined amount performed by Drs. Lillehei and Kirklin in the same time period.[5]

While the bubble oxygenator predominantly was utilized during Dr.

Cooley's surgical procedures to repair congenital heart malformations in children, he and Drs. DeBakey and Morris also implemented the apparatus while performing operations on 32 adult patients with aneurysms of the thoracic aorta. "Observations made in these patients indicate that controlled extracorporeal circulation is a satisfactory method of dealing with problems concerned with excisional therapy of aneurysms of the thoracic aorta," they reported in a paper presented to the American Surgical Association.[6] Also stressed in their presentation was their use of the bubble oxygenator as the perfusion methodology in other surgical procedures for aneurysms: "Successful resection and graft replacement of aneurysms located in the ascending aorta, aortic arch, and entire descending thoracic aorta have been possible using such techniques."[6]

It was during this early clinical use of the heart-lung machine when Dr. DeBakey experienced an epiphany. Having established that heart function could be duplicated by mechanical means during surgery, he found that some patients seemed resistant to being weaned from cardiopulmonary bypass after completion of the procedure but could be weaned after several hours of prolonged support from the heart-lung machine after surgery. "Experience also showed us that a certain proportion of these patients with damaged heart function could not be successfully weaned," he said.[7] "The fact that not all such patients survived led to the obvious search for other methods of more prolonged support of the failing heart, for days or weeks, to give the heart more time to recover."[8]

Inspired that this concept could be used clinically in patients with reversible heart failure following surgical incision of the heart after myocardial infarction, pulmonary embolism, and other causes, Dr. DeBakey established an experimental laboratory to develop the appropriate apparatus. This new laboratory included a machine shop headed by engineer Louis Feldman, whom Dr. DeBakey described as "an excellent machinist to provide the means of fabricating innovative, mechanical technologic develops for cardiovascular surgery."[7] Supported by funds from the Department of Surgery, special grants from grateful patients, and the Houston American Heart Association, the research program in the laboratory was directed toward the development of "mechanical heart pumps that could provide prolonged ventricular assistance," known as ventricular assist devices (VAD), as well as a total artificial heart.[8] It was a research program that ultimately was to dictate the direction of Dr. DeBakey's future pioneering endeavors in the field of cardiovascular surgery.

Of immediate concern to Dr. DeBakey were the postoperative complications that could develop in patients who underwent cardiovascular surgical procedures, particularly those that involved the heart-lung machine. "We had some pretty big cases, and it was during the early days of vascular surgery, so we had a lot of complications," recalled Dr. John Ochsner, a surgical resident from 1956 to 1961 who also was the son of Dr. DeBakey's mentor. "It was very common for us to have grafts and suture lines rupture and people getting ischemia. When we first were doing peripheral vascular work and abdominal aneurysms, we didn't anticoagulate them during the operation, and I can remember more than one patient who was gangrenous from the belly button down. We had a lot of infected grafts that were terrible to deal with. The state of the art was immature, and unfortunately we had to face all of those terrible, terrible things."[9]

The urgent need for specialized postoperative care of cardiovascular patients was a major concern to Dr. DeBakey. Inspired by an idea he previously had implemented for injured soldiers when faced with a shortage of personnel during his military experience, he approached Mr. Bowen with an adaptation of that concept for The Methodist Hospital. He proposed an area near the recovery room for "intense care" of patients following cardiovascular surgery, one in which personnel were specifically hired and trained to work. "The hospital hired the nurses and in those days nurses weren't hired for such duty; they served as private nurses for private patients," Dr. DeBakey explained. When Mr. Bowen agreed to allot six beds and hire the nurses, "I started giving them a little training, and I asked our colleagues in cardiology to give them some training in electrocardiography and other monitoring procedures."[10]

Within a few short years, Dr. DeBakey's concept was to evolve into the first "intensive care unit" for surgery and medicine at The Methodist Hospital. The cardiologist charged with training the newly hired nurses in that unit was Dr. Edward W. Dennis, the first full-time cardiologist from Baylor University College of Medicine on the staff of The Methodist Hospital. Originally named chief of the cardiac clinic at Jefferson Davis Hospital in 1953, the Emory University trained internist and cardiologist had transferred to The Methodist Hospital in 1956 to become head of the new cardiorespiratory laboratory opened on the ninth floor.

Responsible for cardiac catheterizations and performing tests involving the heart, lungs, and peripheral blood vessels, Dr. Dennis was also to become chief of the hospital's electrocardiogram (EKG) department, an area that was growing exponentially. When The Methodist Hospital was on Rosalie Avenue, there had been an average of 60 to 80 EKGs per month; in the Texas Medical Center in 1956, the hospital averaged 325 EKGs per month. Within the following seven years, the monthly number was to escalate to 923. While expertly responding to this growing demand for his services, Dr. Dennis was to become known as a consummate workaholic among his colleagues.

With an ever-increasing need for the services of additional cardiologists for training, teaching, and patient consultations, Drs. DeBakey and Cooley, as well as all the other cardiovascular surgeons, often called upon Dr. Chapman and his colleagues at the Houston Cardiovascular Associates, otherwise known as "The Chapman Group." Participating in his clinical practice in 1956 was Dr. Paul Peterson, a graduate of Baylor University College of Medicine and former resident in cardiology at The Methodist Hospital who had joined Dr. Chapman after returning from his European tour of duty in 1955. Another Baylor University College of Medicine graduate and former resident who trained in cardiology at The Methodist Hospital, Dr. H. Liston Beazley, who had set up practice in Harlingen, was persuaded to join Drs. Chapman and Peterson in 1964.

As the number of members gradually increased in the coming years, The Chapman Group was to become seemingly omnipresent at the hospital throughout the following four decades. Because of an imperative implemented by Dr. DeBakey and the volume of cardiovascular surgical procedures, the services of these volunteer faculty members in cardiology were called upon frequently out of necessity. "I wanted every patient to be seen by a cardiologist," Dr. DeBakey said, acknowledging how taxing the workload was for Dr. Dennis and the other full-time cardiologists on faculty. "You have to remember that I had, in a sense, all private patients so I was in charge of that service completely. It gave me the opportunity to expand the clinical resources for Baylor, so I had all the full-time people I could get to see my patients in consultation. So, many of them, that's all they did; they just took care of me. They were busy as hell."[2]

Though the same hectic pace existed in several other areas of The Methodist Hospital, it was especially evident in the Department of Surgery. The emergence of other surgical specialties throughout the 1950s resulted in stiff competition between each of these surgeons and the cardiovascular surgeons for operating rooms and available beds. When Dr. DeBakey's postoperative intense care area was initiated in 1958, the neurosurgeons, general surgeons, orthopedists, and otolaryngologists collectively voiced their opposition to the innovation. Eventually all of them would be converted from naysayers to believers, a turn of events that subsequently caused Dr. DeBakey to remark, "Not a single one later would admit that he objected to it initially."[10]

When noticeable improvements in the outcomes of postoperative cardiovascular patients began to occur in Dr. DeBakey's newly established intense care area during its first six months, Mr. Bowen began receiving adamant demands from the other surgeons to accommodate their postoperative patients' acute needs. Approaching Dr. DeBakey with this request, the administrator was not rebuffed but told the only possibility of ever accepting more patients depended on immediate expansion of the area. "Let's get some more beds in there," Dr. DeBakey said. "But don't use my beds. I am having a hard time as it is. By Friday, I can't operate because all the beds are filled."[10]

For Mr. Bowen, this booked-to-capacity status in the specialized-care area was not a singular occurrence; it was a situation that existed throughout The Methodist Hospital, which in 1958 was turning away 30 to 35 patients a day for lack of available beds. After experiencing four consecutive months of 102 percent occupancy that year, the board of trustees had appointed a committee of doctors and administrative staff to formulate the projected expansion needs for the future. Expecting the medical staff to be satisfied with 100-bed increments over a succession of years, Mr. Bowen was surprised when the chiefs of service proposed expanding the hospital to "the capacity that we need," a total of 375 additional beds.[1] Even more unexpected by Mr. Bowen was the board's accepting the medical staff's proposal "without any question, and we immediately started planning the west wing."[11]

With a projected completion date of 1963, that 375-bed west wing addition already was on the drawing board in 1958 when Mr. Bowen and Dr. DeBakey finalized plans for the newly expanded and renamed "intensive care unit" to accommodate all surgical patients. In order to expedite this renovation within 90 days, Mr. Bowen conceived the conversion of the medical staff suite and doctors' lounge adjoining the operating rooms on the second floor. Included in his quickly approved $150,000 remodeling and expansion program was not only the 24-bed, intensive care unit for all surgical patients requiring constant nursing service but also a temporary building to house a 35-bed "progressive care" unit for convalescents and patients hospitalized for diagnosis and not afflicted with serious or lingering illnesses. When announcing these plans to the press in September 1958, Mr. Bowen stressed that this interim expansion represented a temporary solution to a permanent need and that "both units will be incorporated in the hospital's permanent expansion program."[12]

When the 24-bed surgical intensive care unit (ICU) at The Methodist Hospital was completed in November 1958, it became the only one of its kind in Houston and one of the first established in the United States. Within a few months, because of the gratifying outcomes experienced therein, Mr. Bowen received a request from the medical area for their own ICU, resulting in the creation in January 1959 of an additional eight-bed unit strictly for acutely sick medical patients. What soon followed was a hasty revision of the proposed expansion plans to include the combination of these two specialized areas into one substantially enlarged 52-bed ICU. "This new unit will enable us to provide better patient care by placing all intense care patients in a geographic location where we can concentrate experienced nursing personnel," Mr. Bowen said, indicating it would be located next to the newly enlarged operating suite on the second floor.[13]

The increased capacity of the newly revised and enlarged ICU was predicated by current experiences in both the surgical and medical ICUs and the projected needs generated by the addition of seven operating rooms to the existing eight-room operating suite. Two of those new rooms were to be especially equipped for cardiovascular surgery, including a special electronics control room equipped with the latest technological equipment to monitor biological functions of the surgical patient. The new equipment was to provide Dr. DeBakey and his team of surgeons with the ability to monitor intra-arterial blood pressure and blood flow and provide electrocardiograms and electroencephalograms during all vascular and open-heart surgeries.[14] With these enhanced facilities and the established reputation of the cardiovascular program at The Methodist Hospital, the estimated increase in the number of cardiovascular surgical patients in the future was sizable, albeit inaccurate—the actual volume of patients was to be far greater than anyone ever could have expected in 1959.

One unexpected area of growth in the field of cardiovascular surgery was directly attributed to a surgical advance introduced by Dr. DeBakey in 1958. It was the first successful patch-graft angioplasty to counteract the narrowing of an artery caused by arteriosclerosis. Though others previously had demonstrated the feasibility of arterial repair experimentally, the successful clinical application of this method by Dr. DeBakey and his team of cardiovascular surgeons at The Methodist Hospital was revolutionary, as was the volume of cases they were to perform during the following four years. "This patch graft method of arterial repair has permitted successful extension of reconstructive surgical treatment of occlusive lesions in small arteries and has simplified operative treatment of certain aortic lesions," he and his surgical team reported in a peer-reviewed journal. "Analysis of our experience with patch graft angioplasty in 619 patients during the past four years reveals that both immediate and long term results are highly gratifying."[15]

This patch-graft method of arterial repair was yet another of the rapidly evolving advances made in cardiovascular surgery at The Methodist Hospital. Having dedicated their main efforts to diseases of the aorta and its major branches, specifically aneurysms and occlusive lesions during the previous seven years, Dr. DeBakey and his associates collectively possessed a surgical experience with more than 3,000 cases by1959.[16-17] Occlusive disease of the abdominal aorta and peripheral arteries accounted for more than 1,600 cases, and numbering more than 1,200 were the cases involving aneurysms of the thoracic aorta, the abdominal aorta, and major peripheral arteries. Cases of acquired injuries to the aorta and major arteries totaled more than 165, and the congenital condition of coarctation of the aorta was addressed in 150.[18]

In the more than 1,600 cases that involved arterial graft replacement with the flexible, knitted, seamless Dacron tube invented by Dr. DeBakey, the results were significantly better than those obtained with homografts and other synthetic grafts. "All aneurysms may now be considered operable, although the method of approach may vary with location," Dr. DeBakey concluded in 1959. "The changing conceptual developments which have taken place in the surgical consideration of occlusive disease are perhaps even more significant than those in aneurysmal disease."[19]

One of the major factors in the conceptual and technical developments of vascular surgery for occlusive diseases at The Methodist Hospital was the availability in the early 1950s of the precise diagnostic procedure of arteriography, the injection of dye through a catheter in order to produce detailed X-rays of the body's blood vessels.[20-21] Combined with his extensive surgical experiences, this ability to view and delineate the complex, segmental involvement and multiple sites of occlusive disease enabled Dr. DeBakey to determine that "arteriosclerosis may be diffuse and extensive, but it may also be highly localized. Although this important feature of the disease was earlier recognized in the arterial bed of the lower extremities, it has since been found to occur in much the same way in other major arterial segments."[19, 22]

Details of this observation and of his team's various other modifications of the previous concept of surgical treatment of occlusive and aneurysmal disease were presented in Dr. DeBakey's presidential address to the International Cardiovascular Society during its September 19, 1959, meeting in Munich, Germany. Having presented similar lectures the previous year in Belgium, Spain, Portugal, Japan, Australia and the Philippines, Dr. DeBakey enhanced his reputation as the expert in the field and continued to attract an inordinate number of referred patients from his peers all over the world.[23]

Achieving the same end results after also traveling throughout Europe, Japan, and South America in 1958 and 1959 was Dr. Cooley. In those multiple speaking engagements and presentations, he reported the largest accumulated experience by any single surgical team, a total of 475 open-heart operations, 75 percent of which were patients with congenital heart defects. Often accompanied by Dr. Dan McNamara, pediatric cardiologist and director of the heart clinic at Texas Children's Hospital, Dr. Cooley detailed his extensive use of the bubble-oxygenator and heart-lung machine during those open-heart surgeries, particularly during the rare operations he performed for the removal of tumors from the inner chambers of the heart.[24-26]

Other members of the cardiovascular team at The Methodist Hospital also generated a vast number of referrals. Recognized as one of the pioneers of cardiovascular and peripheral vascular surgery, Dr. Morris introduced innovative renovascular reconstruction techniques and devoted his research efforts to renal and peripheral vascular conditions, thereby establishing himself as an expert in those fields.[27-29] Though Drs. DeBakey and Cooley were the acknowledged pioneers in innovating various surgical techniques, vascular instruments, and synthetic grafts for aortic aneurysms, Dr. Crawford's inclusion graft techniques and established expertise in treating complex diseases of the aorta resulted in a perpetual, sizable flow of referrals.[30] Often overlooked by the mainstream media as a key factor in establishing the unbridled growth in the number of cardiovascular patients in the late 1950s and subsequent decades at The Methodist Hospital, Dr. Crawford later was to be identified by *Texas Monthly* magazine as one of "the first-rate heart surgeons you've never heard of."[31]

Without question, the one heart surgeon who most everyone in the

United States had heard of in the late 1950s was Dr. DeBakey. He had been interviewed and featured in national magazines, quoted generously in wire-service stories about heart surgery, and credited by experts as being the foremost pioneer in the emerging field of cardiovascular surgery. Often invited by medical organizations, schools, and hospitals around the world to lecture and perhaps give demonstrations of his surgical techniques, Dr. DeBakey was an eloquent speaker and soon found that the demand for his talents at the podium equaled that for his surgical prowess. More often than not, his speaking engagements generated local newspaper coverage in the cities he visited, but one, in particular, was to garner considerably more attention.

It was an invitation he received in 1958 from the Union of Soviet Socialists Republic, the USSR. Since it was during a particularly tense period in the Cold War, the advisability of Dr. DeBakey's making such a visit was debatable. At the time, Premier Nikita Khrushchev was issuing demands for the United States to formally recognize the Soviet Union as a world power by agreeing to a proposed summit meeting. When President Dwight D. Eisenhower remained noncommittal, Premier Khrushchev ratcheted up the saber rattling about the inevitability of Communists' achieving world domination following an American-Soviet clash. Because of his belief that health care was a universal need with no political barriers, Dr. DeBakey immediately accepted and embarked on his first trip to the USSR in December 1958. At the personal request of the Russian Ministry of Health, Dr. DeBakey first stopped in Leningrad to address the All-Russian Congress of Surgeons about recent advances in vascular surgery, particularly the surgical treatment of aneurysms and occlusive disease of the aorta and major peripheral arteries.

The next stop was Moscow, where he had been invited to visit several clinics as the guest of Professor A. A. Vishnevski, a member of the Academy of Medical Sciences of the USSR and director of the Institute of Surgery in Moscow.[32] When Professor Vishnevski expressed a keen interest in learning more about certain aspects presented in his Leningrad speech, particularly the synthetic tubes used for arterial grafts, "Dr. DeBakey left three of the Dacron patches with me when he was in Russia," the professor said. "I used one of them as a replacement part for a large artery in a patient. The patient was doing well when I left three days later for the United States."[33]

Having been told by the Russian Embassy in Washington that several of the Russian surgeons were coming to the United States to attend the

Society of University Surgeons meeting in February 1959, Dr. DeBakey reiterated an invitation he already had extended to Professor Vishnevski during his visit. He invited the Russian to come to Houston for a tour of the cardiovascular facilities at The Methodist Hospital, which Professor Vishnevski immediately accepted, arriving January 20, 1959. During his two-day visit, the Russian surgeon was able to observe Dr. DeBakey and his team in the operating suite as they performed open-heart surgery. His reaction was documented both in local newspapers and wire service stories published around the country. "I am impressed by the excellence of the operations I have seen here," Professor Vishnevski said. "Vascular surgery in Houston is being done better than any place in the world."[33]

An American institution's achieving such recognition in the height of the Cold War from a Soviet scientist was unprecedented as well as indicative of Dr. DeBakey's prowess as an international statesman and diplomat. To one keen observer, the universal and boundless parameters of the Houston surgeon's reputation was directly attributable to his following the advice received years earlier from his mentor at Tulane, an observation to which Dr. DeBakey agreed. "He told me that my father told him, 'If you do more of something than anybody else, then you are the authority,'" recalled the younger Dr. Ochsner, who was a young child during Dr. DeBakey's years with his father at Tulane. "When I was in Houston as a resident, he was invited to go to Mayo Clinic as a visiting professor to show them how to do abdominal aneurysms. He was really thrilled because he was going up to Mecca to show them how to do it. He was going up there as the authority on aneurysms."[9]

As for his becoming one of the most respected authorities on medical issues in Congress in the late 1950s, Dr. DeBakey always gave due credit to the knowledgeable advice he received and followed from his mentor Mrs. Lasker, but his innate ability as a statesman was to play a major role. Appointed to serve as a member of the prestigious National Advisory Heart Council of the National Heart Institute in 1957, Dr. DeBakey joined other council members in considering applications for research and research training grants and cooperative agreements; in recommending funds for those applications that showed promise of making valuable contributions; and in suggesting research programs to be conducted at the National Heart Institute. To contribute meaningfully to the accomplishment of these goals, Dr. DeBakey adapted his busy schedule to attend the council's four meetings a year, one in winter, one in spring, and two in the fall.

While in the nation's capitol for these council meetings, it was not unusual for Dr. DeBakey to also spend time with Mrs. Lasker and her Washington associate Mike Gorman. Together they would conjure up and employ various tactics to lobby Congressional members for increased funding for biomedical research at the National Institute of Health (NIH). On many occasions, Mrs. Lasker's close friend and health-syndicate ally Florence Mahoney would host an intimate gathering at her home, thereby affording Dr. DeBakey the opportunity to interact socially with some of the country's most influential elected officials. That a packet of reading material about biomedical research was the usual party favor came as no surprise to her guests, who were accustomed to her purposeful hospitality. When one federal official identified the perennial hostess and all of "Mary's little lambs" as being members of a "noble conspiracy," Mr. Gorman interjected, saying he preferred to call it a "high class kind of subversion, very high class. We're not second story burglars. We go right in the front door."[34]

One front door in Washington, the one at 1600 Pennsylvania Avenue, had been wide open to Mrs. Lasker and Mrs. Mahoney during the late 1940s and early 1950s during the Truman administration, but they had found the White House during the Republican administration of President Eisenhower not to be as receptive to their Democratic agenda. Throughout the late 1950s, their top priority had become the full-time cultivation of all the appropriations committee members in Congress. They also continued their ongoing efforts to enhance existing relationships with Democratic leaders Senators John F. Kennedy, Lyndon B. Johnson, and Lister Hill. As a result, throughout the Eisenhower administration the Democratic-controlled Congress consistently voted more money for health programs than recommended by the administration.[35] Theirs was a well-honed mission embraced by lifelong, progressive Democrat Dr. DeBakey, who enthusiastically joined their efforts whenever he was in town.

The major thrust of these noble conspirators' efforts to increase federal funding for biomedical research culminated in an area in which Dr. DeBakey was known to excel. As one of the "citizen witnesses" to appear before the appropriations committee in both the House of Representatives and the Senate in 1959, he presented an eloquent plea for increased support of the National Heart Institute's proposed annual budget.

The essence of his testimony was a succinct overview of the research and educational advances made in the field of cardiovascular disease in the previous decade, particularly those made in the development of highly effective methods of surgical treatment in recent years. "Until recently, the various methods of therapy for these conditions were essentially palliative in nature and far from satisfactory," he testified. "In recent years, however, and on the basis of knowledge gained from investigative studies, precise diagnostics as well as effective therapeutic methods have been developed. Thus, a high proportion of patients who formerly would have died or would have been seriously disabled from gangrene of the lower extremities, strokes, and high blood pressure due to arteriosclerosis involving the arteries to the kidneys may now be completely relieved."[36]

Also included in his presentation was a brief summation of the recent developments in the surgical treatment of strokes, a new field of endeavor at The Methodist Hospital. Stating that his team's experience with successful restoration of normal circulation in more than 95 percent of the patients with inconclusive lesions, was gratifying, [37-38] he stressed "there is an urgent need for more intensive research in this field in order to permit wider and more effective application of this new knowledge. In this connection you will be pleased to know that the National Heart Institute has recently established a well coordinated collaborative research program to strengthen and intensify studies in this direction."[36]

Another program of considerable interest to Dr. DeBakey was the proposed budget for establishing centers of cardiovascular research in strategic parts of the country. Emphasizing that the nucleus for such centers already existed in a number of institutions throughout the country, he advised the politicians that "little difficulty would be encountered in putting this proposal into immediate operation." As a valuable addition to the Research Training Grants Program of the National Heart Institute, which Dr. DeBakey credited with the previous expansion and intensification of cardiovascular research in this country, the establishment of these special centers constituted "the wellspring of further cardiovascular research endeavors. Indeed, the whole future of our research efforts in this important disease area is dependent upon the output of the young medical scientists who are receiving their research training through this grant program."[36]

Concluding his brief presentation, Dr. DeBakey said: "The tremendous strides that have been made during the past decade clearly reflect the vigor and intense activity characterizing the current status of cardiovascular research and portend other advances of even greater importance. You have every reason to take pride in the important role you have played in these developments, and with your continuing generous support of these research endeavors only the limits of imagination can restrict their progress."[36]

This was the type of charming finesse Dr. DeBakey was known to deliver in every testimony. Because of his ability to seamlessly combine an infinite knowledge of the medical profession with such subtle political acumen, Mrs. Lasker and Mr. Gorman were inspired to mastermind yet another role for him to play in their benevolent conspiracy. Within a year, their newly hatched plot came to fruition. Announced in May 1960 was the appointment of Dr. DeBakey as chairman and Mrs. Lasker as vice chairman of the newly formed, 21-member Advisory Committee on Health Policy of the Democratic Advisory Council. Its purpose was to develop the health plank for the Democratic Party platform at the 1960 convention in Los Angeles.

The resulting platform plank included a provision for "medical care for older persons" by the use of "the contributory machinery of the Social Security system for insurance covering hospital bills and other high-cost medical services."[39] Eventually known as "Medicare," it was to become one of the most controversial issues of the presidential campaign and throughout the following five years. It would also have a dramatic impact on Dr. DeBakey's standing in the medical community.

Having just received the distinguished service award from the American Medical Association (AMA) in recognition of his major contributions to heart and blood vessel surgery in June 1959, Dr. DeBakey was to be virtually ostracized from that organization for his unwavering advocacy for Medicare in the early 1960s. "I did not consider it to be a step toward national health insurance, as the AMA labeled it, but a worthy humanitarian way of ministering to impoverished or low-income patients," he said, recalling the ongoing "vituperative" debate that evolved following the election of President Kennedy. "The AMA's opposition had become increasingly strident. Members were assessed dues to create a $3.5 million war chest to conduct a public campaign against such legislation."[40]

One result of such an organized opposition was clearly obvious to Dr. DeBakey. "Once it became known that I supported Medicare, when the AMA was strongly opposed to it, I became a kind of pariah, and I had telegrams from some physicians saying that they would never refer another patient to me," he said, noting such a threat was inconsequential since many of his patients came to him on their own. "It concerned me at first because I was sincere in my belief and couldn't understand why anyone would object to Medicare. You just have to accept the fact that if you are going to get out in front on an issue, some are going to shoot you in the back."[10]

While his stance on Medicare was to remain a contentious issue, Dr. DeBakey received unanimous praise from the medical community for his ongoing advocacy with Mrs. Lasker for an annual increase in federal research funds for the NIH. One of the direct beneficiaries of their combined efforts in 1960 was The Methodist Hospital and Baylor University College of Medicine.

Announced October 2, 1960, by Dr. Stanley W. Olson, the dean of Baylor University College of Medicine, was the receipt of a $262,500 grant from the National Heart Institute for the establishment of the country's first Cardiovascular Research Center at The Methodist Hospital. "The grant will be used for the study of the nature, treatment and prevention of hardening of the arteries, the leading cause of death and the major cause of heart attacks, strokes, and poor circulation," Dr. Olson stated, noting there were to be subsequent grants of $396,350 in its second year and $491,325 annually for the following eight years.[41]

Named as the center's principal investigators in developing research studies were Dr. DeBakey and Dr. Raymond D. Pruitt, the newly appointed chairman of the Department of Medicine at Baylor University College of Medicine in 1959. Dr. Pruitt was already recognized as an expert in the field of electrocardiography, coming from the Mayo Graduate School of Medicine where he had established a distinguished career as a cardiologist, investigator, administrator, and educator.

In order to create the ideal location for the Cardiovascular Research Center, Mr. Bowen once again had to reconfigure the oft-revised expansion plans at The Methodist Hospital. After consulting with Dr. DeBakey, he announced that the new center's six-bed research ward was to incorporate the Goldston Cardiovascular Research Unit adjacent to the other research laboratories on the hospital's ninth floor and that construction was to be completed in 1961.

This reconfigured area was foreshadowed in Dr. DeBakey's definition of an ideal cardiovascular center, first articulated in a 1960 testimony to Senator Hill and the appropriations committee of the Senate: "The Center should be housed in a discrete geographic area to permit staff members to work in sufficiently close proximity with one another, and with sufficient integration of their activities, in order that ideas and technical advances can be continuously exchange and critically evaluated and research opportunities immediately recognized and exploited."[42]

Dr. DeBakey's innate ability to recognize and exploit opportunities to further enhance the cardiovascular program at The Methodist Hospital was renowned in 1960, but it soon would garner legendary status. With the subtle power of persuasion he so effectively deployed during congressional testimony, he would be able to both captivate Mrs. Fondren's attention about a mutually desired goal for the future and also produce concrete results.

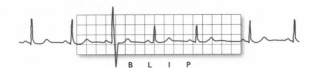

B L I P

POPCORN AND MILK

As a child, Dr. John Ochsner had the opportunity to know Dr. DeBakey not only as a colleague of his father, Dr. Alton Ochsner, but also as his family's favorite babysitter. "When my mother and father would go out of town, Dr. DeBakey and his late wife, Diana, would baby-sit for us," he recalled. "As children, we really loved having them as sitters because they were such nice people. I can remember getting Dr. DeBakey to make a muscle and hanging on his arm and chinning. He and my father worked incessantly. When he was working with my Dad, Dr. DeBakey would come to the house on Sunday afternoons, and they would go into my Dad's study around noon and work on papers and such until 5 o'clock. When they finished, my mother would make them popcorn and pour each of them a big tumbler of milk, after which they'd stuff the popcorn into the milk and eat it with a long spoon, saying how wonderful it was. I'd say it was a good way to ruin a glass of milk and a bowl of popcorn."[1]

---

1. Gregory RT. Childhood memories of giants in vascular surgery: Matas, DeBakey, de Takats, and Ochsner: An interview with Dr. John Ochsner, *Cardiovascular Surgery*. 2003;11(5): 407–411.

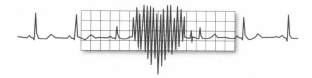

CHAPTER SIX

THE LASKER CONNECTION
1960 - 1964

"Communication—the human connection—is the key to personal and career success."
PAUL J. MEYER

For a period of seven months in 1960, Mrs. Fondren resided on the eighth floor of The Methodist Hospital. Early in the year, while on a visit to Southern Methodist University, the 80-year-old had fallen, broken her hip, and been flown back to Houston to be operated on by Dr. Joe King, chief of the orthopedic service at The Methodist Hospital.

Throughout her recuperation and rehabilitation, she was ensconced in her favorite room, 807, which offered a commanding view of the sprawling landscape directly north of the hospital. At the time, with the exception of the Jesse H. Jones Library, erected in 1954, and the Baylor University College of Medicine's original structure, the Roy and Lillie Cullen Building, erected in 1947, the Texas Medical Center property visible from her window was scarcely populated. Though there were acres of undeveloped land to gaze upon, Mrs. Fondren concentrated her attention on just one, the piece of property adjacent to the hospital that lay right below her window. Quite often she would glance outside and remark, "We've got to build something on that property over there and right away."[1]

With many of her frequent visitors, Mrs. Fondren would follow such an observation with an inquiry about their thoughts on the subject. For Mr. Bowen, who visited every day and catered to her every need, the opportunity to discuss the hospital's needs directly with its major benefactor was not unusual. Having known Mrs. Fondren for more than 12 years, he had been privy to exactly where she stood on each and every

issue since the late 1940s. Recalling how well they worked together in
the early years on Rosalie Avenue, Mr. Bowen said, "It was fun to run the
hospital then; Mrs. Fondren made the decisions and I carried them out."[2]

On many occasions during her residency in room 807, Mrs. Fondren
would discuss the vacant lot next door and ponder its fate with Mr. Bowen.
With the west wing construction plans finalized and groundbreaking
ceremonies imminent, Mrs. Fondren confided she was convinced that
upon the 1963 completion of that expansion, which would double the
hospital's capacity, there nonetheless would be a demand for additional
space. Her envisioned building would be the obvious solution for such a
nebulous need, so she was determined to define a purpose for its existence.

It was a frequent topic of conversation not only with Mr. Bowen but
also with several other visitors. One of them was her orthopedic surgeon,
Dr. King, who often stopped by to check on his patient's recovery progress,
and, when given the opportunity, to express his hopes of establishing an
area for research in orthopedics. Another frequent visitor to Mrs. Fondren's
room was Dr. DeBakey, although his calls were strictly social. Since his
arrival in Houston, Dr. DeBakey found Mrs. Fondren to be one of his
stalwart supporters. In awe of the international recognition generated by
his pioneering efforts in cardiovascular surgery, she often expressed her
gratitude for his elevating the stature of The Methodist Hospital. "We
are so proud because Dr. DeBakey is here and he's known all over the
world," she said, recalling how much he had helped the once little-known
hospital to grow exponentially. "It really is a wonderful thing for us when
you think about such a thing happening in Houston."[3]

Although the many conversations during Dr. DeBakey's visits with Mrs.
Fondren were not documented, they no doubt included some mention of his
travels, particularly those to Washington for his efforts to increase federal
funding for cardiovascular research. One specific outcome of his efforts—
President Eisenhower's September 1960 signing of the appropriations bill
that included $20 million for research construction grants to establish
clinical research centers for cancer and heart research—unquestionably
became an integral part of his proposed possibilities for the vacant lot
viewable from room 807.

Whatever transpired in their conversations with Mrs. Fondren during
those seven months, these three visitors had no expectations of immediate
action. However, a few days following her release from the hospital, after
she, in her own words, "got up and walked out,"[3] she surprised Mr. Bowen
and Drs. King and DeBakey with a request for a formal proposal for what

they needed to build her envisioned building. Invited to attend a meeting of the Fondren Foundation to make their individual presentations within a matter of days, the three gentlemen "frantically conferred," recalled Mr. Bowen, noting their coming to a hasty decision to request the lofty total of one million dollars. "We soon found out we shot too low when one member of the foundation spoke up and said, 'Well, you can't build a good house for that these days.'"[3]

As was expected, no conclusive decisions were made by the foundation that day, but it was this initial meeting that marked the conceptual beginning of the $9 million Fondren-Brown Cardiovascular and Orthopedic Research Center at The Methodist Hospital. When the concept for this complex eventually was formalized, the Fondren Foundation and Trusts contributed $2,750,000 toward the Ella F. Fondren Building; the Brown Foundation, in honor of George R. Brown, contributed $1,000,000 for the Herman Brown Building; the NIH contributed $1,960,000; and Mr. and Mrs. Edgar Brown and the DeBakey Medical Foundation also were major donors. Scheduled for completion in 1968, the new complex officially was to be announced at the October 27, 1964, groundbreaking ceremonies.

During those intervening four years between inspiration, conceptualization, and realization of Mrs. Fondren's vision, more than 93 physicians and scientists worked with architects and administrative personnel to design the ideal complex necessary for research in a wide range of medical disciplines. To provide for future expansion, the two adjoining buildings were structures designed to permit the later addition of floors, but initial plans called for approximately 42 percent of each building to be devoted to research and training facilities. The Fondren Building, originally consisting of a ground floor plus six floors, was to house both orthopedic and cardiovascular research, including 50 beds. The adjacent and attached Brown Building, originally consisting of a ground floor plus four floors, was to house clinical and laboratory areas devoted exclusively to cardiovascular problems. Included were to be eight operating rooms connected to a central monitoring and computer system and laboratories, all exclusively for cardiovascular procedures.

These projected facilities reflected the needs of a far more sophisticated cardiovascular program than the one existing in 1960. Charged with the responsibility of establishing a viable cardiology department to support the needs of the hospital's burgeoning patient population in cardiovascular surgery was the medical college's newly appointed Chairman of the Department of Medicine Dr. Raymond Pruitt. After naming Dr. Edward

Dennis as director of the program, Dr. Pruitt began to recruit additional cardiologists to join him on the full-time faculty.

The first full-time cardiologist recruited by Dr. Dennis to The Methodist Hospital was Dr. Samuel Kinard, a recent graduate of Baylor University College of Medicine who received his training in internal medicine and cardiology at the University of Colorado. Within the next five years, three more cardiologists were to join Drs. Dennis and Kinard: Dr. Benjamin McCall, a graduate of Duke University Medical Center; Dr. John F. Lancaster, a graduate of Tufts University; and Dr. Manus F. O'Donnell, who arrived in 1965 after graduating from the medical school of Queens University in Ireland.

"There were five of us and we were busy as hell, as you can imagine with the volume of Dr. DeBakey's practice," Dr. O'Donnell recalled, noting there was a steady stream of patients for cardiovascular surgery throughout each week. "He would think nothing of admitting 30 to 40 patients in a weekend. A lot of them were aneurysms, but many were for heart valve surgery, aortic valve replacements and mitral valve replacements. No coronary bypasses at that time, but a good deal of valve surgery, as well as aneurysm surgery."[4]

In tandem with the growing complement of full-time cardiologists at The Methodist Hospital from Baylor University College of Medicine, the number of cardiologists in private practice in Houston began to escalate. In addition to Drs. Chapman, Peterson, and Beazley in "The Chapman Group," other private-practice cardiologists at The Methodist Hospital in the early 1960s included Drs. Ray Skaggs, John Lewis, Everett Price, and William Gaston.

The increasing number of cardiovascular surgical procedures for acquired valvular heart disease at The Methodist Hospital reflected the progress made in the field of operative therapy following the advent of open-heart surgery. A prerequisite for attacking cardiovascular diseases was a safe method for clearly visualizing the coronary arteries prior to surgery, and in 1958, pediatric cardiologist F. Mason Sones at the Cleveland Clinic developed the first accurate diagnostic technique for occlusions and coronary lesions. After accidentally hand-injecting contrast media into the right coronary artery of a 28-year-old male with rheumatic heart disease under X-ray visualization, Dr. Sones recorded the image on movie film, thereby performing the first selective cine coronary arteriography.[5] "In many ways the development of arteriography was perhaps the most important key that opened the door to vascular surgery," Dr. DeBakey said, noting that Dr. Sones' technique not only led to the advanced studies of coronary artery disease, but, more importantly, also became the impetus for the development of aortocoronary artery bypass surgery.[6]

With the improved diagnostic capabilities of arteriography, the definitive treatment of aortic and mitral valve disease was to evolve when refinements were made in artificial valve prostheses in the early 1960s.[7-8] After utilizing the newly introduced caged-ball valve prostheses in 607 cases over a period of three years, Dr. DeBakey and his team of surgeons endorsed the procedure as effective, concurring "valve replacement ideally should be performed once a patient with acquired heart disease first demonstrates evidence of decompensation or when angina or syncope develops."[9]

One of the pioneers in developing cardiac valve prostheses was Dr. Arthur C. Beall Jr., a newly recruited member of Dr. DeBakey's team. A graduate of Emory University and the Emory University School of Medicine, Dr. Beall had joined Baylor University College of Medicine as a resident in 1954 but was called to active duty in the United States Navy in 1956. As a naval medical officer, he served as the assistant chief of thoracic surgery at the U.S. Naval Hospital in Oakland, California, and worked with cardiovascular surgeon Dr. Frank Gerbode in his research laboratory at Stanford University Hospital, which was located in San Francisco at that time. Research programs in Dr. Gerbode's laboratory in the late 1950s included the exploration of using homograft valves for cardiac valve replacement, work that would lead to the creation of prosthetic heart valves.[10-11]

Following his return in 1958 to complete his general surgery residency with Dr. DeBakey, Dr. Beall joined the Department of Surgery in 1959. In 1961, he and Dr. Cooley introduced the concept of priming the pump oxygenator with 5 percent dextrose and distilled water for open-heart operations, thereby greatly relieving the pressure on blood bank facilities, a major advance.[12]

Continuing his research efforts, Dr. Beall eventually conceived the Beall-Surgitool Teflon disc valve, which incorporated a seating ring with two parallel wire strut retainers to control the excursions of the disc.[13] After its 1967 introduction, the prosthesis was to undergo five design changes during its 10 years of clinical existence, with each new design bringing increased knowledge and better hemodynamic efficiencies.[14-15] By 1973, more than 10,000 Beall-Surgitool prostheses had been used in mitral valve replacements worldwide,[16] making it one of the most widely used prosthetic valves in the world from 1965 until the mid-1970s.[17]

The pioneering efforts of another new member of Dr. DeBakey's team of surgeons at The Methodist Hospital, Dr. H. Edward Garrett, also was to impact the field of cardiovascular surgery in the early 1960s. A graduate of Emory University School of Medicine who began his general surgery residency at Vanderbilt University before joining the Army Medical Corps for two years in Korea, Dr. Garrett came to Houston to continue his training in general and thoracic surgery under the direction of Dr. DeBakey. Upon completion of his training in 1961, Dr. Garrett was appointed to the faculty of the Baylor University College of Medicine, where he personally directed Dr. DeBakey's clinical service at The Methodist Hospital.

For Dr. DeBakey, who gradually had built the Department of Surgery since 1948, there became a pressing need to expand at a more rapid pace in the 1960s. In tandem with the remarkable progress made in the entire field of cardiovascular surgery, the pioneering advances made at The Methodist Hospital alone continued to attract international attention, resulting in an influx of patients from all over the world. "I had to increase my personnel in my department," Dr. DeBakey explained. "At one time, I would have more than 100 patients in the hospital. It would take me a couple of hours to make rounds."[18]

The shortage in the number of cardiovascular surgeons at The Methodist Hospital in 1962 also reflected the departure of Dr. Cooley, who remained in the Baylor University College of Medicine Department of Surgery but restricted his practice to St. Luke's Episcopal Hospital and Texas Children's Hospital. Since a majority of his patients already were in those two hospitals, Dr. Cooley had suggested the move to Dr. DeBakey, who had concurred, recognizing how the inability to get patient rooms at The Methodist Hospital had become "a very stressful situation" for all concerned.[19]

Within months of Dr. Cooley's relocation to those nearby hospitals in the Texas Medical Center, he was directing the most active open-heart program in the world. Although not consulted about the plans to establish a cardiovascular center in Mrs. Fondren's envisioned building next to The Methodist Hospital, Dr. Cooley had heard the rumors. Stating that he preferred the location for such a facility in the Texas Medical Center to be located closer to Texas Children's Hospital and St. Luke's Episcopal Hospital, Dr. Cooley decided to create a specialized cardiovascular facility of his own in this preferred location.[20] He was anxious to include research and education as part of its overall program and conceived the idea of an institute that relied on philanthropy as opposed to income derived from patient care. Instead of having patients of its own, the envisioned institute would draw patients from its two nearby hospitals for treatment. Approved by the boards of trustees of Texas Children's Hospital and St. Luke's Episcopal Hospital and chartered on August 3, 1962, the Texas Heart Institute was to become what Dr. Cooley would describe as "his greatest achievement."[21]

In retrospect, when recalling the circumstances surrounding the founding of the Texas Heart Institute, as well as the career path choices he made that led to its conception in 1962, Dr. Cooley said, "The best decision I ever made was to give up entirely my participation in the Methodist program and confine myself to Children's Hospital and St. Luke's Hospital. Now, St. Luke's Hospital, at that time, was an institution of 175 beds. The Cardiology Service was indeed very small and not very active. Most of the cardiologists with whom I had been working were at Methodist Hospital and they decided to stay at Methodist Hospital and send patients to me for surgery here."[19]

There would continue to be many patients transferred to Dr. Cooley in the early 1960s. There also were a growing number of cardiologists at The Methodist Hospital who began to practice at both institutions, a practice that continued even after the June 1963 opening of the west wing with its additional 375 beds at The Methodist Hospital. Regardless of the expansion, The Methodist Hospital continued to remain overcrowded with a continually growing patient population of predominantly cardiovascular patients.

Among Dr. DeBakey's patients in 1963 was one of Hollywood's biggest stars whose every move was chronicled by the famed gossip columnists of that era. In her nationally syndicated column, Hedda Hopper reported the details of Clifton Webb's "delicate vascular surgery" along with that star's exclamation that "one of the greatest experiences of his life was meeting that truly dedicated Dr. DeBakey, who invented the rare heart operation. People come from all over the world, and he performs 12 to 14 surgeries daily. While Dr. DeBakey had Clifton on the table, he also removed his appendix and corrected a hernia that Clifton didn't know he had."[22] Another syndicated columnist penned the news of Mr. Webb's framing a sample piece of a Dacron graft, the synthetic material "Dr. DeBakey used to sew up his aorta."[23]

Not as famous as a Hollywood star, but nonetheless garnering newspaper coverage in their hometowns, were many other patients of Dr. DeBakey. Most mentions included a reference to him as either "the internationally known" or simply as "the great" cardiovascular surgeon. Regardless of such recognition, there were few, if any, among his patients who were referred by the nation's physicians who opposed Dr. DeBakey's stance on medical care for the aged under Social Security. Already ostracized by the American Medical Association for his previous advocacy efforts during the 1960 Democratic convention, Dr. DeBakey further exacerbated the situation in 1962.

"President Kennedy was anxious to have a group of medical people come and stand with him on a television presentation he was going to make to the people about Medicare," Dr. DeBakey said, recalling the March 27 event at the White House. "I was asked to help get some medical people to come there, and I was amazed to see how few we could get to stand up, even though some of them were for it. There was great opposition at that time in the medical profession. So, we rather stood alone, some of us, and were targets for their attacks."[24]

While some of his peers were derisive, one of Dr. DeBakey's staunch supporters throughout this period of political turmoil was Mary Lasker, who remained an avid proponent not only of President Kennedy's initiative but also of the failed national health insurance program initially proposed by President Truman in 1945. As a fellow member of Dr. DeBakey's platform committee at the 1960 Democratic convention, she also was concerned about the fate of its recommended and approved committee to improve care of patients with heart disease and cancer in the United States. Though impanelled by President Kennedy in 1960 and chaired by Dr. DeBakey, the committee had yet to present its findings formally due to extenuating circumstances.

According to Dr. DeBakey, President Kennedy requested the committee's report to be delivered to him on April 17, 1961, at the White House. The precise timing of the presentation was in order to facilitate media coverage from the White House press corps. On the designated day and time, Dr. DeBakey and committee members gathered in the old Hay Adams Hotel across the street. "We waited to get the word to come over," he said, recalling that this initial wait lasted more than three hours. "Finally we did get the word to come on over. So we went into the White House where the press usually has its—I've forgotten the name of that particular room—and we sat there and waited and waited. After a while somebody came in and said, 'President Kennedy wants to express his regrets in being delayed meeting with you, but if you'll be kind enough to wait, he's busy with matters of an urgent nature.' We didn't know at the time about the Bay of Pigs until later. So we kept waiting and waiting, and finally we'd been there two or three hours. Finally, someone came in and said he was sorry that the president would have to cancel his meeting with us, so we left the report and never heard another word about it."[25]

Over the years, the inconclusive outcome of Dr. DeBakey's committee was attributed to the "Bay of Pigs Report," a name that often was misinterpreted to mean the entire effort was a failed mission much like its namesake's American-led attempt to overthrow Fidel Castro's government in Cuba. Though such misinformation was intolerable to Mrs. Lasker, it was the lack of government attention to the needs of the nation's patients with cancer and heart disease that ultimately would inspire her to instigate efforts to establish a more formalized commission for that purpose in the future. She believed the next one should also be chaired by the same medical expert, in whom she had great confidence, saying, "Dr. DeBakey is not only a great surgeon; he's really a medical statesman."[26]

Always highly complimentary of her protégé, Mrs. Lasker not only expended efforts to enhance his political stature but also referred patients to his care at The Methodist Hospital.[26] Many were friends, or friends of friends, who were in need of cardiovascular care, but one was a recent acquaintance. Out of the blue, Princess Liliane of Belgium had contacted her to request a favor. The second wife of abdicated King Leopold III of Belgium, she had established a program of flying Belgian patients with congenital heart malformations to the United States for surgical procedures unavailable in Belgium and was seeking a contribution from Mrs. Lasker to help cover the costs. Sympathetic to her cause, Mrs. Lasker explained her interests were predominantly in medical research and suggested she submit a formal request for a grant from the National Heart Council.

After that first meeting with Princess Liliane, Mrs. Lasker conjured up a possible solution to her plight. "I took the matter up with Dr. Michael DeBakey, who was on the Council with me. I said, 'You know, Michael, it's so pitiful about this woman who is trying to do something in Belgium and if you would go there and see her, you could help her and maybe you could show them how to write a request so that they would get their grants instead of being turned down. If she asks you to come, will you go?' Dr. DeBakey said, 'Yes, I'll go,'" Mrs. Lasker recalled. "So I told the Princess that this important heart surgeon, if he were invited, would come to Belgium and talk to them about how to get grants from the United

States if she invited him. Well, very shortly she did invite him. He really became devoted to her and went there frequently. He taught there; he took patients to operate on [whom] she brought from Belgium; he taught people and did operations on television in Brussels and in Leuven and the major medical centers, and he's really made a great work of trying to help her."[26]

For his complete body of work, particularly his pioneering research to solve the problems of cardiovascular disease, Mrs. Lasker was to bestow her highest compliment on October 30, 1963. Awarding Dr. DeBakey the Albert and Mary Lasker Foundation's 1963 Albert Lasker Award for Clinical Research, Mrs. Lasker and Dr. Farber, the chairman of the awards committee, stated: "His laboratory investigations, translated with extraordinary courage and unprecedented technical skill to the patient, have resulted in the correction and cure of previously incurable cardiovascular disease, replacing what would have been lingering, chronic disease and disability, or sudden death, by vigorous, happy and productive life."[27]

Not one to rest on his laurels for past accomplishments, Dr. DeBakey remained focused on the future and his aspirations to create a total artificial heart. In the week preceding the Lasker award presentation in New York, Dr. DeBakey announced the first historic step in achieving his goal at the annual meeting of the American Heart Association in Los Angeles. After speaking about the surgical team led by Dr. Crawford at The Methodist Hospital and their attempt to implant a ventricular assist device (VAD) in a human being, he and his team received worldwide recognition for the technical feat. "Although an entire artificial heart may be as far from medical achievement as man's dream of reaching outer planets, Houston's daring surgeon Michael E. DeBakey described a novel device that for three days took over a great deal of the work of one diseased heart," *Time* magazine reported.[28]

Also reported by that magazine and countless newspapers was the fact that even though the device "worked well enough to restore the patient's blood pressure and electrocardiogram to near normal," the patient only survived three and one-half days, succumbing to previous complications that could not be overcome and not from failure of the "plastic pump."[29] Medically known as an "intrathoracic, pneumatic-driven pump that partly bypassed the left ventricle from the left atrium to the thoracic aorta," it had been developed in the research laboratory Dr. DeBakey established to research and create a total artificial heart in the late 1950s.[30]

The efforts in that research laboratory were enhanced with the arrival of Dr. Domingo Liotta, a 1961 fellow in cardiovascular surgery at Baylor University College of Medicine. Formerly with Dr. Willem J. Kolff in the Department of Artificial Organs at Cleveland Clinic, Dr. Liotta had been involved in that clinic's previous implantation of artificial hearts in dogs. At the request of Dr. DeBakey, he devoted some of his fellowship time to research efforts, working closely with Louis Feldman, Dr. DeBakey's laboratory engineer who had proven expertise in creating innovative mechanical technology. [31]

Joining Dr. Liotta in Dr. DeBakey's laboratory in 1962 was the recently recruited surgeon and physiologist Dr. C. William Hall, who was known to tinker around the kitchen in his home on free evenings and weekends in his quest to create an implantable heart pump. Molding silicone rubber around plaster-of-Paris heart molds and then vulcanizing the creation in his wife's oven, he had produced the prototype of the heart pump. After experimental studies in more than 50 animals demonstrated its efficacy, the pump made medical history when it was implanted in 1963. Universally acclaimed as the first artificial heart, that prototype was to be placed on permanent display at the Museum of Natural Science at the Smithsonian Institution in Washington, D.C.[32] When asked his thoughts about the outcome of the first human recipient, Dr. Hall replied: "We don't really know what he died of. The man had many things wrong with his kidney, brain, liver, and lungs. However, the pump was still working when he expired. It had proved its value in clinical applications."[33]

Pleased with his research team's accomplishments and optimistic about the limitless applications made possible by the implantable heart pump, Dr. DeBakey remained determined to achieve his ultimate goal, a total artificial heart. In search of a funding source for further research in this field of endeavor, Dr. DeBakey lobbied Senator Hill's Subcommittee on Health in 1963, presenting this proposal: "Experimentally, it is possible to replace the heart with an artificial heart, and animals have been known to survive as long as 36 hours. This idea, I am sure, could reach full fruition if we had more funds to support more work, particularly in the bioengineering area."[34]

In response to Dr. DeBakey's testimony and that of other prominent medical and scientific researchers in support of federal funds for the development of an artificial heart, there was consensus in Congress that the program had merit. Following a congressional mandate for an ad hoc advisory group to present a detailed plan, the committee submitted a recommendation to the National Advisory Heart Council of the National Heart Institute (NHI) to pursue the artificial heart "with a sense of urgency," a suggestion council member Dr. DeBakey was to embrace with zeal.[35]

Since the creation of an artificial heart was primarily an engineering task, Dr. DeBakey suggested that someone with hands-on experience serve as the director of the NHI artificial heart program to organize the initial efforts.[36] Approved by the council to fulfill this role was his nominee, Dr. Hall, who took a six-month sabbatical from Dr. DeBakey's surgical research laboratory to serve in that capacity at the NHI. With the intent of developing a totally implantable mechanical heart within five years, Congress appropriated $581,000 in 1964. While later deemed by critics to be "absurdly under-funded and overly ambitious," the Congressional directive marked the official beginning of the artificial heart program in the United States and resulted in the immediate awarding of six contracts for technical development.[37]

To no one's surprise, one of the first recipients of a major NIH grant for artificial heart research in 1964 was Dr. DeBakey. Having already established a working relationship with the biomedical engineering laboratory of Rice University in 1963, Dr. DeBakey knew that the duplication of the heart's pumping action by a mechanical substitute required the collaboration of biologic and physical scientists.[38] Together with Dr. W. W. Akers, professor and chairman of the chemical engineering department at Rice University, Dr. DeBakey planned to use the awarded funds in 1964 to concentrate their joint efforts to bring this ambitious plan for an artificial heart to fruition.

In spite of Dr. DeBakey's optimism about the feasibility of a total artificial heart, some cardiovascular surgeons did not share his view. One, in particular, was Dr. Cooley, who was known to express his disinterest in the concept. "I really don't see that it would have much value now," he said. "There are complications arising for mechanical devices that come in contact with the blood stream, the necessity for external connections for power, and the fact there is no evidence that they can run for considerable lengths of time."[39]

Also skeptical about the total artificial heart were journalists, who described Dr. DeBakey's joint venture to achieve that goal as "fascinating and somewhat unbelievable."[40] Remaining a thorough believer was Mrs. Lasker and her group of noble conspirators who continued to lobby for increased federal funding for the artificial heart program. On more than one occasion during the months following the 1963 assassination of President Kennedy, Mrs. Lasker was to meet with her great friend President Johnson at the White House. During their conversations she discussed not only the need for a national artificial heart program but also the perceived stalemate of Dr. DeBakey's "Bay of Pigs" report on heart disease, cancer, and stroke, the three leading causes of death in the United States.

Since the impetus for that ill-fated report had been the health plank in the 1960 Democratic Party platform, Mrs. Lasker lobbied for a method to help President Johnson achieve its desired purpose during his administration. Stressing the efficacy of reappointing the previous chairman, she suggested that the president impanel a more formalized committee. Her methods of persuasion proved to be effective, because shortly afterward President Johnson announced the President's Commission on Heart Disease, Cancer, and Stroke, headed by Dr. DeBakey. Mrs. Lasker then recommended 27 prominent individuals from the fields of medicine, science, philanthropy, and public affairs to serve as panel members.[41]

When the White House contacted Dr. DeBakey in early spring 1964 with President Johnson's request to chair the commission, he replied that he "was highly honored to accept," but anticipated there would be great pressure to produce results in a timely manner. In his first meeting with the president to discuss the commission, "he told me what he would like to have us do," Dr. DeBakey said, recalling the president's expectation of a finished report in less than a year.[24] "He said, 'I want to be able to include a message from this commission in my address in January.' As a consequence, he wanted to have the report by sometime in October. So we had really to, in a sense, accelerate the whole process."[25]

Shortly thereafter, in a March 7, 1964, presidential news conference at the White House, President Johnson announced the formation of the Commission on Heart Disease, Cancer, and Stroke, saying, "The leading causes of death in the United States are heart disease, cancer, and stroke. They have a greater impact than all other major causes of death in this country. Fifteen million Americans are today suffering from these diseases. Twenty-three million days of work are lost every year because of them. Two-thirds of all Americans now living will ultimately suffer or die from one of these diseases. I have therefore asked the distinguished panel of laymen and doctors to recommend steps that can be taken to reduce the burden and incidence of these diseases. This panel will be chaired by Dr. Michael E. DeBakey of Baylor University College of Medicine in Houston, Texas."[42]

Provided with office space in the Executive Office Building and a staff of 13, Dr. DeBakey was to devote a large portion of his time to working in Washington during the following nine months. At the first meeting of the commission April 17 at the White House, President Johnson said, "There is nothing that really offers more and greater hope to all humanity and to preserving humanity than the challenge in the task that you have undertaken. Somehow, someway, sometime, you are going to find the answers, and I hope it will be soon."[43]

To bring together the concept of the report and the recommendations, Dr. DeBakey divided the commissioners into specific sections, which in turn comprised subcommittees on education, research, and economics. In pursuit of all the facts, he requested and received consultations from various experts in the health field; testimony from groups and organizations; and pertinent information from the National Institutes of Health and the Public Health Service. Watching over this process from the beginning to the end, Dr. DeBakey said, "Once we had all the facts that we could collect, well, then we sifted these, analyzed and reviewed them, and drew certain conclusions."[24]

The involvement of Dr. DeBakey in every aspect of the commission necessitated his making more frequent trips than usual to Washington, all the while maintaining his burgeoning surgical service at The Methodist Hospital. Known to schedule more than ten surgical procedures per day, Dr. DeBakey continued to amass a growing patient population. Since an emergency with any of his patients could arise in his absence, Dr. DeBakey relied heavily on the expertise of Dr. Garrett, who was given the responsibility to resolve any difficulty that occurred by implementing all means possible. In 1964, Dr. Garrett was to do precisely that, resulting in yet another extraordinary breakthrough in cardiovascular surgery at The Methodist Hospital.

The surgical event occurred following the urgent readmittance to the hospital of one of Dr. DeBakey's recent patients. Diagnosed by his cardiologists as having coronary artery arteriosclerotic occlusion and in need of an endarterectomy of the left main coronary artery for angina pectoris, the 42-year-old patient previously had seen Dr. DeBakey, who had discharged him after advising the procedure was too risky and suggesting further medical treatment at home. Within a matter of months, the patient's condition worsened and his cardiologists readmitted him to The Methodist Hospital, demanding that "something, anything" be done to save him. Since Dr. DeBakey was out of town, Dr. Garrett, along with Dr.

Jimmy F. Howell, a former resident who joined the Department of Surgery in 1964, made the decision to attempt a unique procedure to alleviate the debilitating occlusion.[44]

Inspired by the success he had achieved in surgical procedures to bypass occluded leg and kidney arteries with a vein graft, Dr. Garrett believed such a graft should work with the heart as well. Therefore, he and Dr. Howell proceeded to remove a vein from the leg of the patient for that purpose. After connecting the patient to the heart-lung machine, the surgeons sewed one end of the vein to the aorta to provide the necessary source of blood and bypassed the occlusion by sewing the other end of the vein to a healthy area of the left anterior descending coronary artery.

The specifics of this operation were not reported until seven years later, after establishing proof that the bypass procedure was effective and had withstood the test of time. "The operation was accomplished without incident, and convalescence after operation was uncomplicated," Drs. Garrett, Dennis and DeBakey reported in 1972. The purpose of publishing the specifics so long after the fact was attributed to two reasons: "(1) to the best of our knowledge, it represents the first successful aortocoronary bypass with autogenous saphenous vein graft, and (2) it is the longest follow-up of a functioning aortocoronary saphenous vein bypass graft to date."[45]

Since The Cleveland Clinic's Dr. Rene Favaloro performed an aorto-coronary bypass with autogenous saphenous vein graft in May 1967 and published the specifics in 1968,[46] he generally is the surgeon credited for introducing the first coronary artery bypass (CAB) to the clinical arena.[47]

Another newsworthy event in 1964 was to generate immediate recognition for Dr. DeBakey, Dr. King, and The Methodist Hospital. It was the October 27 groundbreaking ceremonies for the cardiovascular and orthopedic centers in the Fondren and Brown Buildings. Presided over by Mr. Bowen and attended by Princess Liliane of Belgium and other dignitaries, the ceremonies featured a simultaneous groundbreaking for the two buildings with silver-finished shovels in the hands of Mrs. Fondren and George Brown. As Dr. DeBakey surveyed the detailed plans of the two buildings to be constructed on the vacant lot that first inspired Mrs. Fondren's vision four years earlier, he stated with confidence, "This is only the beginning," a prophecy that was to be proven true.[48]

Coming to a close in October was the Commission on Heart Disease, Cancer, and Stroke, which had gained a shortened appellation, the "DeBakey Commission."[49] As requested by the president, Dr. DeBakey and his commissioners had completed their assigned task in less than a year, compiling 35 specific recommendations of two general types. The first category included those programs recommended for the frontal assault on problems related to the conquest of heart disease, cancer, and stroke. The second category concerned strengthening the total national resource for advancing scientific knowledge and providing medical services for the broad problems of American science and medicine.

Included in the report was a strong recommendation for increasing federally funded support of the NIH Artificial Heart Research Program, an idea emanating from the chairman.[31] Also attributed to Dr. DeBakey was one of the most innovative aspects of the report, the development of regional medical centers. "The idea behind it was that if we could create regions, both geographic and population regions, in which there existed a complex of medical institutions and at least one major medical center, and create cooperative arrangements among these institutions, that we would be able to enhance the care of these patients," he explained.[25] "I had the advantage as chairman, so to speak, to initiate and push the concept. That is not to say that I want to take full credit for the concept. Don't misunderstand me. But I did have, in a sense, the opportunity and the responsibility. And I have been credited by most of the people with being sort of the architect of the program."[24]

All members of the commission were scheduled to present the published compilation of the commission's recommendations to President Johnson in the Cabinet Room at the White House at 1:00 PM on December 9, 1964.[50] When asked to arrive an hour earlier for a private conference with the president in the Oval Office, Dr. DeBakey did so, only to find his meeting was delayed unavoidably because of a phone call. Such an occurrence might have conjured up a sense of déjà vu about the Bay of Pigs report after Dr. DeBakey's waiting so long for the president were it not for what happened next, which turned out to be an altogether different situation than before.

According to Dr. DeBakey, "Jack Valenti came in and he said, 'There's a long-distance call here that I think you better take. It's from a doctor in New York, and it's about the Duke of Windsor.' So I went to another room and answered the call and talked to the doctor, who told me that the Duke of Windsor had an aneurysm of the aorta and that he wanted to have him come immediately to Houston for me to operate on him. Well, in the meantime, while I was on this call, the president finished his call. Jack Valenti said to the president, 'He's on the telephone. I'll get him right away.' So that's how the story, I think, got out that I made the president wait on me while I was on the phone."[24]

It was not the only time the president would play second fiddle to the Duke of Windsor. Although the news coverage he received after announcing the contents of the report from President Johnson's Commission on Heart Disease, Cancer, and Stroke was robust on December 9, it was to pale in comparison to that of Dr. DeBakey's aneurysm surgery performed on the Duke of Windsor the following week at The Methodist Hospital.

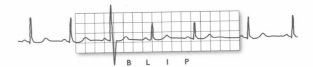

MARY'S LITTLE LAMBS

A s one of Mrs. Lasker's protégés, Dr. DeBakey quickly learned the value of cultivating the media. A noteworthy example was a column penned at her suggestion by Mrs. Lasker's good friend Eppie Lederer, better known as the nationally syndicated advice columnist Ann Landers. After the June 21, 1971, column that implored readers to mail letters to their senators to support passage of a $100 million cancer research bill appeared in more than 1,000 newspapers nationwide, millions of letters from her readers were delivered to Capitol Hill in the following days. Such a "blizzard" of public support had never been experienced before. One secretary in charge of sorting the mail even hung an "Impeach Ann Landers" sign in her office. Within a matter of weeks, the Senate passed the bill by a large majority and, in appreciation of her support, President Richard M. Nixon invited Mrs. Lederer to the signing of the National Cancer Act on December 23, 1971.[1]

---

1. Kogan R. *America's Mom: The Life, Lessons, and Legacy of Ann Landers.* New York, NY: Harper Collins; 2003:104.

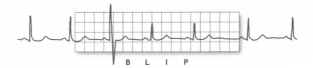

B L I P

THE POWER OF THE PRESS

*T*hrough *his friendship with Mrs. Eppie Lederer, Dr. DeBakey also reaped the benefits of the vast public awareness generated by her nationally syndicated "Ask Ann Landers" columns. Over the decades, she was to include countless references to "my good friend, Dr. Michael DeBakey" as well as his and Dr. Gotto's many books, The Living Heart and The Living Heart Diet, to name a few. She often referred her readers to articles written by Dr. DeBakey, and on one memorable occasion used Dr. Gotto's direct advice in her column:*

> *Dear Ann: My wife and I both have high cholesterol. Last night, she said she read somewhere that frequent sex lowers the cholesterol. We have never heard this before. We decided to ask Ann Landers. How about it? –Idaho Inquirers*
>
> *Dear Idaho: I checked with Dr. Anthony [sic] Gotto, a world recognized authority on cholesterol at the Baylor College of Medicine in Houston. He said the only way frequent sex might help lower cholesterol would be if a couple engaged in sex instead of eating eggs, cheese, ice cream, liver, and caviar."*[1]

---

1. Landers A. Ask Ann Landers column, *Boca Raton News*. September 6, 1988.

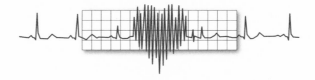

CHAPTER SEVEN

THE PRICE OF FAME
1964 - 1970

"He who has a thousand friends, has not a friend to spare,
and he who has one enemy will meet him everywhere."
RALPH WALDO EMERSON

The official announcement that His Royal Highness Prince Edward Albert Christian George Andrew Patrick David, Duke of Windsor, was to enter The Methodist Hospital in Houston for corrective arterial surgery by Dr. Michael E. DeBakey generated front-page news around the world on Saturday, December 11, 1964.

Simultaneously announced a day earlier by an aide to the duke in New York and a spokesman for The Methodist Hospital in Houston, the news startled members of the incredulous New York media. "Why did the duke's New York physician, Dr. Arthur Antenucci, choose an out-of-town surgeon and hospital for the surgical procedure?" they asked the duke's aide, who replied: "It's very simple. The No. 1 man in the field is Dr. DeBakey and he wants to operate in his own hospital with his own team."[1]

Though there was no sense of urgency implied by either spokesman, the announcement came within 24 hours of the initial call Dr. DeBakey received at the White House regarding the duke. Pressed into immediate action at The Methodist Hospital by Dr. DeBakey were Mr. Bowen and his new assistant administrator, Thomas Fourqurean, who began to implement the extensive preparations requested by the royal patient and his entourage.

Accompanying the 70-year-old former King Edward VIII of England would be his wife, the Duchess of Windsor, the American divorcee Wallis Warfield Simpson, for whom he had abdicated his throne 28 years earlier. In the six rooms on the fourth floor of The Methodist Hospital set aside for his use, one was to be the duke's room, another was for the attending doctors and nurses, the third was for consultation, the fourth was for the duchess's aide, and the final two were a suite of rooms especially decorated in French provincial furniture for the duchess.

Adequate space also had to be provided for the countless journalists expected from around the world, the first of whom began descending on the hospital shortly after the official announcement was made. While the constant presence of the media might have been disruptive to normal activities at The Methodist Hospital, it was an aberration tolerated with bemusement. In a personal letter to his mentor Dr. Ochsner in New Orleans, Dr. DeBakey wrote, "You may have read that the Duke of Windsor is here for resection of an aneurysm of the abdominal aorta. His visit is causing quite a lot of excitement among the members of the world press and we seem to face a continual barrage of reporters and photographers."[2]

Eager to be told each and every detail about the duke's upcoming stay, the persistent reporters began to pepper the hospital staff with endless questions. When one asked whether the duke would be treated like any other patient in the hospital, an unidentified employee responded, "We certainly hope that we can be able to give him that privilege."[3]

One unique service provided by Mr. Bowen for the duke and duchess was a full-time private secretary. Stationed on the fourth floor near their suite of rooms was Betty Hahneman, a native of the United Kingdom who also was Dr. King's administrative assistant in orthopedics. For the duration of their visit, Mrs. Hahneman handled all their incoming letters, post cards, and telegrams sent from around the world, the receipt of hundreds of bouquets of flowers and gifts, and the scheduling and screening of approved visitors.

Another service implemented by Mr. Bowen was created to address the demands of the growing number of journalists who literally camped out at the hospital throughout the 18-day stay of the Duke and Duchess of Windsor. On a daily basis the administration office issued a detailed advisory to update the duke's condition and progress. As a result, beginning with his arrival in Houston by train on December 14, 1964, and continuing until he departed the hospital on December 31 for the Warwick Hotel, there was unprecedented daily news coverage in the print media throughout the United States and Europe.

Often sharing this perpetual limelight with the duke and duchess was Dr. DeBakey, whose previous accomplishments and established expertise in the field of cardiovascular surgery received abundant recognition from his peers, particularly his pioneering efforts in the surgical treatment of aneurysms.[4-5-6-7] In the mainstream media, entire feature articles concentrated solely on Dr.

DeBakey or his pioneering surgical procedures for aneurysms, each with only a passing mention of the Duke of Windsor's particular case.

As in most newsworthy events covered by multiple reporters, some of the pertinent facts became garbled in the transmission. One published newspaper story mistakenly credited Dr. DeBakey and his operating team's performance of 5,600 major cardiovascular procedures "in the past six weeks" instead of the accurate timeframe of "the past six years," a Herculean accomplishment in either case. However, the same report correctly stated the operating team's "95 percent recovery record."[8]

In order to avoid misinformation about the precise details of the duke's December 16 surgical procedure, Mr. Bowen designated administrative assistant Tom Fourqurean to disseminate the information to the awaiting press. Immediately following the successful "67-minute surgery" to remove the reported "orange-sized" aneurysm of the abdominal aorta and replace the weakened section with a Dacron tube, Mr. Fourqurean advised the press: "His Royal Highness tolerated surgery well and Dr. DeBakey was pleased with the operation. For Dr. DeBakey, this was routine. The duke is regaining consciousness and will be going back to his room about noon."[9]

Since each reporter was in search of a unique angle to differentiate each daily dispatch, no detail of the duke's surgery and subsequent recovery was deemed insignificant. No matter how obscure the information, the newsmen were in pursuit of the answers. They repeatedly asked questions about what music was played in the operating room during the procedure; when the duke asked for his first cigarette after the procedure; where the duchess was during the operation; which food items on the soft diet were the duke's favorites; and countless other trivial questions. All of the available answers ended up in print, along with such newsworthy events as "the duke walked from his bed to his chair" two days after the operation;[10] the duke, "feeling in good spirits, took a walk down the hall from his fourth floor suite;" and, the duke enjoyed a traditional Christmas dinner of "stewed prunes and squash" with the duchess.[11]

For the former king's subjects in Australia, the front-page news stories about his surgery and recovery at The Methodist Hospital contained otherwise unknown details, specifically the flowers sent by Queen Elizabeth II and her sister Princess Margaret "to their favorite uncle." According to the *Sydney Morning Herald*, the flowers were "believed to be Royal Family's first public recognition in recent years of the 70-year-old Duke of Windsor" since his abdication of the throne in 1938, and the duke "was visibly touched by the Queen's warm gesture" of sending "white chrysanthemums and yellow Texas roses" and Princess Margaret's arrangement of "bronze chrysanthemums and red carnations."[12]

Several other previously unpublished details appeared in the Christmas day edition of *Time* magazine. In an article titled "Repairing the royal aorta," the magazine credited "famed surgeon Dr. Michael DeBakey" with developing the aneurysm operation performed on the Duke of Windsor. The feature article documented the heretofore elusive fact that the music playing in the operating room during the duke's surgery was *"Two Sleepy People* and *So Beats My Heart for You,"* noting that Dr. DeBakey "was scarcely listening as he performed an operation that only a few years ago would have seemed dangerous indeed." In addition to that scoop, the two-page article included another one, this one directly attributed to Dr. DeBakey, who told the magazine that the duke's aneurysm was not the size of an orange, as reported, but bigger than expected, "the size of a small cantaloupe or large grapefruit."[13]

What remained unknown to the public after such intense media scrutiny were many of the private details about the interactions of the Duke and Duchess of Windsor with the personnel at The Methodist Hospital. Two years after the operation, the Duke of Windsor penned an article for the *Chicago Tribune* in which he detailed how, while convalescing, he and the duchess sometimes had lunch in the board room of the hospital with Dr. DeBakey and his staff.

On several such occasions, the duke dined with "a remarkable, spry old lady of 83, Mrs. W. W. Fondren, widow of one of the men who struck oil at Spindletop at the turn of the century. Except for an air of definite self-assurance about her, a stranger would scarcely mark her as a woman of great wealth."[14] After learning from Dr. DeBakey of her generous donations to The Methodist Hospital, the duke was stunned to hear Mrs. Fondren say, "I'm not interested in making money; only in giving it away." Reflecting on her altruistic mission, the duke said he was "in debt to that experience for the insight it gave me into the charitable instincts of the American character."[14]

Unbeknown at the time to the press, the duke and duchess also left the hospital to make a brief visit to Mrs. Fondren in her stately mansion in Houston's privileged River Oaks neighborhood. Decades later, Mr. Fourqurean recalled how the personnel at The Methodist Hospital, who found the royal couple to be charming, were greatly amused by the duke's reaction to that excursion. Upon returning to the hospital, the duke said he was especially pleased because he rarely had the opportunity to see "an average American home."[15]

What was made available to the press and reported worldwide was the appreciative duke's expression of gratitude moments before he was released from The Methodist Hospital on December 31, 1964: "I am very glad to be able to give this brief New Year's message from The Methodist Hospital in Houston, Texas. As you know, I am now convalescing from vascular surgery performed by Dr. Michael DeBakey, the greatest expert in this field today. Thanks to his unique skill and experience and the wonderful, devoted, round-the-clock care of his team of surgeons, doctors, and nurses, I have come through his quite serious ordeal with a minimum of pain and discomfort."[16]

As photographers and journalists documented Dr. DeBakey's and Mr. Bowen's escorting the Duke and Duchess of Windsor to their awaiting limousine for the short trip to the Warwick Hotel, the hospital's administration office issued its final advisory: "Dr. Michael DeBakey, the prominent cardiovascular surgeon, was pleased with the duke's progress since the 67-minute, Dec. 16 operation for removal of an abdominal artery segment that had ballooned to the size of a large grapefruit. The duke is well on his way to recovery."[17]

Also on the road to recovery was the entire staff at The Methodist Hospital, which happily watched the throng of news media pack up and move to the Warwick Hotel to continue its vigil of reporting any and every imaginable news item about the Duke and Duchess of Windsor. Thinking that a sense of normalcy once again would return to their daily activities, the hospital workers were certain that the media frenzy experienced was a once-in-a-lifetime event. To the contrary, they would soon discover it was only the dress rehearsal for what was to become commonplace for Dr. DeBakey and his cardiovascular surgical and cardiology colleagues at The Methodist Hospital.

Already recognized by his peers as one of the leading cardiovascular surgeons in the world, Dr. DeBakey had been thrust even more into the public's general awareness via the media's incessant coverage of the Duke of Windsor's surgery and recovery. Throughout 1965, whenever Dr. DeBakey's name was mentioned in the press, he was identified not only as the "famous cardiovascular surgeon," but also "the surgeon who operated on the Duke of Windsor." This label would continue to be his trademark in all future news stories regarding his patients, whether they be famous like the beloved Hollywood singing star Miss Jeannette MacDonald, who succumbed to congestive heart failure at The Methodist Hospital on January 14, 1965, and the flamboyant New York producer Billy Rose, who survived an operation to correct a blocked artery in his leg the following December, or simply a previously unknown and penniless patient with vascular disease who hitchhiked his way to Houston to see Dr. DeBakey.

What's more, as chairman of the Commission for Heart Disease, Cancer, and Stroke, Dr. DeBakey received further nationwide recognition when President Johnson included the commission's recommendations in his proposed "Great Society" program presented during the January 4, 1965, State of the Union address to Congress. When the commission's suggested formation of "regional medical centers" became a contentious issue among medical professionals, who labeled it "socialized medicine,"[18] subsequent news coverage about the ongoing debate invariably included a quotation in support of the original concept from Dr. DeBakey, accompanied by the ubiquitous identifying phrase, "the surgeon who operated on the Duke of Windsor."

On May 2, 1965, Dr. DeBakey appeared in the first live television program broadcast on all three national networks and simultaneously around the world via the Early Bird satellite. For 18 minutes of the hour-long program, cameras were focused on Dr. DeBakey's inserting an artificial aortic valve in the left chamber of a patient's heart in the operating room at The Methodist Hospital. During the open-heart operation, doctors who were watching the surgery via satellite on television screens in Geneva asked several questions that Dr. DeBakey answered. This incredible feat of technology was described by wire service stories afterward as follows: "DeBakey, who operated on the Duke of Windsor last year, spoke in casual tones muffled by his surgical mask."[19]

Reflecting on this phenomenon decades later, *Texas Monthly* magazine would attribute Dr. DeBakey's elevated status not to the acclaim he received for the successful surgery on the Duke of Windsor but to the resultant public recognition of his countless contributions to the surgical treatment of heart diseases. Much like Dr. Jonas Salk, who created the spectacular advances in immunization for poliomyelitis in the 1950s and became known as the last hero of the acute disease era, the magazine stated that Dr. DeBakey had become known as the first hero of the chronic disease era in the 1960s.[20]

In the wake of his designation as the "hero of the chronic disease era" came a color portrait of Dr. DeBakey on the cover of the May 28, 1965, issue of *Time*. The accompanying in-depth feature article, entitled "The Texas Tornado," included the obligatory identifying royal reference clause in the opening paragraphs: "To Dr. DeBakey went H.R.H. the Duke of

Windsor to have a potentially fatal, grapefruit-sized aneurysm removed from his abdominal aorta." Thereafter, the article chronicled "the versatility and variety" of Dr. DeBakey's past accomplishments as both a cardiovascular surgeon and medical statesman; detailed the innovations he introduced for the surgical treatment of heart diseases; described his inexhaustible energy while working 20-hour days at the hospital; outlined his typical operating room schedule of eight to ten procedures a day followed by meetings, office work, and correspondence; documented his enthusiasm and confidence about creating an artificial heart; and attributed the Texas Tornado nickname to his having "the incredible drive for perfection, the unending concern for his patients, and the utter domination of his life by his profession."[21]

Also addressed in the article was Dr. DeBakey's dizzying travel schedule, with a comment that he had called such far-flung excursions "his major relaxation." Within the coming weeks he had scheduled trips to Italy to accept the St. Vincent Award of the Turin Academy of Medicine; to Brussels for a visit with Princess Liliane of Belgium; to Paris to see the Duke and Duchess of Windsor; to Athens to visit with Queen Mother Frederica; and to Washington, D.C., to continue his efforts in support of increased federal funding for medical research, another of his passions. "The Federal Government has already put a lot of money into medicine," Dr. DeBakey explained. "And every physician in the United States is better off for it– better off than he ever was before."[21]

In a brief reference to his chairing the president's Commission on Heart Disease, Cancer, and Stroke,[22-23] the article noted that the American Medical Association and Dr. DeBakey were in "violent" disagreement over the commission's proposed federal funding of regional research centers. While it was a well-known fact, the magazine did not address the other areas of contention between the AMA and Dr. DeBakey, particularly its vehement objections to the pending legislation for medical care for the aged through Social Security known as Medicare, of which Dr. DeBakey vociferously favored. A hotly debated subject in both medical and political arenas at the time of the magazine's publication in May, the Medicare bill was under discussion in the Senate Finance Committee, having already been passed by the House of Representatives in April. On July 30, 1965, President Johnson signed Medicare into law as part of the Social Security Amendments of 1965, with an implementation date of July 1966.

One subject that was covered in depth by *Time* was artificial hearts and left ventricular assist devices. With skeptics reportedly wary of the feasibility of either invention, Dr. DeBakey seized this opportunity to present his optimistic opinion, echoing testimony he recently had delivered to the congressional appropriation committees: "It is deficiencies in materials and our lack of knowledge about how they will work over a long period that are holding us up. The materials we have, good as they are, still damage the blood to some extent, and they may become rigid after long use. I am confident that if $50 million were made available today for just this kind of research, an artificial heart, or the vital parts of one, could be ready for permanent implantation within three to five years. If artificial hearts can work, as they have, for 40 hours or more, is it presumptuous to say that it could be done for 40 days or 40 years? Today it may be only a dream; tomorrow it will be a reality."[21]

Such unbridled enthusiasm about the future no doubt influenced the editors' decision to superimpose a "Toward An Artificial Heart" banner across the uppermost corner of *Time*'s cover portrait of "Surgeon Michael DeBakey." It was a gesture that would reverberate from the date of the magazine's publication forward. During the following months in the newspaper and magazine articles in which Dr. DeBakey was either featured or simply quoted, there invariably would now be two ubiquitous identifiers: the surgeon who operated on the Duke of Windsor and also the "Texas Tornado" who was dedicating his research efforts to the creation of a totally artificial heart.

In addition, there was also increased media awareness of the incremental advances made under the auspices of Dr. DeBakey's federally funded research into the feasibility of artificial hearts. As a result of the joint efforts expended by his surgery department and the engineering department of Rice University, after several unreported attempts in the previous year, Drs. C. William Hall and Liotta successfully implanted a "man-made heart" into a dog that lived until the experiment was terminated several hours later.

This accomplishment was duly noted by the national media in the spring of 1965. Wire service reports indicated the experimental operation was deemed a success by both surgeons and that "the device mimicked the action of the dog's heart" and was made of "a silicone-like material called silastic." However, Dr. Hall was cautioned, "The device presents several problems yet to be solved. One of them is the heat generated by the device. Another is the radiation given off by a nuclear power supply."[24]

These were shortcomings that required solutions found only through protracted, extensive research, an indication that the achievement of the ultimate goal of an artificial heart would take an indefinite period of time and much longer than originally hoped. Having already received more than

$1 million in grants from the U.S. Public Health Service since 1964 for research on the total artificial heart, Dr. DeBakey redirected his research team's attention to another goal, that of perfecting the left ventricular bypass pump originally created and implemented in 1963. To achieve that goal, he requested that Dr. Hall apply for a federal research grant from the National Institutes of Health (NIH), the recent recipient of a substantial increase in its budget for artificial heart research.

As recommended by the Commission on Heart Disease, Cancer, and Stroke, the congressional appropriation committees increased the research budget for artificial heart research during the summer of 1965. The precise amount of the increase came as a result of Congressman Fogarty's inviting representatives of the NIH to "supply a statement for the record as to how much money you would need in 1966, in addition to your budget, to start a real planning program to develop an artificial heart." Enthusiastic proponents, including Dr. DeBakey, replied to that request with unabashed gusto, submitting a request for $40 million for fiscal years 1965-1968. Even though NIH Director Dr. James Shannon was not a fervent supporter of the program, Dr. DeBakey and other eager heart surgeons presented a four-phase "master plan" that would conclude with the implantation of "the first artificial heart on February 14, 1970–the first Valentine's Day of the new decade."[25] When there was no voiced opposition to the ambitious plan, the funds were allocated, much to the chagrin of Dr. Shannon. "Jim Shannon was opposed to the concept and NIH's involvement in it because he thought there was not enough basic knowledge and that it was not scientifically sound," Dr. DeBakey recalled decades later. "I went over his head, to Congress."[26]

As one of the strongest advocates for increased federal funding for artificial heart research, Dr. DeBakey understandably was confident that Dr. Hall's request for one of the first grants for artificial heart research would be awarded without opposition. In addition, he knew Dr. Hall also was a recognized proponent of the program, having previously devoted six months of his time as the "loaned" expert to create the contracting policies of the NIH Artificial Heart Program. As its first project director, he had instituted the policy that only contracts to industrial organizations were awarded by the program. Therefore, the recently funded research grants for artificial hearts were to be awarded by the National Heart Institute (NHI).

The only possible drawback to the foregone conclusion about the immediate awarding of Dr. Hall's grant proposal was the fact that he had never written one before. Undaunted by the challenge, he compiled a list of the myriad research projects he could foresee; tallied the possible costs involved in each; and incorporated all of the information in his first grant proposals. Pleased that he could propose a vast amount of research for a somewhat limited sum, he confidently awaited Dr. DeBakey's approval before submitting them to the NHI.

The initial reaction of Dr. DeBakey to his proposals was not what Dr. Hall expected. Upon reading that the requested grants totaled only $25,000, "he almost threw them at me," Dr. Hall recalled with amusement. "In fact, I think he actually did. For Dr. DeBakey was thinking on a much bigger plane. He was considering a whole range of problems that might be studied in connection with the development of the artificial heart. He had decided to solve the whole problem, and not just build a little pump. When Dr. DeBakey got finished with the grant proposal, it totaled $4.5 million, which was awarded."[27]

The receipt of the first of those funds in the summer of 1965 marked the formal beginning of the Baylor-Rice Artificial Heart Program set up under the strict guidelines dictated by the NIH and the NHI for all federally funded research projects. Serving as principal investigator was Dr. DeBakey, who was assisted by coprogram directors Dr. W.W. Akers, the chairman of the engineering department at Rice, and Dr. Hall, with Dr. Liotta named as full-time assistant. With guarded enthusiasm about the continuation of their collaborative efforts, Dr. DeBakey stated in an article jointly published with Dr. Hall, "We are convinced that devices for partial or temporary assistance to a failing heart or even a total implantable replacement are desirable objectives to pursue. The artificial heart will not come as a breakthrough but will develop progressively as the inherent difficulties are defined and overcome."[28]

As research testing and implantation of various pump devices in animals progressed in the laboratories, Dr. DeBakey continued to fine tune his cardiovascular surgery service at The Methodist Hospital. Designated as his chief assistant was Dr. Jimmy F. Howell, while serving as head surgeons were Drs. Cooley, Garrett, Beall, Morris, and Crawford. Two of the newly arrived thoracic surgery residents in 1965, Dr. Edward B. Diethrich and Dr. George P. Noon, proved to be exceptional during residency, later becoming integral members of Dr. DeBakey's cardiovascular team upon completion of their training.

Under Dr. DeBakey's direction, this team of specialists performed the various cardiovascular surgical procedures at The Methodist Hospital. Each team in an operating room comprised a head surgeon, a chief assistant, an assistant surgeon, one or two anesthesiologists, two or three heart-lung machine technicians, and three specially trained nurses.[29] Cardiologists and pathologists were available on call, if needed. In order for the head surgeons to perform ten or more operations in a day, which more often than not was the case in 1965, they spent only the time necessary to complete the specific cardiovascular procedure, leaving the opening and closing of the patient to the assistants. With multiple procedures to perform in a single day, the head surgeon's arriving in each operating room at the exact moment of need was a prerequisite that demanded exceptional teamwork.

Such precise timing was but one of the established mandates in the operating room. Known to be a perfectionist, Dr. DeBakey required strict adherence to the exacting standards of surgical practice, particularly by his residents. Legendary for dispensing harsh criticism of a resident's abilities, education, and competence, Dr. DeBakey was both feared and revered by his trainees. All of them would relish their memories of their experiences with him at The Methodist Hospital. One such former resident was Dr. Edward Diethrich, who described his first three months of surgical residency with Dr. DeBakey as "the worst experience of my whole life." Remembering how the surgeon's withering words affected him at the time, he recalled, "It got to a point that I lost all my confidence; he can shatter you, absolutely shatter you. I never answered back to him. I never raised my voice, because this was what provoked him the most."[30]

After several months the constant criticism suddenly stopped. Out of the blue, Dr. DeBakey began to trust Dr. Diethrich's abilities and respect his judgment, further astonishing the young man by suddenly assigning him to perform operations without his supervision. Months later, still curious about such a dramatic turn of events, Dr. Diethrich observed that one of the current surgery residents had become the latest recipient of his relentless wrath in the operating room. In a casual conversation with Dr. DeBakey outside of the hospital, he took the opportunity to ask why he was so critical of that resident, to which Dr. DeBakey replied: "Ted, you know, I test people. I see what people can do under fire and under pressure. I must know what these people are made of."[31]

For those residents who passed Dr. DeBakey's demands, like Dr. Diethrich, there remained the ongoing challenge of fulfilling his expectations of excellence. "Unless you were there, it is impossible to understand the enormous impact Dr. DeBakey had on young trainees and his associates," Dr. Diethrich said. "His demand for perfection in every aspect of cardiovascular medicine, research, teaching, and clinical care set the standards that are followed to this day. He was a tough mentor but an awesome inspiration."[32]

With his steadily growing reputation as an uncompromising "taskmaster with lofty standards" who had no tolerance for "incompetence, sloppy thinking, and laziness," Dr. DeBakey often was asked by the media to justify his strict training tactics. It was a question he answered succinctly: "I'm accused of being a perfectionist and, in the way it's usually defined, I guess I am. In medicine, and certainly in surgery, you have to be as perfect as possible. There is no room for mistakes. They're all bad, some even fatal. We're not infallible, but you certainly make an effort. And that's what I ask."[33]

Regardless of his justifiable motivation, he achieved the nickname of "Black Mike" from surgical residents for his dark moods in the operating room. Conversely, Dr. DeBakey was held in high esteem by his patients for his gentle display of compassion and concern about their welfare. "He treated each of his patients as if they were royalty," Mr. Bowen said, recalling that in addition to the celebrities and heads of state, Dr. DeBakey also had patients from every walk of life. To Dr. DeBakey, there was very little difference between his patients, be they rich or poor. As he once famously said, "Once you incise the skin, you find they are all very similar."[34]

Because of the large number of patients Dr. DeBakey had on a daily basis, he rarely had time to spend more than a few minutes with each one while making daily rounds. To avoid undo wear and tear on his attending staff, pre-round conferences were held in his office around X-ray viewing screens, where all pertinent information on the patients to be seen was reviewed. Everyone rounding was expected to attend, and it became a ritual long remembered by those participating.

Accompanied by his usual entourage of assistant surgeons, surgical residents, cardiologists, and medical students, Dr. DeBakey depended on his resident to supply the necessary information about each patient before entering the patient's room. Should the information be incorrect or incomplete, the resident knew that the usual unpleasant consequences would be forthcoming from Dr. DeBakey but always out of sight of the patient. "He could be sweet as dripping honey when it came to patients and medical students," recalled Dr. Jeremy R. Morton, a former surgical resident who participated in this ritual. "But he could be brutal with surgical residents. I guess he was just trying to make us tough."[35]

Without question, one patient reciprocated the royal treatment he received from Dr. DeBakey in a memorable way. Returning to The Methodist Hospital for a scheduled checkup in October 1965, the Duke of Windsor arrived at the same time a television crew from the British Broadcasting Corporation (BBC) was filming a special about Dr. DeBakey's "spare-part surgery" and one of his major goals "to perfect the artificial heart."[36] Unexpectedly, when the producer asked whether the duke might say a few words on camera, the duke agreed.

It was to be the first recorded occasion in which the duke permitted a television interview since his 1936 abdication as King Edward VIII, in itself a newsworthy occasion. The first question presented by the BBC interviewer to the duke on camera concerned the reason for his coming to Houston for his abdominal aneurysm surgery the previous December. When the duke's short reply was, "To see Dr. DeBakey," the interviewer reminded him that there were many other surgeons trained by Dr. DeBakey who were closer to home and wondered why he had not chosen one that was more conveniently located. "Well," said the Duke, "I came direct to the maestro."[36]

It was an "unprecedented tribute" that was to be reported in newspapers throughout the United States and all over the world.[37] The aftermath was predictable, but not quantifiable. The Methodist Hospital was already inundated with international patients who had read about Dr. DeBakey in previous news reports, or seen him perform surgery on the satellite broadcast, or read about him in *Time*'s feature article. The simple fact was that whoever became inspired by the duke's praise of Dr. DeBakey and traveled to Houston to seek his care would simply have to join the crowd of others who shared that inspiration. A great many of those were not in the hospital but waiting in Houston hotels for the opportunity to be admitted.

The Methodist Hospital was full, turning away between 50 and 75 patients a day in 1965. "We had patients from all over the world on the waiting list to get into the hospital; they were cardiovascular patients," recalled Margaret McElhany, who supervised both the switchboard and admissions office. "Everybody wanted to come; there was no other place for them to go to but here in Houston, to The Methodist Hospital, and Dr. DeBakey was all they knew to come to. So we really had a time getting all the patients admitted because of Dr. DeBakey."[38]

It was becoming a chronic situation that required an immediate remedy. Since the recently expanded hospital facilities were utilized to capacity, Mr. Bowen had no other recourse than to arrange for additional space to accommodate the overflow. To accomplish this, he leased the Glen Eagle Convalescent Home, a facility located approximately one mile away from the Texas Medical Center. Located at 1130 Earle Street and between Fannin

Street and Bertner Avenue near the Old Spanish Trail, the renovated and renamed The Methodist Hospital Annex provided an additional 180 beds, bringing the total bed capacity of The Methodist Hospital to 908 in November 1965.[39]

Beginning its first day of operation, the Annex experienced land-office business. "It was opened on Saturday and I came in that Saturday and I worked all day long," recalled Mrs. McElhany, whose husband, L. H. "Mac" McElhany, served as the newly appointed director of transportation. "Mac was in charge of the bus that brought the patients back and forth from the Annex. I filled every bed up that Saturday at the Annex with people who were on the waiting list to get into the hospital, at least, every patient that was on my waiting list. Our bed situation was horrible."[38]

Since a predominant number of patients admitted to the Annex were Dr. DeBakey's, he incorporated a visit to that facility into his daily activities. Followed by his usual entourage at The Methodist Hospital, "we used to finish our rounds here and jump in the car and drive over there to see patients," he said, recalling how some of the trips required breakneck speed. "I had one resident who said to me, flat out, 'I'll never ride with you again.'"[40]

The fast lane had become the norm for Dr. DeBakey, not only in his Alfa Romeo as he sped to the annex but also in every other aspect of his professional life. At the age of 57 in 1965, he was at the peak of his surgical career, averaging more than 1,000 operations per year. With an average four or five hours sleep each night, he had an established work ethic that seemed superhuman to others. Beginning at 6:00 AM, he operated hour after hour. "I've been fortunate in that I need very little sleep; I can get along well on four or five hours," he would often explain to those who marveled at his relentless pace in the operating room. Reminiscing about the 1960s decades later, Dr. DeBakey said, "I used to start operating at six in the morning. Sometimes I wouldn't finish until 10 or 11 at night."[41]

A similar schedule was the rule for his surgical colleagues as well as the cardiology consultants at The Methodist Hospital. While referrals to the surgical community grew exponentially from physician-referrals, patient-referrals, and others, so did the number of similar referrals to the cardiologists. Those in private practice led by The Chapman Group saw patients arriving from throughout the southwest as well as nearby Louisiana, New Mexico, Arkansas, and Oklahoma. A large contingent came from Mexico, Central, and South America.

For some of the cardiovascular patients who found The Methodist Hospital geographically inconvenient, a unique solution was created. At the request of Saudi Arabia, Dr. DeBakey and his surgical colleagues had set up and established a center for cardiovascular training and patient care in Riyadh in the late 1970s and early 1980s, the King Faisal Specialist Hospital and Research Centre. Cardiovascular surgeons from The Methodist Hospital and Baylor College of Medicine rotated to Riyadh on a three-month schedule for several years while the center was being established. Among those from Houston who rotated through that service at one time or another were Drs. Charles McCollum, Gerald Lawrie, Kenneth Mattox, Hartwell Whisennand, and Arthur Beall.

A consequence of that program was the referral of large numbers of Saudi Arabian patients primarily to the service of Dr. DeBakey and colleagues, but there were a few exceptions. One internal medicine physician at The Methodist Hospital established a large referral practice directly through a prominent Saudi family.

Large referral practices in cardiology had been the norm at The Methodist Hospital since the early 1970s when The Chapman Group was rounding on more than 120 patients daily. Half of those were seen in consultation with surgical colleagues and the other half had been directly referred to cardiologists.. At that time, since there were few, if any, cardiologists in communities in the southwest due to few cardiology training programs, physicians in Texas towns and neighboring states sent their patients to Houston.

Following the subsequent establishment of cardiology fellowship training programs in the early 1970s at places like Baylor College of Medicine, The Methodist Hospital, and Texas Heart Institute in Houston and later in San Antonio and Dallas, the cardiology community grew rapidly. In 1968, the number of cardiologists practicing adult cardiology in Houston could be counted on two hands. By 2012, they numbered well over 500, encompassing all cardiovascular specialties that have developed over the years: interventional cardiologists, heart failure specialists, electrophysiologists, and cardiologists specializing in imaging. At the same time, the cardiovascular surgical population grew from a handful in the 1960s to about 200 practicing cardiovascular surgeons with training as cardiothoracic, transplant, vascular, or cardiac surgeons.

Since there was only Dr. DeBakey and a handful of practicing cardiovascular surgeons at The Methodist Hospital in the 1960s, the demand for services often exceeded the supply available, resulting in back-to-back operations all day long and often into the night. On the rare days when only a few operations were performed, Dr. DeBakey was not idle.

Instead, he devoted the available afternoon and evening hours to conferring with his surgical team, cardiologists, and researchers; scrutinizing patients' arteriograms and X-rays for the following day's operations; attending to the business of managing the surgical department; returning phone calls from physicians and patients from all over the world; dictating memos and letters; meeting with visiting surgeons; and juggling his already tight schedule to accommodate the ever-increasing number of out-of-town speaking engagements, award presentations, and congressional testimonies—all the while serving as Chairman of the Department of Surgery at Baylor University College of Medicine.

Regardless of the number of operations scheduled, he always took the time each day to visit with each of his patients in both the hospital and annex. In deference to his exacting schedule, the unwritten rule at The Methodist Hospital was for all employees to exit an elevator should Dr. DeBakey enter it, allowing him the exclusive use of express service. This rarely happened because Dr. DeBakey avoided the elevators, usually running up or down the stairs to the next floor. More likely than not, his detours included his entourage, who would be huffing and puffing to keep up with their indefatigable leader.

The end of a usual workday for Dr. DeBakey at the hospital usually came in the early evening, barring any emergency surgery or postoperative complication that might arise. Having deliberately chosen a home close to the hospital, he was able to drive there in a matter of minutes. The close proximity also was necessary to fulfill his need to have immediate access to his patients, an omnipresent concern. To enable him to stay close to critically ill patients, a suite was established at the hospital where he could spend the night if necessary. "If I get a call in the middle of the night, I don't want to use the telephone, I want to see that patient," he said.[42]

Since there were no medical residents or cardiology fellows in the 1960s, it was the cardiologists' responsibility to take care of the cardiovascular surgical patients after surgery. "One of the least pleasant things was to get a call at 3:00 AM," Dr. Manus O'Donnell said, recalling the dreaded message he would hear. "'Hi. I'm Mike DeBakey. I'm here with so and so.' The reference was, 'I'm taking care of this patient and you'd better come in too.' That led to some amusing situations."[43]

Dr. DeBakey required that each surgical resident at The Methodist Hospital take a two-month rotation in the Fondren Surgical ICU. Forbidden to leave the ICU during the two-month period, each resident worked 24-hour days while covering 30 beds of newly operated cardiovascular patients.

It was a daunting challenge, enumerated in tales heard from former residents.

During uninterrupted evenings at home, Dr. DeBakey ate a light meal and then spent time reading, both the latest medical literature and various other books about his myriad interests, and writing editorials and medical manuscripts before retiring at midnight. Arising at 4 or 5 AM each day, he read the *Wall Street Journal* and *The New York Times* in 30 minutes, continued to work on his medical manuscripts and other various literary responsibilities, and returned to The Methodist Hospital to arrive in time for his first surgical procedure at 6:30 AM. It was a schedule he adhered to religiously, with rare amendments for certain other obligations. "I try to conserve whatever time I can for the things I need to do, most of which are in my professional sphere of interest," he said. "I try to use my time as efficiently as I can."[42]

His astonishing ability to adhere to such a structured lifestyle invariably generated curiosity from peers, patients, and journalists. After observing Dr. DeBakey during a typical day, one fascinated journalist described him thusly: "By his nature, he is restless, kinetic, ambitious, curious, an intellectual with an insatiable hunger for knowledge."[44]

To that journalist and any and all others who asked the origin of his regimented lifestyle, Dr. DeBakey credited his parents with instilling in him the determination to achieve perfection. As for the early-rising habits and abhorrence of wasted time, those were specific traits he emulated from his father Shaker Morris DeBakey. From his mother, Raheeja Zorba DeBakey, "the most compassionate and sweetest person I've ever known," came not only all of the most important life lessons but also expert instructions in the art of sewing with precision, an integral part of his profession.[42] His voracious appetite for knowledge was attributed to his childhood upbringing when he was required to read at least one book a week, culminating in his voluntarily reading the entire *World Book Encyclopedia* before he entered college. All of these contributing factors led Dr. DeBakey to believe both of his parents were responsible for his ability to maintain such a demanding schedule. "You are not born with self-discipline, you have to develop that, and someone has to help you," he said. "They have to teach you right from wrong."[45]

Journalists also learned while interviewing Dr. DeBakey that he was not one to dwell on his early life or discuss at any length his past accomplishments. Without fail, Dr. DeBakey always steered the subject to the future. No matter the major thrust of any story written about him or broadcast on television in 1965, there was often some mention of his research team's ongoing efforts to perfect an artificial heart. "It is a feasible objective now," he declared during a BBC broadcast in November 1965. "I am convinced it can be done."[36]

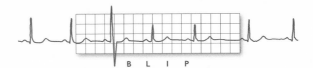

DANNY KAYE - 1965

A mong the noted guests gathered at Mary Lasker's Manhattan townhouse for a New Year's Eve celebration in 1965 was her good friend Danny Kaye, a talented and versatile entertainer known not only for his starring roles on stage and in films but also for his desire to be a doctor instead. Because of his interests, Mr. Kaye devoted his attention that evening to two other guests, Dr. Isadore Rosenfeld, a well-known cardiologist who was Mrs. Lasker's physician, and the "Texas Tornado" who had been featured on the cover of *Time* magazine six months earlier, Dr. DeBakey. During the festivities, when Dr. DeBakey issued an open invitation for Mr. Kaye to observe heart surgery in Houston, the star needed no further urging. When he heard Dr. Rosenfeld was giving a lecture in Houston in the coming week, he decided he would join him for the trip. While in Houston, rather than attend Dr. Rosenfeld's lecture, Mr. Kaye joined Dr. DeBakey in the operating room. Scrubbed and dressed in a surgical gown, mask, and gloves like the doctor he always wanted to be, Mr. Kaye proudly stood next to Dr. DeBakey as he stitched up the patient. A photograph capturing this moment became one of the star's most treasured possessions. "It remained on his bedside table until the day he died," Dr. Rosenfeld said.[1]

---

1. Rosenfeld I. *Doctor of the Heart, My Life in Medicine.* New Rochelle, NY: Mary Ann Liebert, Inc.; 2010:153.

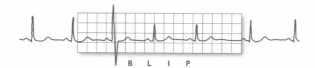

DANNY KAYE – ENCORE - 1980

An evening to remember occurred in early 1980 when Dr. Gotto entertained Danny Kaye and Dr. Isadore Rosenfeld at a dinner at the River Oaks Country Club in Houston. Dr. Winters was privileged to attend with about a dozen other guests. "Our host, sat at the end of the table next to Danny Kaye with Isadore Rosenfeld at the other end," Dr. Winters said. "The repartee between Kaye and Rosenfeld, often with Dr. Gotto as the foil, will be forever remembered. Danny Kaye was given the honor of sampling the first bottle of wine. He announced it 'corked,' precipitating an endless array of wine and dinner stories. At the end of dinner, Danny Kaye attempted to pull the tablecloth off the table and leave the dishes in place. He was not successful, leaving Dr. Gotto to wonder aloud if we would ever be allowed back in River Oaks Country Club."

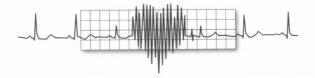

CHAPTER EIGHT

A NEW ERA OF HEART TRANSPLANTATION
1966 - 1968

"Dear Humpty Dumpty, You are not the only one who falls and breaks into pieces.
Sincerely, The Heart."
ZARIAHH RENEE

In the two years since Congress mandated federal funding of the Artificial Heart Program at the National Heart Institute in 1964, research into the feasibility of implanting an artificial heart into a human being was taking place in at least three U.S. surgical research laboratories.

In addition to the Baylor-Rice collaborative research program, in which substantial progress had been made through the collaborative efforts of Dr. Akers at Rice University and Dr. DeBakey's team of researchers, [1-2-3-4-5-6] similarly funded programs existed at the Cleveland Clinic, under the direction of Dr. Willem J. Kolff, and at Maimonides Medical Center in Brooklyn, under the direction of Dr. Adrian Kantrowitz in 1964. First among them to indicate publicly the imminent implantation of such a device in a human was Dr. DeBakey. Unlike the majority of his colleagues in the medical profession who abhorred publicity of any sort, Dr. DeBakey believed the public was entitled to know what was being achieved in federally funded research.[7] Capitalizing on the unprecedented media attention he continued to receive as a result of the *Time* magazine cover story about the Duke of Windsor's operation, Dr. DeBakey embraced every opportunity to document his research team's progress.

At a medical conference sponsored by the New York Heart Association and held in New York City on January 27, 1966, Dr. DeBakey stated in a news conference that "an artificial heart, powered by an air pump, should be ready for use by a human within a month and should be placed in a human within the year."[8] While addressing the journalists, Dr. DeBakey also displayed a working model of the Baylor-Rice device, described by one member of the New York media as being "hardly bigger than a Texas grapefruit" and one that "does not replace the entire heart" but "takes over for the left and powerful side of the great pumping organ." [8]

Within a week, another working model of the Baylor-Rice left ventricular bypass device was delivered to the White House. At the personal request of President Johnson, the device was presented to Congressman John E. Fogarty, the recipient of the American Heart Association's "Heart-of-the-Year Award" on February 3, 1966. "When we read that a fully functioning artificial heart is possible within five years, we pay tribute to congressional leadership, and particularly to Congressman John Fogarty of Rhode Island," the president said during that presentation to him. "And when we finally call a halt to the wholesale murder of heart disease, all of us will bless the day that Congress took effective action."[9]

Shortly after the White House event, Drs. Liotta and Hall successfully implanted one of the Baylor-Rice left ventricular bypass devices into the chest of a 285-pound Hereford calf that lived for 18 days. Since the calf's heart resumed its normal activity following the removal of the device, Dr. Hall believed the calf would have lived indefinitely were it not an experiment that required an immediate autopsy to verify research criteria. Dr. Hall told one newspaper reporter, "We'll have one of these pumps in the operating room waiting for a patient in a very, very short time, perhaps a matter of weeks."[10]

Buoyed by his research team's recent accomplishments and confident left ventricular and right ventricular pumps were to become a mainstay in the future, Dr. DeBakey capitalized on the moment. Designated "Man of the Month" by Walter Cronkite's CBS documentary series "The Twentieth Century" and featured in a 30-minute, nationally televised program on February 27, 1966, Dr. DeBakey was shown operating on a patient with an aneurysm, overseeing his surgical patients in the intensive care unit, and talking with patients' families. When the opportunity to discuss the future was presented, he reiterated his belief that the Baylor-Rice artificial heart would be implanted in the near future.

After speaking to the media about the artificial heart in general terms the following two months during his travels throughout the United States, Dr. DeBakey began to discuss specific details at an April 17 meeting of the Tulane University board of visitors in New Orleans. During an interview with a newspaper reporter, he discussed plans for implementing the Baylor-Rice artificial heart within the month. He described how it would be placed in the chest wall, close to the patient's own heart, and operated by an electric motor outside the body. It would be "only a temporary arrangement" to perform "the heart's functions until the patient's heart was strong enough to take over," he explained.[11]

The specificity of his comments generated a media frenzy reminiscent of the one that occurred during the Duke of Windsor's aneurysm surgery. Within 24 hours of the national publication of Dr. DeBakey's announcement, journalists from all over the world began camping out at The Methodist Hospital. To address the growing demand for further information regarding the imminent implantation of an artificial heart, and concerned that publication of the details "might upset some patients awaiting heart surgery," Dr. DeBakey gathered his team to conduct a "two hour, off-the-record news conference" at the hospital on Tuesday, April 19.[12]

Asserting that the first patient to receive the Baylor-Rice device had not been selected, Dr. DeBakey said, "We are waiting on the best-conditioned patient who needs the artificial heart." He also stated that the decision to use the artificial heart would not be made until after an operation was under way, and therefore there would be no advance notice given to the gathered media. In his conclusion, he stated the obvious, "The team is ready."[13]

Identified to the media as members of Dr. DeBakey's surgical team were Drs. Howell, Liotta, and Diethrich. Also introduced was Dr. Hall, the consultant to the surgical team, and Rice University's Dr. Akers, the engineering specialist. The operating team was to comprise a cardiologist, a pathologist, one or two anesthesiologists, two or three lung machine technicians, and three specially trained nurses. Dr. DeBakey also announced that still and motion pictures of the operation would be available as soon as possible, as "special messengers stood by to rush film to processing laboratories."[13]

The availability of surgical films was a recent innovation championed by Dr. DeBakey. One of the first to have his surgeries recorded on film for educational purposes, Dr. DeBakey worked closely with the audiovisual education department of Baylor University College of Medicine to create the necessary equipment to provide the highest quality films. Unlike other operating rooms, where the cameraman used a tripod in a fixed position near the operating arena, a unique apparatus above the arena was used at The Methodist Hospital. Perched high above the operating table on a 1,500-pound hydraulic stainless steel film stand equipped with lights, the camera operator would lie prone on a padded flat bed to record a surgeon's eye-view. "I would be up, out of the way, with a better view," recalled its operator Joe Zwer, the inventor of the apparatus in the early 1960s. "I was glad that this machine did a better job than anything else we had seen."[14]

Also promising to be superb were the promised color photographs of the surgical procedure. In addition to a staff photographer, the award-winning Ralph Morse from *Life* magazine was to document the procedure exclusively for Dr. DeBakey. Assigned by the magazine to photograph the everyday lives of the original seven astronauts and their families in Houston for the previous six years, he was dubbed the "eighth astronaut" by John Glenn, a frequent observer of cardiovascular operations performed by Dr. DeBakey at The Methodist Hospital. When Mr. Morse learned firsthand of Dr. DeBakey's desire to implant an artificial heart, he requested permission to be in the operating room whenever that procedure might occur. Unable to allow his presence as a bystander, Dr. DeBakey offered to pay him a token fee of one dollar in order to hire him as his personal photographer. Their mutually accepted agreement included Morse's giving Dr. DeBakey the exclusive distribution rights of all photographs taken during the procedure, along with the stipulation they also be made available for publication in *Life*.

The off-the-record briefing also included clarification that there would not be a total heart replacement but an installation of a "half heart," a pump to substitute for the left ventricle, which normally does most of the heart's pumping. Designed to give temporary but sustained relief to a damaged heart, the new device was similar to, but far more sophisticated than, the world's first left ventricular bypass pump implanted by his team in 1963 to keep a dying man alive.[3-12] During the three years following that patient's subsequent cardiac arrest and death on the fourth postoperative day, Dr. DeBakey said the Baylor-Rice collaboration intensified efforts to fabricate a new pump, one that proved to be safe and effective in experiments of several hundred calves.

Supported by the $4.5-million federally funded research project, "this pump consisted in a gas-energized, hemispherical, synchronized pump made of Dacron-reinforced Silastic, with a molded diaphragm separating the gas chamber from the blood chamber," Dr. DeBakey said. "By pulsing pressurized CO_2 into the gas chamber, the diaphragm collapsed the blood chamber and thereby emptied it. The energizing and controlling system consists in a Teflon bellows driven by an electric motor. The pump could be controlled manually or by an electrocardiographic triggering mechanism."[15]

The journalists also were told that the energizing and controlling machine would emit pulses of compressed air to the pump. It would not be implanted in the patient's chest. Instead, it was to be located bedside, where it could easily be disconnected when no longer needed. Should the patient's heart begin to fail afterward, the machine quickly could be put back to work again.[13]

More precise details of the implantation of the "partial heart" were to be available for publication both during and after the procedure. Journalists were told that whenever the decision to implant the device was made, the observation dome above the operating theater would be reserved for the media and that a cardiologist would be there to commentate about the procedure in progress. Aware that all the necessary equipment already had been moved into the operating area that day, the journalists sensed that the procedure was to occur in the immediate future and did not depart the hospital at the conclusion of the press briefing, choosing to camp out there instead.

Theirs was not a long wait. Forty-eight hours after the news briefing, Dr. DeBakey's team implanted the Baylor-Rice device into the chest wall of Marcel L. DeRudder, who was originally scheduled for mitral valve replacement surgery at 7:40 AM on Thursday, April 21, 1966. Unable to work for more than 21 years because of the debilitating effects of rheumatic heart disease, the 65-year-old retired miner had discussed with Dr. DeBakey the extreme frailty of his diseased heart the night before the procedure. Afraid Mr. DeRudder would not live long enough to undergo the valve procedure, Dr. DeBakey discussed the possibility of his team's implanting the artificial heart and thus, perhaps give him a chance to live longer. After explaining that previous attempts to implant such a device had not been successful, but without it he would be doomed, Dr. DeBakey said that Mr. DeRudder understood the odds: "He was quite eager and he said, 'Let's go ahead with it tomorrow morning.'"[16]

Mr. DeRudder declined to advise his wife in Illinois of the possibility of the implantation because he didn't want to worry her but nonetheless granted permission to disclose his identity to the media. "That sounds just like him, worried about me at a time like that," Edna DeRudder said several days later.[16] She went on to explain that when she and her husband first became aware of the new techniques of open-heart surgery developed by Dr. DeBakey several months earlier, they began to share a cautious optimism about the possibilities of his benefiting from such expertise. "My husband told me he was willing to be a human guinea pig," she said. "That way, he said, maybe they would learn something that would save someone else."[17]

Since the possibility of Mr. DeRudder's surviving the valve operation without the implantation of the Baylor-Rice device was dependent on what could be observed during open-heart surgery, Dr. DeBakey gave no advance notice to the media. When Mr. DeRudder's condition began to deteriorate immediately following valve replacement, the decision to implant the device was made at 10:14 AM and the journalists were alerted to convene in the observation deck above the operating area. As the assigned photographers captured every step on film and Dr. John Lancaster, a cardiologist, described each moment to the gathered press, Dr. DeBakey and his team removed one of Mr. DeRudder's ribs and implanted the device, switching it on at 11:15 AM. Within moments, the pump seemed to overburden Mr. DeRudder's weakened arterial system and his heart failed. After the surgical team applied hand massage to Mr. DeRudder's heart, the heart revived and the procedure continued uninterrupted. At its conclusion at 1:45 PM, the external pump successfully had assumed 60 percent of the workload of Mr. DeRudder's heart.[18]

Immediately following the procedure's completion, there was a press conference in which Dr. DeBakey advised that any success was due "to the importance of teamwork." Saying it was too early to evaluate the "left ventricular bypass pump" at that time since it was the first time, "to my knowledge," that such a device had ever been used in a human being, Dr. DeBakey concluded, "We can only speculate and hope."[19]

Along with the resulting laudatory front-page news stories and nationally televised news coverage came an editorial from *The New York Times* that questioned the "ethics of publicizing a highly experimental procedure, with its concomitant raising of possibly unjustified hopes among thousands suffering from heart ailments."[20] It was an opinion shared by Dr. Kantrowitz, who announced that he had used an artificial heart two months earlier at Maimonides Medical Center in Brooklyn, but the patient died of a liver ailment. He had not planned to make the news of the operation public, he said, but changed his mind after learning of Dr. DeBakey's efforts. "We don't do things the way Dr. DeBakey does–television cameras and all," he told a reporter from the *St. Petersburg Times*. "We do things differently in Brooklyn. I did everything possible to keep this out of the newspapers." The following day, to a query from a *New York Times* reporter about that procedure, Dr. Kantrowitz responded, "We chose to study our attempt carefully and analyze the results before making any public statement."[21]

In agreement with such sentiments, other surgeons around the country, as well as disgruntled members of the Harris County Medical Society, began to voice their objections, albeit anonymously in most reported cases, to the "circus-like" conditions surrounding the DeRudder operation. Also printed in newspapers around the country were accusations of Dr. DeBakey's being a "publicity seeker," courtesy of the members of an unidentified organization of chest surgeons who reportedly felt he should be ostracized by the profession.[22]

Impervious to such criticism from his peers, Dr. DeBakey concentrated his attention on Mr. DeRudder, who remained unconscious 24 hours after the implantation. A medical bulletin released to the media at 6:00 AM on April 22 stated "physicians fear there may be some brain damage," advising it was too early to ascertain what effect this would have. This bulletin, as well as all subsequent ones issued about Mr. DeRudder's biological complications developed during the following four days, generated additional press coverage daily. Advising the press that Mr. DeRudder's complications could be overcome, but his heart "still can't assume quite half the workload of a normal heart," Dr. DeBakey concluded, "Without the pump he would have died."[23]

Five days after the implantation, with Dr. DeBakey at his bedside in the early morning hours of April 26, the still unconscious Mr. DeRudder died suddenly from a rupture in his left lung. Up until the moment of his death, the pump continued to perform normally, the last issued medical advisory stated. Following the autopsy, Dr. DeBakey told the gathered press that the cause of the rupture was unknown, a complication "over which we had no control."[24] What was discovered during the autopsy was the fact that "the pump did what we thought it would do," Dr. DeBakey said. "The patient's heart was already showing improvement. With this important encouragement, we look forward to using the device again in the near future."[25]

The future also held the promise of a "permanently implanted artificial heart," Dr. DeBakey said, estimating that the total artificial heart, an ongoing project of the Baylor-Rice collaborative research team, might be available within ten years or sooner.[26] Noting that such a device "might save the lives of an estimated 300,000 U.S. heart-attack victims each year," he also advised that the implantation of a partial or total artificial heart "must be considered only a stopgap, until preventative measures against heart disease are perfected."[25]

Also predictable following the DeRudder case was the immediate increased media interest in Dr. DeBakey, no doubt to the consternation of the medical colleagues already perturbed about his excessive publicity. Appearing as the solo guest on the nationally televised "Meet the Press" on April 29, Dr. DeBakey stated that a total artificial heart could be available by 1971 but "will depend on future developments" in research and funding.[27] It was a belief he reiterated in the "Death of a patient" article published in the May 6 issue of *Time*. Also published that week was "A patient's gift to the future of heart repair," a nine-page feature story in *Life* relating step-by-step details of Mr. DeRudder's procedure, postoperative coma, biological complications, and subsequent death. Saluting Mr. DeRudder for performing "a supreme act of usefulness to the science of medicine and to future generations of his fellow man," the article was accompanied by the dramatic color photographs taken in the operating arena by Mr. Morse, the magazine's award-winning photographer.[28]

Such coverage produced an unexpected outcome. While continuing to espouse the educational benefits of publicizing the advances made in federally funded research in speeches and interviews, Dr. DeBakey nonetheless deferred to his critics both during and after his second attempt to implant the left ventricular bypass pump. On May 17, less than a month after Mr. DeRudder's death, "the cardiovascular team at The Methodist Hospital" implanted the device into Walter L. McCans. When a single Houston newspaper reported the operation after the fact, the national news media responded by descending on the hospital in search of detailed information. There were no news conferences held for the large number of reporters gathered, and a spokesman for the hospital issued "tersely worded" bulletins in which Dr. DeBakey's name never appeared. When McCans, a 61-year-old retired Naval petty officer, died within three days of uncontrollable chest bleeding, Dr. DeBakey was out of town. Upon his return the following day, he remained unavailable to the media.[22]

Similar efforts to constrain media access to Dr. DeBakey were employed by hospital administration for the August 8, 1968 insertion of a left ventricular bypass pump during a procedure to replace a 37-year-old woman's mitral and aortic valves. This third attempt at successful implantation of the Baylor-Rice device was announced after the fact in a short statement issued by Mr. Bowen, the hospital administrator, who refused to disclose the patient's name. Advising the media that Dr. DeBakey was not available for comment, hospital officials also announced that there were to be no press conferences and updated information would be released in "official hospital bulletins" only.[29]

The patient, subsequently identified by hospital administration as Esperanza del Valle Vazquez, a Mexico City beauty parlor operator, was to make medical history. After the left ventricular assist bypass pump supported her for ten days, she recovered sufficiently and was able to have the device removed, becoming the world's first known survivor of an implanted artificial heart. Throughout her 29-postoperative days at The Methodist Hospital, only minimal details were made available to the media, resulting in daily news coverage about the patient's subsequent recovery. Even though the names of the members of the cardiovascular team involved were not identified by the hospital and Dr. DeBakey never spoke publicly about this history-making patient, the majority of the news accounts published included not only his name but also the identifying phrase "the famed cardiovascular surgeon."[30]

This became a recognized pattern in the news coverage of subsequent implantations of the left ventricular bypass pump in three additional patients at The Methodist Hospital in 1966. As before, news accounts included a reference to "the surgical team, headed by DeBakey" with no direct quotes attributed to him. Even though none of these patients survived, the pump reportedly had done the job it "was designed to do in all three cases" and the "deaths came from causes other than heart disease."[31]

The cumulative result of Dr. DeBakey's omnipresence in the media was his being named by an *Associated Press* poll as one of the top newsmakers of 1966. Journalists who participated in the poll chose President Johnson as newsmaker of the year for the congressional implementation of Great Society bills such as Medicare. Recognized by the poll as the leading figure in the field of science for his implantation of "the first artificial heart in a human," the 57-year-old Dr. DeBakey appeared on the nationally published list along with other designated luminaries in their respective fields, such as Truman Capote in literature, Ralph Nadar in business, Sandy Koufax in sports, and Bruce Wayne, Batman, in entertainment.[32]

This national recognition of Dr. DeBakey further enhanced the public's knowledge of the history-making advances in cardiovascular surgery made in Houston at The Methodist Hospital in the Texas Medical Center. The impact of such exposure was measurable. By the conclusion of 1966, the cardiovascular teams at The Methodist Hospital, St. Luke's Episcopal Hospital, and Texas Children's Hospital continued to experience a steadily increasing number of patients referred by either a family physician or specialist for cardiovascular care. More often than not, each member of the team was performing as many as 8 to 10 operations a day, collectively maintaining a 95 percent recovery rate.[33]

At St. Luke's Episcopal Hospital and Texas Children's Hospital, Dr. Cooley and his team of cardiac surgeons at the Texas Heart Institute maintained their already established reputation for performing more open-heart surgeries than any other surgical team in the world. Having operated predominantly on children with congenital heart defects since 1956, Dr. Cooley and his team began in 1966 to concentrate efforts on adults with acquired heart disease. After collectively performing more than 652 open-heart procedures on adults that year, Dr. Cooley's surgical team effectively had made the transition to adult cardiac surgery.[34] According to Dr. Cooley, this evolution was inevitable following the pioneering advances introduced by pediatric cardiac surgeons throughout the previous decade. "After congenital heart disease yielded to surgical correction, progress in cardiac surgery became unstoppable," he explained. "The advances necessitated more accurate diagnoses, thereby stimulating the advent of improved diagnostic instruments and methods"[35]

Heretofore, the only tools available to cardiologists for the diagnosis of various forms of heart disease had been limited to those obtained by clinical observation plus stethoscope, chest X-ray, and electrocardiogram. With the development of cardiac catheterization and the serendipitous discovery of coronary angiography by Dr. Mason Sones in 1958,[36] selection of patients for cardiac surgery was becoming a more scientific process in delineating a road map to help plan the appropriate operation.[37]

For the deadliest heart disease problem, heart attacks, there remained a "lack of solid, scientifically valid information to guide the physician."[38] Long identified as the leading single cause of death in the United States, killing more than 400,000 Americans annually, heart attacks nonetheless had remained a perpetual enigma to medical scientists. Believing the answers only could be found in extensive research, Dr. Shannon, the director of the National Institutes of Health (NIH), seized an opportunity in 1966 to devise an extensive federally funded research program, one that directly impacted Dr. DeBakey.

Without discussing his plan with participants in the Artificial Heart Program, the NIH director unilaterally allocated the additional $10 million appropriation mandated from Congress for the Artificial Heart Program into the newly renamed "Artificial Heart Myocardial Infarction Program." After the fact, Dr. Shannon explained to Congress the necessity of diverting approximately half the original program's funding to other heart research, specifically programs for the study and treatment of heart attacks.[15] In addition, instead of supporting research for a total artificial heart, as appropriated, the remaining funds were to be allocated for the development of "auxiliary heart-pumping devices as a means of helping Americans recover from heart attacks."[39]

For Dr. DeBakey, who successfully had lobbied Congress in 1964 for the increased funding to develop a total artificial heart, this circumvention of his efforts two years later came as no surprise. "Although the leadership of the NIH accepted this mandate from Congress, there was considerable lack of enthusiasm," he said, recalling how the director questioned the feasibility of launching such a major effort from the beginning.[15] Since Dr. Shannon earlier had warned artificial heart researchers and lobbyists "if too much money was authorized, we wouldn't spend it," Dr. DeBakey had planned accordingly.[40] Albeit without increased funding and at a much slower pace, the Baylor-Rice collaborative team was to continue its laboratory research on the left ventricular bypass pump throughout 1967.[41-42-43-44-45]

It was the world's first human heart transplantation by South African Dr. Christiaan N. Barnard in December 1967 that prompted the renewal of Dr. DeBakey's and his collaborative research team's vigorous efforts to develop an implantable total artificial heart. Having initially responded to the news of the transplant with cautious optimism, saying Dr. Barnard's transplant "certainly would be a great achievement if they're able to overcome the rejection," Dr. DeBakey also joined other physicians in praising the physician for his accomplishment.[46]

Upon the death of Dr. Barnard's first heart transplant patient 18 days later, Dr. DeBakey joined other physicians around the world in predicting that the frequency of future heart transplants would be dependent on the availability of donated hearts. This foreseen problem of supply and demand was "why we should work more vigorously towards the development of proper and effectively functioning artificial organs" for all future transplants, Dr. DeBakey said, emphasizing the fact that rejection problems with biological transplants remained to be solved.[47] In Dr. DeBakey's opinion, there was an urgent need for a total artificial heart that permanently could take over if a biological heart transplant failed.

With that renewed purpose, Drs. DeBakey, Liotta, Hall, and Akers and the Baylor-Rice collaborative research team immediately began further development of the total artificial heart. Medically known as an orthotopic cardiac prosthesis, the pneumatically controlled, biventricular cardiac prosthesis was to be totally implantable and based on the principle of the team's left ventricular bypass pump. The team continuously had modified that prototype following its implantation in seven patients since 1966. Since only two of the seven patients survived, the existing pump, albeit far more sophisticated than the first, remained in the investigative phase in 1968.

It was the experimental aspects of transplanting human hearts that captured the attention of the leading heart specialists who attended the January 1968 meeting of the American Heart Association in New York. Joining his colleagues in qualifying the approval of the practice of transplanting human hearts only if the operation was performed on patients "with no other possible hope for survival," Dr. DeBakey also expressed his personal opinion to the press. "Indications for the operation must be carefully delineated," he said. "Such assessment requires the sagest, most deliberative judgment."[48]

Apprehensive about how little was known about the patient's immunological reaction to an implanted human heart, Dr. DeBakey indeed was deliberative when his surgical team at The Methodist Hospital expressed a desire to begin heart-transplanting procedures in early 1968. While Dr. DeBakey adopted a wait-and-see policy, Dr. Cooley did not hesitate, seizing an opportunity to launch his own heart-transplant program at the Texas Heart Institute at St. Luke's Episcopal Hospital in May 1968.

After performing the ninth heart transplant worldwide and the first successful one in the United States on May 2, Dr. Cooley created not only the most aggressive program in existence but also a nonstop media frenzy that was to catapult him into public awareness. By the end of 1968, he had performed 17 heart transplants, the most performed by any surgeon in the world. "It really was the most exciting period we've ever seen in surgery for those of us who were fortunate enough to be actively involved," Dr. Cooley said. "We were put on a pedestal. People sought our opinions in or out of medicine."[49]

While the initial media accounts of Dr. Cooley's transplant operations identified him as a colleague of Dr. DeBakey's at Baylor University College of Medicine in the Texas Medical Center, subsequent news coverage often included the identifications of him as the "heart-transplant man" and Dr. DeBakey as the "artificial-heart man."[50] This differentiation was obsolesced on August 31, 1968, when Dr. DeBakey and his five surgical teams at The Methodist Hospital performed the world's first multi-organ transplant two kidneys, a lung, and a heart from the same donor to four different patients. That historic surgery was the 11th heart transplant in Houston but only the first at The Methodist Hospital. Afterward, when asked by the media about Dr. Cooley's ten transplants compared to his one, Dr. DeBakey said, "His success has been helpful to reassure all of us."[51]

During the following four months, there were to be nine more heart transplants at The Methodist Hospital and seven more at St. Luke's Episcopal Hospital. By December 1968, only four of Dr. DeBakey's 10 heart transplant patients and three of Dr. Cooley's 17 were still living. As Dr. DeBakey initially had feared, the body's innate rejection of foreign tissue was not sufficiently controllable, making chronic rejection of the trans-planted heart inevitable in each patient. Even though successful heart transplantations eventually turned out to be short-lived without effective immunosuppressants, it was an era of seemingly miraculous moments. Re-called Dr. DeBakey, "You had a patient in heart failure who could hardly get out of bed, and with a heart transplant you could convert him into a fellow who goes out and plays golf."[49]

Such a possibility instilled great expectations in untold numbers of ter-minally ill heart patients around the world, many of whom came to either Drs. DeBakey or Cooley in search of a new heart in 1968. At the conclusion of the year, both surgeons lamented the fact that dozens of potential recip-ients had died while futilely waiting for a donor heart in Houston. In Dr. Cooley's opinion, cardiac transplantations were "close to being perfected, if they have not already," but the most serious limitation "seems to be the scarcity of donors."[52]

This was precisely the supply-and-demand problem Dr. DeBakey predict-ed at the beginning of the heart transplant era in 1967. While he continued to believe the easy accessibility of a total artificial heart would alleviate the shortage situation in the near future, the newly designed Baylor-Rice biven-tricular pump had yet to be sufficiently tested in the laboratory. The feasi-bility of the total artificial heart had been established in the fall of 1968, Dr. DeBakey said, but "it was not ready for human implantation."[15]

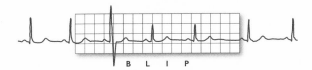

TRANSPLANTED HUMOR
FROM SOUTH AFRICA

On March 2, 1968, a few months after he performed the world's first human heart transplant in South Africa, Dr. Christiaan Barnard prefaced his presentation to the American College of Cardiology at its annual meeting in San Francisco with a brief story. Before his talk, "Is Human Cardiac Transplantation Premature?" he told of how he and his chauffeur had traveled all over South Africa in recent months as he gave lectures on various aspects of heart transplantation. At each event, the chauffeur would sit at the back of the hall, where he absorbed all of the information. "I realized after a few weeks that my chauffeur had learned quite a lot about heart transplantation," Dr. Barnard said. "One night we were driving to this little town where I was sure they didn't even know what I looked like. I was very tired and wanted to relax. I asked him, 'Van, do you think you could impersonate me and give the lecture tonight?' Without hesitation he said, 'Sure, Professor, I know your lecture by heart.'"

Swapping his Italian suit with the chauffeur and donning his uniform, Dr. Barnard entered the town hall and took his seat in the back row as his chauffeur took the stage. Fascinated by the chauffeur's lecture, he said he watched him "open-mouthed in admiration" and joined the audience in applauding him at the end of his presentation. When the moderator asked if he would take questions from the floor, the chauffeur happily agreed. "He was a little weak on the medical questions, but much better on the political questions," Dr. Barnard said.

Continued on page 132

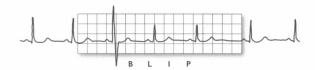

"Then catastrophe struck. A gentleman in the audience stood up. I recognized him even from the back and went cold. It was Michael DeBakey, who asked a convoluted question about immunology and rejection. I was just about to jump up and admit everything when my chauffer smiled, cleared his throat, and pulling himself up to his full height, said, 'Excuse me, sir, but aren't you Dr. DeBakey from Houston?' And when Dr. DeBakey acknowledged that he was, the chauffer never flinched. Instead of continuing the charade at that point, he simply indicated the question was so easy that even his "chauffeur at the back of the hall will answer it for you."

    While a majority of the San Francisco audience roared with laughter at Dr. Barnard's expertly delivered punch line, Dr. DeBakey, who was sitting in the front row, only "smiled thinly," it was reported.[1]

---

1. McRae D. *Every Second Counts: The Race To Transplant the First Human Heart*. New York, NY: Penguin; 2007:269.

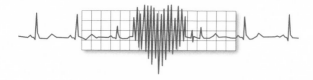

CHAPTER NINE

SCHISM
1968 - 1970

"Fate ordains that dearest friends must part."
ANONYMOUS

Since 1964, the National Heart Institute's lofty goal to implant a total artificial heart into a human being within 10 years had been compared to President John F. Kennedy's 1962 pledge to land a man on the moon before the end of the decade. Both accomplishments were to take place in 1969. As a result, "Houston" was to become the first word spoken from the moon and the last word in heart surgery.

The city already had established itself as the undisputed Mecca for heart transplant patients. Twenty-six of the world's 89 heart transplants in 1968 had been performed in the Texas Medical Center, a volume unmatched by any other center. Because of the incessant media coverage of each procedure performed, heart transplants dominated the news, becoming one of the most reported stories in 1968. At year's end, in recognition of his performing more heart transplants than any other surgeon, Dr. Cooley was singled out by the *Associated Press* as one of the top newsmakers of the year. In less than one year, he had been catapulted out of obscurity in the shadow of Dr. DeBakey and onto the front pages of newspapers around the world.

While the media's interest in 1968 was concentrated primarily on heart transplants, the rapt attention of those in the medical profession remained devoted to the volume of cardiovascular procedures performed in Houston. Of the 25,000 open-heart operations performed annually in the United States' 7,000 hospitals, close to 10 percent of those procedures took place in The Methodist Hospital, Texas Children's Hospital, and St. Luke's Episcopal Hospital in Houston's Texas Medical Center.

What's more, the official Medicare records for 1968 indicated that the two highest paid physicians in the United Sates practiced in Houston. The nationally published news stories about the recently instigated government program included the following breakdown of its highest payments ever made: $202,959 to Dr. DeBakey for 604 operations and $193,124 to Dr. Cooley for 408 operations. Included in the resulting news coverage was Dr. DeBakey's explanation that all Medicare payments were deposited in a fund at the medical college and not to the surgeons personally. Furthermore, he said, the operations in question had been performed by his team, "rather than himself alone," and involved "the whole range of cardiovascular operations and open heart surgery–the most complicated and the most difficult type of operations."

At the time, it was not common knowledge that Drs. DeBakey and Cooley, as well as all full-time faculty members of the Department of Surgery, donated a large percentage of their surgical fees to a general fund at Baylor University College of Medicine. Under confidential contractual agreements, each surgeon in turn received a portion of the pooled fees. In addition to those surgical procedures covered by Medicare and the nine heart transplants in 1968, Dr. DeBakey and his surgical team at The Methodist Hospital performed more than 4,800 cardiovascular procedures and maintained a daily census of 155 cardiovascular patients. The resulting surgical fees collected in the Baylor University College of Medicine's special fund covered all the operating expenses of the Department of Surgery as well as a major portion of the college's other expenses.

With the ever increasing demand for surgical treatment, Dr. DeBakey and his surgical team moved into the newly opened Herman Brown Building—with eight major operating rooms for cardiovascular patients—in October 1968. Also opening in October was the adjacent Fondren Intensive Care Unit, specially designed to meet the needs of 50 cardiovascular patients. Included in its facilities was a Special Organ Transplant Unit designed to allow maximum isolation of the patient and strict sterile technique.

Four of the new operating rooms were for the exclusive use of Dr. DeBakey and his two assistants, Drs. Diethrich and Noon, who continued their established, high-volume pattern of averaging more than 12 procedures a day. In any given month in 1968, their number of highly sophisticated operations on aneurysms and vascular repair alone exceeded the amount some surgeons performed annually.

Also performed in those operating rooms were kidney transplants, a program initiated in 1963 by Dr. DeBakey and his associates, The Methodist Hospital, and Baylor University College of Medicine. "The heart and lung transplant programs were begun in those operating rooms August 31, 1968," Dr. Noon said. "This was a historic day. The donor was the first multi-organ donor. The heart, lung, and two kidneys were transplanted in four different recipients."

Unprecedented volume also was maintained in the remaining four cardiovascular operating rooms, the shared domain of Drs. Howell, Crawford, and Morris. When the steadily increasing numbers of one particular procedure occurred in 1968, these three cardiovascular surgeons accurately noted its probable impact. It was the procedure pioneered at The Methodist Hospital in 1964 for coronary artery revascularization but not published until the February 12, 1973, issue of the Journal of the American Medical Association (JAMA). Drs. Garrett, Dennis, and DeBakey stated in that publication, "To our knowledge, this is the first successful case of a saphenous vein-coronary artery bypass with the longest follow-up of a functioning coronary vein bypass graft."[8] The report, Aortocoronary Bypass With Saphenous Vein Graft: Seven-Year Follow-up, was to be declared a landmark article by the editors of JAMA November 13, 1996.[9]

The procedure entailed forming bypasses of reversed saphenous veins connecting the ascending thoracic aorta to the more distal undiseased areas of the three coronary arteries. Because Dr. Rene Favaloro, working at the Cleveland Clinic, previously published a report about the first series of patients undergoing myocardial revascularization by internal mammary artery implant procedures in 1964, he generally has been credited for the introduction and dissemination of the procedure into clinical practice.[10] Known at the time as the "distal coronary bypass," the procedure "became a daily routine" for Drs. Howell, Crawford, and Morris in 1968. Within two years, after a series of more than 317 distal coronary bypasses had been performed, the surgeons reported in a peer-reviewed journal: "The greatest problems that we foresee are logistic and related to the capacity of catheterization laboratories and operating rooms to manage the number of patients with coronary artery disease."[11] Theirs was to be a prescient view of what was destined to become the most frequently performed heart operation in the world.

In the collective eight operating rooms, the surgical teams performed many procedures pioneered at The Methodist Hospital as well as those perfected there. Among these were operations for valve replacement or repair, carotid artery insufficiency, carotid artery reconstruction, left ventricular aneurysm repair, aneurysm resection, pulmonary resection, great vessel aortic resections, and surgical reconstruction for both aortic and peripheral vascular occlusive disease.

At St. Luke's Episcopal Hospital, Dr. Cooley and his surgical team performed an equally impressive volume of surgical procedures within the Texas Heart Institute. While Dr. Cooley's unmatched number of heart transplants garnered the world's attention, the medical community was aware that he had amassed a cumulative total of more than 4,000 open-heart operations since the institute's founding in 1962. Maintaining his record of performing more open-heart surgeries than any other surgeon in 1968, Dr. Cooley also embellished his reputation for being "fast," often completing heart transplant operations, known to last more than four or five hours elsewhere, in less than two hours.[12]

The operating technique employed by Dr. Cooley was similar to the one effectively established by Dr. DeBakey. "One way I was able to maintain a high volume of cases was to let other surgeons do the routine parts of the operation—opening the patient's chest, retracting the ribs, establishing connections to the heart-lung machine, and closing the chest postoperatively—while I performed only the repair itself," Dr. Cooley explained. "Although this approach reminded some observers of an assembly line, it allowed me to benefit the most patients within the time available."[13]

This was a technique in which Dr. DeBakey excelled, as exemplified when 35 operations were scheduled in four different operating rooms at The Methodist Hospital on one day. "We started at 7:30 in the morning, and sometime in the evening we sent out for food," recalled one former surgical resident who participated in the marathon. "By 12:30 AM the next morning we were really dragging. DeBakey stuck his head outside the operating room and yelled to no one, 'Does anyone else need surgery? We're just getting warmed up!'"[14]

Such time-management skills were applied to every aspect of Dr. DeBakey's professional and personal life and never more so than during his afternoon rounds. On one documented occasion, Dr. DeBakey and his entourage visited 47 patients in 32 minutes.[15]

Even though these daily encounters with his patients were brief out of necessity, Dr. DeBakey developed long-lasting relationships with each. Known to stay in touch with his patients in the years following each of their individual surgical procedures, Dr. DeBakey always was interested in knowing any little change in the patient's condition, meticulously documenting each for research purposes.

The efficiency of Dr. DeBakey's established pattern of frequent travels around the world astounded his colleagues and friends. Often sandwiched in between his extensive travels to and from Europe were visits to New York to perform his duties as chairman of the Albert Lasker Research Awards Jury.

"He doesn't get tired traveling to Europe," Mrs. Lasker said. "For him to go to Paris is like my going down to Lord & Taylor's or Bergdorf Goodman's. He went to Europe and back. He went to get a prize in Turin. He stopped in Paris and was taken to some great party by the Duke and Duchess of Windsor. He came home and he does as many as 12 operations in a day. Then he went to Boston and then Washington and the next week to Israel. He is the most extraordinary person."[16]

The seemingly indefatigable Dr. DeBakey predominantly devoted his travels to meetings with heads of state, visits to medical facilities, speaking engagements, award presentations, medical consultations, and lobbying for increased funding for medical research. Each of his trips was planned to his exacting specifications by his office staff, who oversaw all of his professional affairs.

In Dr. DeBakey's absence, his staff had the authority to arrange for the admittance and examination of new patients, thereby allowing the expediency of any patient's required surgical treatment immediately upon Dr. DeBakey's return.

As illustrated in his multifaceted interests, Dr. DeBakey relied on his innate ability to process several tasks simultaneously. He was known for mastering the art of "multitasking" decades before the computer engineering industry coined that word in the late 1980s. After convincingly demonstrating this skill throughout his previous 20 years as the chairman of Department of Surgery at Baylor University College of Medicine, Dr. DeBakey assumed another formidable task at that institution, that of also serving as its president and chief executive officer.

In assuming those leadership responsibilities in May 1968, Dr. DeBakey was to oversee the creation of an environment conducive to future expansion, an effort that heretofore had been stymied by extenuating circumstances. Even though its research programs were among the largest of those at any medical school or university in the nation and its international reputation was established with the cardiovascular advances made by Dr. DeBakey and his colleagues, the Baylor University College of Medicine was in the midst of a financial conundrum in 1968.

From the mid-1960s, Baylor University College of Medicine had been operating on an increasing deficit amounting to several hundred thousand dollars a year.[17] As the only independent medical school in Texas and an integral part of Baylor University, the nonsectarian college was sponsored by the Baptist General Convention in Texas, which contributed less than one percent of the annual operating budget of $20 million. Prohibited from accepting certain state and federal funding available for medical education because of this sectarian affiliation, the college relied heavily on the private sector for the monetary support of its programs.

With a capacity enrollment of 84 medical students in each entering class, predominantly from out-of-state, the college had positioned itself to be a national institution rather than a state resource for future physicians like the other two medical schools in Texas. Those state-supported branches of the University of Texas in Austin, located in Galveston and Dallas, were slightly larger in size than the Houston college but catered to an overwhelming majority of Texans whose medical education was subsidized by the state, a restricted source of revenue at Baylor University College of Medicine.

Another impediment to the college's growth was its inability to accept state or federal funds for any physical expansion of its facilities. This type of funding also had to be generated strictly from within the private sector. To skirt that specific issue during the planning phase of the Fondren–Brown Building in the early 1960s, it was The Methodist Hospital and not Baylor University College of Medicine who applied for and received the federal funds required to complete that building's construction. This makeshift maneuvering was acceptable at the time, but, for the future, a permanent solution was required.

Already set into motion when Dr. DeBakey assumed his leadership responsibilities was a two-pronged plan to address both of these shortcomings. The cumulative result of these efforts was to alter the future immeasurably at both the college and The Methodist Hospital. In response to the acute shortage of physicians projected for the state of Texas, particularly in the rural areas, the Baylor University College of Medicine's dean of academic affairs had submitted a proposal to the Texas College and University System Coordinating Board in Austin. Requesting direct appropriation of state funds to subsidize the education of in-state residents, the dean advised that such funding would allow the doubling of the college's enrollment to include a substantial increase in the proportion of Texans in the entering classes. Since new classroom facilities for the expanded student population would have to be erected at the projected cost of eight million dollars, the dean advised this was a "sum to be derived from private resources."[18]

When word was received of the coordinating board's approval of this request for inclusion in its "A Proposal for the Development of Medical Education in Texas, 1969 -1980" to the Texas Legislature in early 1969, Dr. DeBakey and the Houston Executive Committee of the Baylor University board of trustees sprung into action. Submitted to the Baptist General Convention of Texas and Baylor University was the executive committee's formal request to form a separate, nondenominational, nonprofit corporation to assume ownership and control of Baylor University College of Medicine.

Utilizing the coordinating board's planned recommendations to the Texas Legislature as the basis for its written request, the Houston trustees of Baylor University College of Medicine stated there was "a grave shortage of physicians" and "to meet that great public need without sacrificing excellence" required enlargement of the college through use of state and federal funds without restriction from the Baptist General Convention of Texas. Noting that under Baptist control the college had "flourished and attained a pinnacle of excellence of which Texas Baptists can be justly proud," the trustees concluded the proposal by stating, "This institution should not be subject to any conditions which would hamper its growth or cause it to lose the high standards which it has attained."[17]

The formalities of the Texas Baptists' accepting this proposal were lengthy, consuming the months of October and November. Presented for consideration to the full Baylor University board of trustees, the Christian Education Commission, and the executive board of the Baptist General Convention of Texas, the proposal also required approval by the full convention in annual session, convening November in Fort Worth. After session delegates there voted 2,960 to 40 to cut its official ties with Baylor University College of Medicine, the dye was cast.[19] Announcing the formal separation in December 1968, Baylor University president Abner V. McCall stated that the university's board of trustees concurred with the majority of delegates at the annual session, concluding it was "the only reasonable and practical course under the present circumstances."[17]

One month later, in January 1969, President McCall and the Baylor University board of trustees unanimously voted to grant independent status to the medical college in order "to allow receipt of government funds without violating Baptists principles of separation of church and state."[23] Ratifying a charter establishing a nonprofit corporation to operate the medical college under the name of Baylor College of Medicine, the university board appointed the new entity's nondenominational board of trustees. Within a matter of days, those newly named trustees announced the election of L. F. McCollum, chairman of the Continental Oil Company, to serve as chairman and Dr. DeBakey to serve as president.[21]

In so doing, the founding trustees enthusiastically endorsed Dr. DeBakey's fully articulated vision of making Baylor College of Medicine one of the top medical and graduate schools in the United States. All were aware that the college's newfound independent status allowed not only eligibility for federal and state funding but also the opportunity to capitalize on its already established reputation. With the state subsidization of in-state medical students and the subsequent doubling of enrollment, an overriding priority became the recruitment of other top scientists to serve on its faculty and to improve the existing research and clinical components. "One of Dr. DeBakey's strongest themes was that in a true academic health center, you have to integrate teaching, research and patient care; you can't separate them, and they've got to be under unified control," said Dr. William T. Butler, who later served as the college's second president from 1979 to 1996 and its interim president from 2008 to 2010.[22]

In addition to the internationally published stories about the newly named Baylor College of Medicine in January 1969 were those documenting the simultaneous accomplishments of its newly elected president. First was the January 20th awarding of the Presidential Medal of Freedom to the "famed Texas surgeon" by President Johnson, one of his last official acts of office on the day of President Richard Nixon's inauguration.[23] The second, which was deemed by the media to be just as impressive as the first, if not more so, was the news that "Martin Sinatra, father of singer Frank Sinatra, was admitted to Methodist Hospital Sunday for observation and tests under the direction of famed heart surgeon Dr. Michael DeBakey."[24]

While his treating such famous patients was to be frequently acknowledged by the media throughout his career, what continued to dominate the media's attention in 1969 was Dr. DeBakey's heart transplants. Superseding all news coverage of his other accomplishments in the month of January were the internationally published reports of his surgical team performing its 10th heart transplant—the 27th such procedure performed in Houston and the 118th in the world.[25]

Included in that coverage was the ubiquitous mention of Dr. Cooley's record-holding 17 heart transplants, even though he had not performed one since November 1968 due to a lack of donors.[26] According to Dr. James J. Nora, a cardiologist and immunologist at the Texas Heart Institute in 1969, this shortage gradually had become acute: "Initially, we had a big flood of donors because we were doing so well, but donor families got discouraged because so few patients survived beyond a few weeks or months."[27]

Only three of Dr. Cooley's 17 heart-transplant recipients were still alive in February 1969, but the critics who chose to emphasize the mortality rate rather than the other aspects of heart transplantation frustrated him. Appearing with Dr. DeBakey at a news conference following the annual meeting of the American College of Cardiology in New York, Dr. Cooley said, "We are taking dying people and prolonging life, and improving the quality of those lives. You have to put this in perspective."[28]

After stating that there were those in the medical profession who "have become faint hearted in the face of a few initial defeats," Dr. Cooley lamented the profession's lack of interest and support as well as that of the lay people.[26] He defined his critics as being members of both groups who collectively were in three separate categories: "'Ignoramuses,' who write abusive and uninformed letters; 'reactionary scientists,' and the 'envious' who think that individual surgeons are getting too much publicity."[28]

Not concurring with his Houston colleague's assessments regarding who was to blame for the perceived disinterest in heart transplantation was Dr. DeBakey, who also addressed the gathered press. Casting no aspersion on either the critics or the medical profession, he acknowledged that there had been "a certain amount of discouragement, concern over the high mortality rate that's occurred," but stated his belief was that heart transplantation was still a form of clinical investigation in which it would take time to ascertain all the answers.[26]

Transplant surgeons worldwide already had determined one of the key factors in the discouraging results of heart transplantation was the heart's vulnerability to rejection. Even though immunologists made incremental advances in crossmatching tissues of the donor's heart with the recipient, the question as to whether rejection was due to technique or to incompatibility remained unanswered in 1969.

Nonetheless, Dr. Cooley continued in his mission to increase awareness of the shortage of donors, well-matched or otherwise. Traveling throughout the country to make this predicament more evident to his peers, he was one of the featured speakers at various medical conferences. In an effort to draw public attention to his cause in early 1969, he and members of his transplant team at the Texas Heart Institute created an event worthy of news coverage. After registering as donors at Houston's newly established "living bank" for persons wishing to donate their organs for transplant operations, Dr. Cooley announced, "Today we got together and became card-carrying cadavers."[29]

With the publication of that newly coined phrase, Dr. Cooley successfully increased the general public's awareness of the need for organ donors and also his leading role in the year-long era of heart transplantations. Even though the constant media attention he enjoyed only began in 1968, he had been recognized by his peers as one of the acknowledged pioneers in heart surgery since the mid-1950s. Co-publishing with Dr. DeBakey more than 82 scientific papers in peer-reviewed journals, Dr. Cooley often appeared with him to present programs at medical conferences. Since those in the medical profession knew him to be a full-time faculty member in the Baylor College of Medicine Department of Surgery chaired by Dr. DeBakey, he and his equally accomplished associates rarely were identified by their hierarchical ranking therein. Instead, they collectively became known as simply the "Houston Group."[30]

Because of its unparalleled experience in heart surgery, the "Houston Group" was much in demand at medical conferences. Fourteen members were invited to present their clinical experiences with heart transplants at the March 31, 1969, annual meeting of The American Association for Thoracic Surgeons in San Francisco. Appearing first in the two-part presentation were Dr. DeBakey and his surgical team followed by Dr. Cooley and his. Unbeknownst to all parties concerned, this was to be the last joint appearance of these two famed heart surgeons at a medical conference, or anywhere else for that matter, for decades to come. Four days later, the status quo of the "Houston Group" was to undergo an unexpected and irreparable change.

The rupture was caused by "one of the most extraordinary episodes in the history of medicine," the first implantation of a total artificial heart into a human being.[31] News of Dr. Cooley's April 4, 1969 implantation of a total artificial heart into Haskell Karp came as a surprise to those in the medical community who had expected Dr. DeBakey, one of the recognized pioneers in artificial heart research, to be the first to accomplish such a feat. Just as bewildered, if not more so, was Dr. DeBakey, who was in Washington to attend a National Heart Institute committee meeting to evaluate artificial heart research.[32-33]

Having flown to Washington the day of the procedure, Dr. DeBakey knew nothing about it until the next day. "I was in Washington when I read in the morning papers there about the use of this artificial heart that Dr. Cooley had put in a patient, and I was shocked," he was to recall years later. "Now Dr. Cooley had no experience with the artificial heart program at all. He didn't do any laboratory work. I didn't know that he had done all of this surreptitiously."[34]

The secretive nature of both the planning and execution of Mr. Karp's operation was by design. Assisting Dr. Cooley not only in the implantation but also in the creation of the implanted artificial heart was Dr. Liotta, an investigator for Dr. DeBakey in the federally funded Baylor-Rice Artificial Heart Program. By their own admission, neither surgeon sought Dr. DeBakey's permission to perform the procedure because they thought he would deny their request. Accordingly, all aspects of their advance preparations had to be clandestine.[32]

The specifics of their collusion were disclosed in a press release and reiterated during a press conference immediately following Mr. Karp's implantation. The release stated that Drs. Cooley and Liotta designed and developed the "orthotopic cardiac prosthesis," constructing and testing it over a four-month period at Baylor College of Medicine; the construction of its pneumatic control system, developed by off-duty engineers at Rice University, was by Texas Medical Instruments; and the funding for the development of the heart device "came from private foundations, and research activities for the study were aided by grants from heart associations of Alice, Huntsville, and Weimer, Texas."[32]

Referring to the historic importance of being the first time a man-made device completely took over a human heart's function, Dr. Cooley stated, "I was concerned because it had never been done before. We had to put up one Sputnik to start the space program. We had to start here somewhere."[32] Emphasizing that the priority for implanting the device into Mr. Karp was to keep him alive while awaiting a donor heart, Dr. Cooley said, "The operations I do are designed to save a person's life. This was the purpose of my effort with Mr. Karp. He would have been dead Friday afternoon if I hadn't operated. It was a desperate effort to save a person's life."[36]

After being kept alive by the artificial heart for 65 hours, Mr. Karp underwent another surgical procedure April 7 in which Dr. Cooley replaced the mechanical substitute with a human heart. Thirty hours later, Mr. Karp died, succumbing to pneumonia and kidney failure. The news of Mr. Karp's death coincided with that of the National Heart Institute's formal request for a Baylor College of Medicine investigation into the artificial heart implantation. This published announcement generated a great deal of speculation in the academic world, much of which was chronicled in nationally syndicated newspapers. Though there were repeated references to Dr. DeBakey's expressed opinions of the implantation, he was to make no public comments throughout the ensuing controversy.

Others, however, spoke freely, albeit anonymously. In one widely distributed copyrighted story in the *New York Daily News*, unidentified "informed sources" in Washington were described "as understanding that the artificial heart used in the operation was 'largely, if not entirely, developed by Dr. DeBakey's research team under a federal research grant,'" while other anonymous sources were reportedly claiming "Dr. Cooley went ahead with his sensational operation without getting a go-ahead either from Dr. DeBakey or a medical school committee that is supposed to pass on human experimentation."[37]

No such allegations were evident in the official statements released by the National Heart Institute. Officials there indicated that Dr. DeBakey, as president of Baylor College of Medicine, had requested the investigation, but its purpose was to ascertain whether federal funds had been utilized in the development of the artificial heart implanted into Mr. Karp. These were appropriate questions based on the premise of its issuance of more than the $1,500,000 in grants for artificial heart research to Baylor College of Medicine since 1964. As an investigator in the Baylor-Rice Artificial Heart Program, funded by those grants, Dr. Liotta was subject to the federal guidelines for medical experiments on humans. The penalty for noncompliance with these guidelines was a cutoff in federal funding at Baylor College of Medicine.

Emphasizing that there was no evidence that any violation by Dr. DeBakey had occurred and his request for detailed information was a routine procedure, Dr. Theodore Cooper, director of the National Heart Institute, stated: "If experiments are going to be carried out on man, every effort must be made to insure the experiment is safely conceived, that the procedure is done with informed consent (of the patient), and that scientific matters involved be reviewed by scientists and physicians at the hospital not involved themselves in the experiments."[36]

Such reviews at Baylor College of Medicine were the responsibility of the Committee on Research Involving Human Beings, chaired by Dr. Harold Brown, who first learned of Mr. Karp's operation from a newscast afterward. An emergency meeting of Dr. Brown's committee occurred following Dr. Liotta's public confirmation of the deliberate secrecy of the procedure. Reportedly stating that the artificial heart used was never presented to this committee for approval, Dr. Liotta also admitted that Dr. DeBakey was "not even aware the device existed."[38]

In addition to Dr. Brown's committee, another of the college's standing committees had embarked on its own fact-finding mission about Mr. Karp's operation. Charged with the supervision of the Baylor-Rice Artificial Heart Program and fully aware that its federal funding may have been jeopardized, this committee had convened before the receipt of Dr. Cooper's written request for a formal inquiry. To address the specific questions posed by the National Heart Institute, Mr. McCollum, chairman of the Baylor College of Medicine board of trustees, appointed a "special committee." Because he was expected to testify before each, Dr. DeBakey did not serve as a member of any of these committees. Since his testimonies, as well as those of all others, were deemed confidential by the college's board of trustees, there was to be no public record of the various committees' deliberations.

Since details of the ongoing investigation were inaccessible and Dr. DeBakey remained incommunicado on the subject, journalists turned elsewhere for answers. During a press conference held for Dr. Cooley during his April 10 visit to Baltimore, Maryland, he was asked if he felt like he had violated any federal regulations. "I have done more heart surgery than anyone else in the world," he replied. "Based on this experience, I believe I am qualified on what is right and proper for my patient. The decisions are made by me with the permission of the patient. I don't see how I violated any government regulations."[39]

In various other published reports, Drs. Cooley and Liotta continued to assert what previously had been stated at the press conference following Mr. Karp's operation. Both doctors adamantly maintained that the privately funded implanted artificial heart was independently developed in four months and differed from Dr. DeBakey's device.[40] "This particular heart was developed through Dr. Cooley's Institute," Dr. Liotta told the *Associated Press*. "We have used federal funds through the years to gain experience and knowledge, but this heart was not financed by the government."[33]

A very different opinion was held by Dr. Hall, who served as director of the Baylor-Rice Artificial Heart Program for five years. Having successfully implanted the program's first two-chamber artificial heart into a dog in 1965, he possessed institutional knowledge of its design and development. Since extensive research into artificial hearts had been taking place both in Houston and elsewhere for more than a decade, he reasoned, "It's unusual, if not impossible, to develop a whole artificial heart system in four months." As to whether Mr. Karp's artificial heart differed from Dr. DeBakey's prototype, Dr. Hall stated, "It's the same one."[41]

Precise details about the Baylor-Rice artificial heart were published in the April-June 1969 issue of the peer-reviewed *Cardiovascular Research Center Bulletin*. Titled *Special Article: Orthotopic Cardiac Prosthesis: Preliminary Experiments in Animals with Biventricular Artificial Heart* and coauthored by Drs. Hall, DeBakey, and eight other colleagues, the manuscript recounted the technical and physiological problems encountered by the seven calves implanted with the Baylor-Rice artificial heart during the first three months of 1969. In the ten coauthors' opinion, "Results of these preliminary experiments suggest that a biventricular pump of this design can be developed to duplicate the functions of the two ventricles of the heart, but much work needs to be done before it will be possible to obtain proper control of the mechanism for adequate perfusion and viability of vital organs. Although two calves survived a short time, functional viability was adequate . . . Human experimentation must await unequivocal evidence of the safety and effectiveness of such a device in humans."[42]

Whatever impact these findings had on the Baylor College of Medicine special committee's investigation of Mr. Karp's implantation was not publicly documented. In two letters sent to Dr. Cooper at the National Heart Institute in May, board chairman Mr. McCollum stated that the committee found sufficient supporting evidence that federal funds were involved in the development of the artificial heart implanted. Based on these findings, Dr. Liotta was suspended from the Baylor-Rice Artificial Heart Program April 18 and his salary from the federally funded grant discontinued. According to a spokesperson at the institute, Dr. Liotta's participation in the Karp operation was "the first instance anybody knows of involving a violation" of the federal guidelines in the research or use of artificial organs.[43]

The special committee at Baylor College of Medicine also found the artificial heart had been implanted without prior review by the Committee on Research Involving Human Beings at the college, representing another noncompliance with a requirement for federally funded experimental devices. Since Dr. Cooley received no federal funds, his name did not appear in Mr. McCollum's report, nor was any indication given as to whether there would be disciplinary action against him. Instead of detailing the particulars of Dr. Cooley's, or any of the participants' indiscretions, Mr. McCollum looked forward, submitting the college's proposed plan to eliminate the possibility of a similar reoccurrence. "To insure that guidelines for experimentation established by the National Heart Institute and this college shall be followed in the future," he advised Dr. Cooper that the Baylor College of Medicine faculty was to implement the mandatory signing of all new appointees and present staff of an agreement to observe the college's regulations and bylaws with the understanding that failure to comply with these guidelines was to lead to a "consideration of disciplinary proceedings."[44]

After reviewing Mr. McCollum's letters and the proposed plan of action, the National Heart Institute released the following comments from Dr. Cooper on May 15: "The National Institutes of Health system of guidelines governing clinical research relies heavily on the good will and integrity of the recipient institution. The National Heart Institute believes that the action taken by Baylor in this matter is evidence of its intention and its ability to enforce these guidelines."[45]

The importance of this vote of confidence from the National Heart Institute "would be hard to overemphasize," Mr. McCollum announced. "Our college of medicine currently receives approximately $3 million a year for its cardiovascular research, including the Artificial Heart Program. Not only were these grants in jeopardy, but also other substantial federal grants might have been endangered had Baylor been held responsible for this violation of federal guidelines. The Board of Trustees has asked me to express its gratification for Dr. Cooper's statement and wishes to express complete confidence in Dr. DeBakey and deep appreciation of the dedication of a faculty and staff who made Baylor a great medical school."[46]

Regardless of the reported findings of the special committee to the National Heart Institute, Dr. Cooley continued to maintain his position in the matter. "I still consider it my heart," he told a reporter from *United Press International* on May 17. "I will use it again if the occasion arises. I have a heart available to use. Let the record show we tried and also let the doubting ones know we will try again." As to whether he would sign the college's proposed mandatory agreement to comply with its regulations and bylaws, Dr. Cooley indicated his reticence, saying, "Before agreeing to do so, I must study the guidelines to determine whether they permit me to continue to serve my patients in their best interests." On the subject of Dr. Liotta, who remained on staff at the Baylor College of Medicine following his suspension from the Baylor-Rice Artificial Heart Program, Dr. Cooley said he planned to hire him to work at the Texas Heart Institute.[47]

There was to be no public statement made by Dr. DeBakey, who continued to conduct himself with dignity and composure. For the edification of those in the medical profession, he and his colleagues affixed an addendum to their already published research paper in the *Cardiovascular Research Center Bulletin*.[46] Dated May 15, 1969, the statement read: "This is a true and accurate account of the development and testing of the orthotopic cardiac prosthesis."[44]

Within the following month, the Baylor College of Medicine board of trustees had approved the revised rules of the Committee on Research Involving Human Beings, entitled "Protection of the Individual as a Research Subject."[44] These guidelines required Baylor faculty to follow NIH guidelines for research and to submit research protocols to the Committee on Human Research for approval before proceeding with any clinical trials, including surgical ones. On June 27, while plans to implement these rules into the college's new appointment form were being finalized, Dr. Cooley and Texas Heart Institute associate Dr. Grady L. Hallman resigned from the academic faculty of Baylor College of Medicine. Doctor Cooley announced that his serving as an unpaid clinical professor at the college was contingent on his acceptance of the newly mandated rules and regulations regarding research.[48]

Shortly thereafter, Dr. Cooley submitted a proposal for the continuation of his independent research at the Texas Heart Institute in the field of cardiac replacement. When that request was accepted at St. Luke's Episcopal Hospital but denied by the research committee at Baylor College of Medicine, Dr. Cooley refused to sign the college's appointment form. He then tendered his resignation from the unpaid position of clinical professor of surgery, effective September 2, 1969, which was accepted by the board of trustees.

In the resulting news coverage of Dr. Cooley's departure from Baylor College of Medicine, noticeably absent was any reference to his former mentor. In turn, Dr. DeBakey did not publicly acknowledge Dr. Cooley's resignation, nor did he mention his name. After an interview published in the April 1970 *Life* magazine in which Dr. Cooley was asked if he had used Dr. DeBakey's heart and he replied, "Well, I guess, in effect I took it,"[49] Dr. DeBakey remained silent. Several months later, when speaking publicly about the implantation of the artificial heart into Mr. Karp, Dr. DeBakey did not mention Dr. Cooley. The omission occurred while Dr. DeBakey was addressing the National Academy of Sciences on October 20, 1970. During his speech, he showed a slide of the Baylor-Rice artificial heart and said: "Some of you may recall this was publicized on television as having been put in a patient. But, of course, it is the same pump that was developed in our experimental laboratory and was just simply taken from the laboratory without our knowledge and done the way it was."[49]

When journalists asked Dr. DeBakey afterward to identify who had taken the heart from his laboratory, he declined, saying: "I've made this statement in previous talks before scientific groups while discussing the history and development of the artificial heart. I've never mentioned any names and don't intend to. Any inferences that are drawn will have to be drawn by someone else."[50]

One thorough analysis of this entire episode, obtained by personal interviews conducted in Houston of all the protagonists by two noted bioethicists, Renee C. Fox and Judith P. Swazey, appeared in *The Courage to Fail*, published in 1974.[51] In "The Case of the Artificial Heart," the coauthors state: "Sufficient documentary evidence has already been presented to indicate the device Dr. Cooley implanted in Mr. Karp was, except for minor modifications, identical to the orthotopic cardiac device designed and tested in DeBakey's laboratory under a National Heart Institute grant, awarded to DeBakey as principal investigator . . . What does need to be examined is what led Cooley and (Dr. Domingo) Liotta to covertly take the artificial heart model from the Baylor Laboratories to St. Luke's Hospital, secretly work on it, and at first claim that the pump unit they implanted in Mr. Karp was made entirely by them, financed by private funds."[52]

Although Dr. Cooley was censured by the Harris County Medical Society, for excessive publicity, and the American College of Surgeons, for not following the rules of Baylor College of Medicine and the American Heart Institute, both bioethicists stated the strongest action taken in the case of the artificial heart was a lawsuit, later dismissed by a federal court, filed by Mrs. Karp, who sued Dr. Cooley and two others for malpractice. "The formal and informal sanctions that been brought to bear upon the defendants have been mild," the authors continued. "Cooley and Liotta's professional activities have been restricted only in a relatively minor way. . . . Their relative immunity has also been fostered by the mass communication system. The media paid far more attention to the fact that for the first time in medical history an artificial heart was implanted in a man . . . than to the serious moral issues the case raised."[53]

In conclusion, the authors stated: "In our view, this case and its outcome show that the medical and law professions, and the larger society to which they belong, have not satisfactorily dealt with the social, moral, and legal issues involved in therapeutic innovation with human subjects."[53]

When each surgeon went his separate way in 1969, their established identities as two of the most famous members of the "Houston Group" remained unchanged. As before, their unprecedented volume of patients combined with their individual pioneering surgical accomplishments were to continue unabated. Together or apart, each possessed the capability to inspire awe.

Remarking on this phenomenon in 1970 was Dr. James D. Hardy, the noted surgeon who was one of the founders of the University of Mississippi School of Medicine. As the former president of the American Surgical Association, the American College of Surgeons, and the International Society of Surgery, he had a unique perspective of the Houston surgeons' previous 18-year association. "You have to hand it to Mike and Denton," he said. "Denton is the technician and Mike knew how to spread the news. They've made Houston the heart capital of the world."[54]

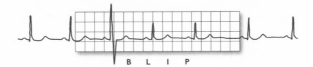

B   L   I   P

SINATRA DID IT HIS WAY

*F*rom the moment Dr. DeBakey and Mr. Frank Sinatra met in 1969, they became kindred spirits and lifelong friends. "Dr. DeBakey told me that in all the years he'd spent watching people deal with their parents' grave illnesses, he had never seen anything like my father's devotion," Nancy Sinatra said. "He was moved by such concern, and especially by the unashamed displays of affection and tender love."[1] Over the following years, Mr. Sinatra referred countless friends and acquaintances to Dr. DeBakey for medical care, paying all the expenses incurred for many of them as well as annually contributing to the DeBakey Medical Foundation.[2] When The Martin Anthony Sinatra Medical Education Center, named in honor of Mr. Sinatra's late father, opened in Palm Springs in 1971, Dr. DeBakey took part in the opening ceremony. While a houseguest of Mr. Sinatra in Palm Springs in 1974, Dr. DeBakey attended an 80th birthday party thrown by his host for Jack Benny; it was there that he met his future wife, German actress Katrin Fehlhaber. He also was one of the few invited guests to Mr. Sinatra's July 11, 1976, wedding to Barbara Marx, and he served as a pallbearer when Mr. Sinatra's mother died in 1977.

1. Sinatra N. Frank Sinatra: An American Legend. Frank Sinatra Biography website. http://sinatrafamily.com/biography. Accessed October 1, 2013.
2. Lemann N. Super medicine. *Texas Monthly*. April 1979; 126.

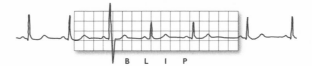

IMPORTING EXPERTISE

*R*eturning home from his worldly travels, Dr. DeBakey became known for surprising his colleagues at The Methodist Hospital and Baylor College of Medicine with an unconventional souvenir from his trips, a new recruit. While in London in the late 1960s to give a lecture, Dr. DeBakey met a young British cardiologist with an interest in the relatively new concept of postoperative cardiovascular intensive care medicine. His name was Dr. David Brooks of St. Mary's and Westminster Hospitals. Persuaded by Dr. DeBakey to oversee the new Fondren intensive care unit (ICU) at The Methodist Hospital, Dr. Brooks accepted the offer sight unseen. He did come and stay for several years, but his position and responsibilities in the ICU were never clearly delineated. The disappointing result was his leaving that post and entering private practice after several years. "Shortly thereafter, Dr. Brooks opted to return to London and his position at St. Mary's Hospital, where he remained for the rest of his career," Dr. Winters said. "Although his Houston career was short, we were to have a long professional and personal friendship, and he was instrumental in my being admitted to the Royal Society of Medicine."

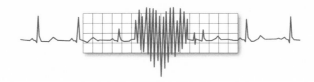

CHAPTER TEN

THE PILGRIMAGE
1960 - 1970

"There are no days in life so memorable as those
which vibrated to some stroke of the imagination."
RALPH WALDO EMERSON

Beginning with the advent of open-heart surgery in the 1950s, and escalating with each cardiovascular surgical advance made during the 1960s,
heart-disease patients migrated to Houston from all over the world.

Among this eclectic cross section of the celebrated and the unknown,
the wealthy and the indigent, and the young and the old, was a distinct sim-
ilarity: Each had hope of benefiting from one of the miraculous treatments
indigenous to the heart capital of the world. By the early 1970s, when thousands of such hopefuls had begun to arrive in the Texas Medical Center on an
annual basis, the migration became a phenomenon likened to the pilgrimages
made to the religious shrine of Lourdes.[1-2]

Hundreds of hopeful patients consistently arrived each week at The
Methodist Hospital throughout the 1950s and 1960s. While some came in
limousines accompanied by an entourage, there also were those who had
hitchhiked alone. A majority of the patients were referred by a physician to
either Dr. DeBakey or another specific surgeon on staff, although an increasing number of patients were referred directly to a private cardiologist. Many
others came without a medical referral or even an appointment, including individuals who had written to Dr. DeBakey about not only their affliction but
also their insufficient funds to seek treatment. After he responded, "If you can
come to Houston, there will be no charge for the hospital or the operation,"
many of these recipients arrived unannounced, clutching his written promise
in hand.[3]

Regardless of an arriving cardiovascular patient's motivating circumstances, socioeconomic status, or medical condition, each underwent a cardiology consultation, a prerequisite initiated by Dr. DeBakey. "There were five cardiologists on the Baylor University College of Medicine Cardiology Service at The Methodist Hospital: Ed Dennis, Sam Kinard, Ben McCall, John Lancaster, and me," recalled Dr. O'Donnell, who joined the hospital's cardiology staff in 1967. "It was not unusual for Dr. DeBakey to have 100 patients at any given time, so we had plenty to do. He would assign all the patients to the cardiologists who worked them up and got them ready for surgery and took care of them afterwards. That is the way it was done."[4]

For the limited number of Baylor cardiologists on staff at The Methodist Hospital in the 1960s, the growing number of patients in Dr. DeBakey's service began to impact their already stretched-to-the-limit schedule. In addition to managing the daily treatment and care of hundreds of Dr. DeBakey's patients and their other daily responsibilities, they also had to interpret each of the electrocardiograms generated in the hospital each month. The resulting time constraints eventually necessitated an increase in the number of hospital patients who received cardiology consultations by cardiologists in private practice. Providing a majority of these consultations were the four members of The Chapman Group, Drs. Chapman, Peterson, Beazley, and Marvin Brook.

Recalling his hectic cardiology rotation with Dr. Beazley in this time period, former Baylor College of Medicine student Dr. John Flake Anderson said, "He was a kind, gentle guy and great teacher and had wonderful bedside skills. He worked primarily with Dr. Jimmy F. Howell, a busy cardiac surgeon on Dr. DeBakey's service. The way in which they cranked cardiovascular patients through that system was phenomenal. Patients came through by the hundreds. The Methodist Hospital Annex on Fannin Street, a mile or two away from the Medical Center, served as the cardiovascular admitting hospital. Patients would trek in there, probably a couple hundred on Sunday afternoon. They'd also come every day of the week, but Sunday afternoon was the busiest time. That was the first stop into the system."[5]

The average number of patients on Dr. DeBakey's service was 200, including 70 on his preoperative list. In addition, an increasing number of patients began to accumulate on the services of both Drs. Crawford and Morris. "It was like a surgical factory," said Dr. George Kennedy Hempel Jr., a thoracic surgery fellow at The Methodist Hospital in 1965. Having rotated on Dr. Morris' service, Dr. Hempel experienced the genesis of that surgeon's inevitable surge in patient population: "George did a lot of the small-vessel work–tibial, artery vein graft (below the knee), renal artery grafting, etc. When coronary bypass started, he was one of the early and best surgeons doing that procedure because he was already good working with small vessels."[6]

Already established in the field of vascular surgery as one of the leading authorities in thoracoabdominal aneurysms and aortic disease was Dr. Stanley Crawford. Having been praised internationally by his peers as a "superb abdominal surgeon" who also was "the world's best when it comes to the aorta," Dr. Crawford also experienced a growing number of referred patients throughout the 1960s.[7] When his service grew to a size rivaling those of Drs. DeBakey and Cooley, he embraced his third-place standing behind the cardiovascular giants with trademark wit. To associates who would ask his plans for further increasing his share of the market, he was known to quip, "I'll give Cooley everything on the top, DeBakey everything on the bottom and I'll take what's left in between."[8]

As one of the world's leading heart surgeons during the early 1960s, Dr. Cooley had amassed an all-encompassing patient population. While the majority comprised individuals with congenital heart defects, by mid-decade there was a continuing increase in the number of patients with acquired heart disease. Since moving in1956 into St. Luke's Episcopal Hospital and Texas Children's Hospital, Dr. Cooley and his team of heart surgeons had performed more open-heart procedures, predominantly on children, than any other surgical team in the world. At the conclusion of 1966, in addition to pediatric procedures, more than 652 open-heart surgeries had been performed on adults with acquired heart disease. Like all of Dr. DeBakey's cardiovascular patients, each was also under the care of a cardiologist.

For Dr. Cooley, a medical-surgical coalition was essential in the treatment of patients with operable congenital heart defects. As an assistant to the surgeon-pediatric-cardiologist team responsible for the first Blalock-Taussig anastomosis in 1944 at Johns Hopkins Hospital, he had witnessed the benefits of such a coalition firsthand. Beginning in 1954 and continuing throughout his career at Texas Children's Hospital, he entrusted the diagnosis, treatment, and follow-up care of his patients with congenital heart defects to the hospital's staff of pediatric cardiologists, Dr. Dan McNamara and colleagues. He also established and maintained a close working relationship with Houston cardiologists in private practice, particularly Dr. Chapman. Referred to Dr. Cooley by The Chapman Group in 1956 was the first patient to undergo open-heart surgery in Houston. Twelve years later, Dr. Cooley's first recipient of a heart transplant also was a patient referred by Dr. Chapman.[9]

In addition to being actively involved with Dr. Cooley's pioneering innovations in heart surgery at The Methodist Hospital and St. Luke's Episcopal Hospital in the 1950s and 1960s, Dr. Chapman also shared the surgeon's outside interests, tennis and music. A coronet player, he played in "The Heart-beats" band with Dr. Cooley, who played the double bass. Founded by Drs. Cooley and Hallman in 1965, the all-physicians' volunteer band originally formed to play for their own enjoyment but throughout the following decade could be found performing for fundraisers and medical events not only in Houston but also nationally. "In New York we played for the American Thoracic Surgical Society, with ten of the most outstanding cardiovascular surgeons in the world playing the percussion instruments," Dr. Chapman said. "Playing in this band provided a great source of release and relaxation for each member, as well as creating an effective fund-raising tool for many local charities."[10]

Of a completely different nature was the harmonic relationship Dr. Chapman forged with Dr. DeBakey. Lasting more than five decades, their mutual admiration had begun shortly after Dr. DeBakey's 1948 arrival in Houston. Demonstrating pioneering skills in the early days of cardiology that were complimentary to those of Dr. DeBakey in surgery, Dr. Chapman and his innovative "Dawn Patrol" had created the first cardiac catheterization laboratory in the South in 1946 and subsequently was instrumental in securing the funding for The Methodist Hospital's first catheterization laboratory through Walter Goldston.

As the only cardiologist on staff in the early 1950s, Dr. Chapman often could be found together with Dr. DeBakey and a patient. In so doing, they established not only a lasting bond but also the foundation for Dr. DeBakey's championing the coalition of cardiology and cardiovascular surgery in the diagnosis, treatment, and follow-up care of cardiovascular patients.

As professional associates during those beginning years at The Methodist Hospital in the 1950s, Dr. Chapman often joined Dr. DeBakey in his recreational activities before Dr. DeBakey began "to conserve whatever time I can for the things I need to do, most of which are in my professional sphere of interest."[10] Dr. Chapman recalled, "Just as I enjoyed playing in The Heartbeats with Dr. Cooley as well as our numerous tennis matches, with Dr. DeBakey I learned of another side to this illustrious surgeon. Occasionally we joined with Ben Taub and Webb Mading, owner of a drugstore chain. The four of us motored to Seabrook to Ben Taub's yacht. There we spent the weekend talking, eating, wade fishing, playing countless games of gin rummy, and long-range dreaming about the future of the Texas Medical Center."[11]

Unforeseeable at that time was the extraordinary growth of the field of cardiology, particularly at The Methodist Hospital. Dr. Chapman belonged to a select group of trained cardiologists, "heart specialists" in a subspecialty of internal medicine first recognized in the 1940s. He became one of the first members of the American College of Cardiology, founded in 1949. In its first decade of existence, with the exception of cardiac catheterization, there had been few other technological innovations introduced in the field.

In the early 1950s, Dr. Chapman and all heart specialists depended on their clinical observation of the patient and on instruments and technology introduced decades earlier—the stethoscope, sphygmomanometer, electrocardiogram, chest X-ray, and fluoroscope. The prognosis for patients diagnosed with coronary heart disease or a myocardial infarction (MI), known as a heart attack, before the advent of open-heart surgery was grim, at best. Heretofore, medical therapy espoused by Dr. Chapman, and other cardiologists in the early 1950s, comprised a brief list that included digitalis, nitroglycerine, morphine, quinidine, anticoagulants, penicillin, diuretics (Mercuhydrin), oxygen, sedatives, rest, special diets, and noradrenaline for shock.[12]

There were no special care units, defibrillators, cardioverters, implantable pacemakers, potent antihypertensive agents or diuretics to treat patients with rheumatic or syphilitic heart disease, hypertension, or coronary artery disease. Since the concept of a coronary care unit had yet to be introduced for specialized care, the mortality rate in hospitals for MI was more than 25 percent.[13]

For surviving MI patients, the cardiologists' recommended treatment was documented in the fourth edition of Dr. Paul Dudley White's authoritative textbook *Heart Disease,* published in 1951: "As the result of experience during the last twenty-five years, I have found that a very satisfactory plan of treatment for the average case of acute MI is one month of full (bed) rest . . . (followed by) one month of gradually increasing activity, the first week in a chair a little more each day, the second week walking on the level increasing distances, the third week going slowly over the stairs once a day, and the fourth week going out for short daily rides . . . and a third month if possible to consolidate recovery."[14]

Many MI patients developed acquired "heart block," an arrhythmia diagnosable by electrocardiogram. Caused by damage to the heart muscle and its electrical system, it was a condition associated with ischemic heart disease. Before the advent of implantable pacemakers in the 1960s, restoration of the normal cardiac activity required external mechanical stimulation to temporarily pace the heart. In the early 1950s, the alternate current-powered "portable pacemakers" were large, bulky boxes filled with vacuum tubes. Wheeled around and plugged into the wall, this equipment was portable in name only. By the mid-1950s, as a temporary assist to maintain the heart's ability to conduct the electrical impulses, it had become indispensable to the heart surgeons who performed pioneering procedures in congenital heart surgery.

The advances made in acquired coronary heart disease during the 1960s created an urgent need for more sophisticated diagnostic techniques for patients with such known or suspected conditions. When one such technique, arteriography, the X-ray study of the coronary blood vessels, was introduced at the Cleveland Clinic by a pediatric cardiologist in 1958, one of the first cardiologists in the country to fly to Cleveland to observe this procedure was Dr. Chapman. "Dr. Mason Sones of the Cleveland Clinic invited me to visit his clinic to see his technique of selective cine coronary aortography and left ventricular angiography," Dr. Chapman recalled. "He injected dye into the coronary artery and, by taking a series of cine coronary arteriograms, revealed by visualization of the dye, whether the artery was open with unobstructed flow, or varying degrees of stenosis, or even complete obstruction. Selective cine coronary arteriograms have allowed pinpoint delineation of the abnormalities in the coronary arteries, which led to the development of coronary artery bypasses and angioplasty."[15]

Within months of Dr. Chapman's visit with Dr. Sones, this newly invented method of percutaneous angiography was being performed at The Methodist Hospital. "In those days there were two cath labs on the ninth floor of the hospital and Dr. Dennis was in charge," Dr. O'Donnell said, recalling how he and the other four cardiologists on staff first implemented the new diagnostic technique in the early 1960s. "It was ordinary fluoroscopy and you had to put on red glasses as you had a limited time exposure, 20 minutes at most, because the radiation was too much for the patient and the physicians."[16]

As the number of diagnostic angiographic procedures performed in each catheterization laboratory increased exponentially, the cardiologists soon were faced with another time constraint, this one imposed by Dr. Dennis. "He loved to make rules," Dr. O'Donnell said. "One of the rules was if you didn't have a patient on the table by 2:00 PM, you couldn't proceed with it that day. In those days, the lab closed at 3:00 PM.; we weren't open 24 hours like today. When the lab closed, it was closed until the next day. If there was an emergency in the middle of the night, we did angiography in the X-ray department and believe me, that was an ordeal. We used the Sones method and it was an ordeal."[16]

Also taking place in the X-ray department were other angiographic procedures performed primarily by the surgeons. The most frequent, translumbar aortography, was a percutaneous needle-puncture technique conceived in 1929 by a Portuguese urologist to study lower-limb arterial circulation. The surgeons inserted rapier-length aortogram needles into an anesthetized patient to inject the contrast dye directly into the target arteries via the lumbar region.

Although Dr. Sven-Ivar Seldinger had invented an alternative technique in 1953,[17] proving it was possible to catheterize the aorta from a percutaneous puncture of the femoral artery, Dr. DeBakey and his team of surgeons preferred direct puncture by the lumbar route. Catheter studies were used in selected instances, but predominantly it was "the use of direct percutaneous needle arteriography in most patients for evaluation of the peripheral arterial vascular system."[18] Believing this preferred technique was necessary for "careful mapping of the vascular supply of the abdomen and lower extremities," Dr. DeBakey and his staff of cardiovascular surgeons had performed more than 3,000 translumbar aortograms by the mid-1960s.[19]

Among those surgeons at The Methodist Hospital was a consensus regarding their participation in these arteriographic studies: "We believe arteriography should be performed by a member of the surgical team," reported one group of surgeons. "This is the person who can most accurately correlate the arteriographic findings with the clinical examination. It is the members of the surgical team who must determine if the arteriograms obtained give proper and sufficient information to determine the status of the vascular tree and be prepared to perform the indicated surgical procedure. This does not imply that the participation of a radiologist is not encouraged. His help in interpretation and advice regarding radiologic techniques are invaluable."[18]

The surgeon who performed the majority of Dr. DeBakey's translumbar aortograms in the early 1960s was Dr. W. Sam Henly, a former surgical resident who after training joined Dr. DeBakey's surgical staff. While translumbar aortography at other medical facilities gained a reputation for being extremely difficult, often requiring the assignment of three or four members of the surgical and radiology team to physically restrain the patient to prevent damage to the aorta during injection of the radiopaque dye, this was definitely not the case at The Methodist Hospital. To avoid pain and apprehension for the patient, the surgeons' arteriographic studies were performed with the patient under anesthesia.

"Aortography was fairly easy," Dr. Henly explained, pointing out that the patient was put to sleep beforehand. There was an X-ray table used specifically designed for these arteriographic procedures called a "Bucky table." This table was a movable steel plate that covered one-half of the underlying X-ray cassette. As the injected contrast dye traveled distally in the patient's vascular system, the surgeons simultaneously moved the steel plate to expose the distal portions of the X-ray cassette. "The head of radiology, Dr. Curtis Burge, had brought down a technician from Minneapolis with him. His name was Murphy and he devised that sliding panel with which we could take two pictures, one of the abdomen, and then he would pull a string and expose the lower frame to show the legs and we would take a second picture."[20]

This sliding panel also was used for the surgeons' percutaneous needle arteriograms of the carotid and peripherals in the X-ray department. If a patient were undergoing all three procedures, he would lay prone on his stomach atop the sliding panel and the surgeons first would inject a seven-inch needle through the left flank into the aorta opposite the twelfth thoracic to first lumbar vertebra. With the needle in the aorta, they would inject, get two X-rays, one of the abdomen, one of the pelvis. Next, they would turn the patient over, put needles in each femoral artery, and get one exposure of the thigh and one of the calves. Then the surgeons would put needles in each carotid artery and get a single X-ray of each and then often do intrafollicular punctures of the subclavian arteries to see the vertibrals. "We used to call it the 'voodoo doll technique' because the patient ended up with seven different needle sticks into seven different arteries," said Dr. Roehm, a cardiovascular interventional radiologist recruited by Dr. DeBakey in 1965.[20]

Having been trained at the University of Minnesota by Dr. Kurt Amplatz, one of the pioneers in the emerging field of interventional radiology, Dr. Roehm was anxious to demonstrate the latest radiologic techniques to both the cardiologists and surgeons at The Methodist Hospital. He mistakenly thought he would be welcomed with open arms, but "everybody ignored me," he said, recalling his desire to share his newfound knowledge about the benefits of catheterization techniques in needle arteriography. "When I got here in 1965, no one was using the Seldinger technique, which was artery puncture, take out the needle, put in a guide wire, take out the needle, and then replace it with a catheter."[20]

To implement this revolutionary technique at The Methodist Hospital, Dr. Roehm patiently waited for the opportunity to demonstrate its advantages over the surgeons' existing techniques. In anticipation of that opportunity and because the required guide wires were yet to be commercially available, Dr. Roehm ordered only one at a time from a gentleman he knew in Minneapolis who made them in his basement. Within a few months, he had established his "fame" in employing the technique with a couple of Dr. Crawford's cases.

Thereafter "Dr. Crawford sent me all his patients," Dr. Roehm said. "Stanley was the first and then George Morris and Jimmy Howell stopped doing translumbars and sent me patients when they realized I knew what I was doing."[20] However, the last of the surgeons to relinquish their arteriographic patients to Dr. Roehm were Drs. DeBakey, Noon, and McCollum, who, to Dr. Roehm's dismay, were to continue doing their "multiple puncture techniques" throughout the coming decade.[18]

Angiographic studies, both by catheterization and direct needle puncture, were to become one of the most used diagnostic tools for acquired heart disease at The Methodist Hospital during the 1960s. In both catheterization laboratories, an increasing number of patients were scheduled for diagnostic procedures performed by both the Baylor cardiologists and members of The Chapman Group. "We got our first image intensifier in the early part of 1968," Dr. O'Donnell said, recalling the impact of that technological advance on daily activities. "That made an enormous difference. First of all, the images were much better and you were not limited in time, as with fluoroscopy."[16]

The efficient use of cardiologists' time and resources became a necessity with the ever-increasing stream of cardiovascular patients flowing daily through The Methodist Hospital Annex. In order to conduct the growing number of in-depth cardiologic evaluations required, the hospital cardiologists and members of The Chapman Group often found themselves to be needed in two places at the same time. Since an integral part of each cardiology evaluation was coronary angiography, the established gold standard of diagnostic tests for coronary artery disease, each patient at the annex had to be transported to one of the two catheterization laboratories at The Methodist Hospital for this procedure.

Before the advent of coronary bypass procedures in the mid-1960s, the only existing operation for coronary artery disease was the Vineberg procedure, the implantation of mammary arteries directly into the left ventricular myocardium.[21-22] At The Methodist Hospital, "because all patients coming to Houston got worked up angiographically for coronary artery disease, Ed Garrett and I did 50 Vineberg procedures in 3 months, half the number that Arthur Vineberg had done in 10 years," Dr. Hempel said, recalling his fellowship studies while on Dr. DeBakey's service. "Because we had over 200 patients in the hospital, there were many candidates for all these procedures. It was a great time to be involved in cardiovascular surgery."[6]

The Vineberg procedure was but one of the many cardiovascular operations performed in unprecedented volume during the mid-1960s at The Methodist Hospital. These phenomenal accomplishments captured the attention of the medical profession and triggered a never-ending influx of not only visiting surgeons from all over the world but also quite a few curious cardiologists. Many came in groups, having made advance arrangements to observe specific surgeons in the operating arena before taking guided tours of the cardiovascular center. Others arrived in Houston purely by happenstance, as was the case with Dr. William L. Winters Jr., who landed in Houston in 1968.

Having been the first cardiology fellow at the Temple University School of Medicine in Philadelphia in 1958, Dr. Winters had been a cardiology faculty member there for 10 years, serving as the director of the Cardiovascular and General Clinical Research Centers and the Cardiac Care Unit. By 1968 he had become one of the pioneering investigators in the embryo years of echocardiography, the method for continuously recording movements of the components of the heart by means of high frequency ultrasound.

Technologically developed as Sonar during World War II, reflective ultrasound was used for the measurement of distances underwater and detection of enemy submarines. The subsequent successful use of reflected ultrasound for nondestructive flaw detection in metals in 1945 inspired a Swedish physicist and cardiologist in 1953, Dr. C. Hellmuth Hertz and Dr. Inge Edler, to investigate medical uses of pulse-reflected ultrasound, specifically for the evaluation of mitral valve disease, and to better select patients for mitral valve commissurotomy.[23-24] Nine years later, efforts to build echo-ranging equipment to further evaluate cardiac diagnosis commenced in the United States at the University of Pennsylvania Medical School in Philadelphia with Drs. Claude Joyner and John Reid. Unfathomable at that time, echocardiography was destined to revolutionize diagnostic cardiology.[25]

As they began to establish this new field, Dr. Winters was a contributing author to one of the first peer-reviewed articles written about the clinical application of ultrasound in the analysis of prosthetic ball valve function in 1965. The contribution of echocardiography in the diagnosis of mitral valve disease and the subsequent confirmation of its clinical utility in the detection of pericardial effusion became an enormous stimulus to broaden the development and interest of the technique in this country. However, it remained a very labor-intensive and technically difficult procedure, to the extent that many initial operators lost their enthusiasm when it became apparent how much time it took to obtain accurate, readable records.

It was Dr. Winters' echocardiographic investigations of the pericardium that inadvertently resulted in his unexpected trip to Houston. At a March 1968 American College of Cardiology meeting in San Francisco, he participated in a panel discussion about pericardial disease with one of the well-known cardiovascular surgeons in the "Houston Group," Dr. Grady Hallman, who worked at St. Luke's with Dr. Denton Cooley. This chance encounter turned out to be serendipitous. Right at that time, the Texas Medical Center with Drs. DeBakey and Cooley was the envy of the cardiovascular community in this country, maybe in the world. When they started talking about Houston, Dr. Hallman suggested that Dr. Winters stop by to visit on his way back to Philadelphia and he accepted his invitation.

After flying directly from San Francisco to Houston, Dr. Winters spent two days with Dr. Hallman, who personally gave him a tour of the cardiovascular facilities at The Methodist Hospital and St. Luke's Episcopal Hospital. Dr. Winters was introduced to Drs. DeBakey and Cooley and fellow cardiologists Drs. Dennis and O'Donnell. Somehow or other, he missed meeting Dr. Don Chapman, but about a week or ten days after his return to Philadelphia, he received a letter from him saying, "I heard you were in Houston looking around, would you be interested in moving to Houston?" Dr. Winters recalls, "Well, I hadn't thought about it at all, but it was so exciting down here in that field that I said to myself, 'I better come back and take a look.'"

Although he only planned to stay in Houston for three days on his return visit, he changed his mind and stayed for six. In making rounds with Drs. Peterson and Beazley, Dr. Winters discovered why they were seeking a new colleague. The fourth member of The Chapman Group was Dr. Marvin Brook, a nephrologist who was recently invited to join them. They thought he would add a new dimension to their services, but soon afterward he received orders to enter the army, therefore opening a space for a new member to care for the rapidly growing practice.

After a fascinating, whirlwind six-day visit, Dr. Winters finally had the opportunity to spend time with Dr. Chapman. Because he was in private practice with a clinical appointment at Baylor, Dr. Winters believed Dr. Chapman was in an ideal circumstance—both private practice and teaching in the medical school. After showing him around, Dr. Chapman said, "We would love to have you come join us here in Houston." Dr. Winters immediately replied, "If I come, there is one request I would make and that is that you buy me an echocardiographic machine." Having worked in echocardiography for three or four years in Philadelphia, Dr. Winters could count the number of echocardiographers in the country on one hand. "Three were in Philadelphia, one was in Indiana, and one was in Rochester, New York," Dr. Winters recalled. "There may have been two or three others."

Even though Dr. Chapman promised to provide an echocardiographic machine at The Methodist Hospital, Dr. Winters nonetheless was apprehensive about making the move, recalling, "This is an exciting place but I am not sure I want to live in Houston." Upon returning home, he spoke at length with his wife, Barbara, about the prospect of leaving Philadelphia, but they couldn't quite come to grips with the decision. "Then Don called me one night and said, 'We want to know what you are going to do.' So I looked at Barbara, and she looked at me, and we said, 'Let's go,' and we did," Dr. Winters recalls.

"To this day I give full credit for the move to my wife," says Dr. Winters. "We were moving our three young sons a long way to a whole new world and leaving friends and family behind. However, I did have a promise in my back pocket that we could return to Philadelphia if the move did not work out."

By the time he joined The Chapman Group in August of 1968, the influx of new cardiovascular patients had reached a new level in the Texas Medical Center. Among the hundreds of patients who were seeking treatment for coronary heart disease were two new groups: the first included those desperate to become the recipient of a heart transplant, and the second comprised those referred for coronary artery bypass grafts. Since Dr. Chapman had already made the decision that The Chapman Group would not become involved in the initial consultation and postoperative treatment of heart transplant patients, the coronary artery bypass patients gained their undivided attention.

As a surgical treatment of coronary artery occlusive disease, the coronary artery bypass graft (CABG), previously known as "distal coronary bypass," was evolving in 1968. Similar to the other cardiovascular procedures performed at The Methodist Hospital, the volume of these revascularization surgical procedures steadily increased monthly. In the beginning years Dr. Morris was to become prolific, performing coronary artery bypass surgery on 1,698 patients at The Methodist Hospital between 1967 and 1975.[26]

"When all the cardiovascular surgeons began to perform the procedure, there was an era of 10 or 15 years where we were just swamped with patients being referred for bypass surgery," Dr. Winters remembers. In the late 1960s and early 1970s, anyone who had angina symptoms and any obstruction in one or more arteries received a bypass. Except for nitroglycerin and then beta-blockers, there was little else with which to treat them, and no one else in the region was doing them except down in New Orleans. "So we had many patients coming here referred from all over the state, all over the Southwest," Dr. Winters stated. "The early fruits of the surgeons' labor were reported in 1972 in *The American Journal of Cardiology*."[27]

To cope with the sudden increase in patients at The Methodist Hospital in the 1960s, "Ed Dennis was without a doubt the most driven individual I ever met," Dr. O'Donnell said, recalling the frenzied pace maintained by the cardiologists. "We all worked hard in those days, but Ed outdid everybody else. Ed was in the hospital every morning at 5:30 AM. In those days we also read all the electrocardiograms at The Methodist Hospital, which was about

2,000 a month. The five of us did that and it wasn't that big of a chore. But when John Lancaster and Ben McCall left to set up the cardiology service at St. Joseph Hospital in the late 1960s, there were only three of us in our group to do all those electrocardiographs and everything else."[16]

With only three Baylor University College of Medicine cardiologists on staff in the late 1960s, The Chapman Group began to consult a larger number of cardiovascular patients at The Methodist Hospital. Recalls Dr. Winters, "I remember one time when the five of us in The Chapman Group had a hospital census of 120, second only to Dr. DeBakey's service. One night I remember being on call when we had 27 admissions. We didn't have residents or fellows in those days, we did it all ourselves. It was a huge volume with eight, ten, twelve catheterizations a day and we would be working till 12 or 1 o'clock in the morning."

Eager to begin echocardiographic investigations, Dr. Winters patiently awaited the delivery of the promised echocardiographic equipment purchased with funds obtained by Dr. Chapman from the Anderson-Clayton Foundation. Delivered in 1970 was one of the first commercially available machines, a Smith Kline instrument. Later, a Tectronix light-sensitive paper recorder became available.[28] The Smith Kline instrument afforded, at most, a four-beat image of the heart on an oscilloscopic screen. A similar instrument was in the possession of the neurology department, being used by Dr. Meyer Proler, a neurologist, for identifying the midline structures of the brain with ultrasound. "A year or two later when the Unirad instrument arrived in cardiology, a continuous paper recording became available," says Dr. Winters.

As Dr. Winters facilitated his pursuit of clinical research with echocardiography, the Medical Center Cardiovascular Research Foundation was established and perpetuated over the years with philanthropic funds. It ultimately was to be converted in the late 1990s to the Winters Center for Heart Failure Research.

In 1970, finding the appropriate space to establish the hospital's first echocardiograph laboratory in cardiology was a challenge, even when assisted in their search by Mr. Bowen, the hospital administrator. For a modality that was to become the most commonly used cardiac imaging technique in the world, its eventual Houston debut was humble, located under the stairs in the back of the basement of the Fondren Building.

Available space simply did not exist at The Methodist Hospital in 1970. The 1,040-bed facility maintained an impressive occupancy rate, primarily attributed to the cardiovascular surgeons' large number of bypass patients. The process for admitting, treating, and releasing each bypass patient was vastly different from what was to be in the future. In the late 1960s and early 1970s, bypass patients were admitted to the hospital three or four days before the surgical procedure so that the cardiologists could perform the necessary diagnostic tests. "We were very leisurely about it," recalls Dr. Winters. "There was no great rush. In those days the patients would stay 10, 12, 14 days after surgery."

To most of these patients, Mr. Bowen became a familiar face. Believing "the patient always comes first," he worked seven days a week and religiously made patient rounds each morning to make sure each received the best nursing care. "There was no telling where he would show up on those rounds–in the kitchen, laundry, or maintenance," said Michael V. Williamson, a former executive vice president. "As a result of these rounds, he knew everything that was going on in the hospital."[29]

Whatever Mr. Bowen did not know about the day-to-day activities in the hospital, his assistant did. A registered nurse who previously served on the surgical floor, Pat Temple was placed in charge of the VIP patients, of which there were many. Always with a smile, Ms. Temple had the ability to defuse any explosive situation and usually did. According to Dr. Winters, "I used to call Pat Temple our personal 'Radio Shack' because of her outstanding ability to respond quickly and accurately to any and all inquiries. She was the epitome of that electronics store's advertising slogan, 'You've got questions? We've got answers.'"

She also was known for efficiently handling the special arrangements, no matter how outrageous, that often were requested by the hospital's VIP patients. Because of her ability to achieve the seemingly impossible, and with the utmost discretion, Ms. Temple became almost as well known as Mr. Bowen among not only the patients and hospital staff but also Houston community leaders.

Since both Mr. Bowen and Ms. Temple had established an excellent working relationship with all members of the clinical and academic staffs at The Methodist Hospital, they were well aware of the major concerns of each. In 1970, of paramount importance to both staffs were the changes taking place at the newly independent Baylor College of Medicine and the unavoidable difficulties inherent with any and all possible changes in the affiliation agreement between the college and hospital.

For all concerned, there were many unknowns about the future in 1970, but for The Methodist Hospital there was one certainty—come rain or shine, hundreds of cardiovascular patients would continue to be en route there every day.

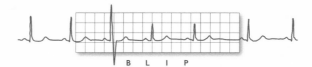

MISTAKEN IDENTITIES

*F*rom its inception, the American College of Cardiology (ACC) showcased its annual March meeting in various venues around the country. In the early days, when smaller convention centers were all that was required, a local cardiologist was selected as chairman to oversee the facilities provided for the professional meetings. When attendance at this meeting grew exponentially in the late 1970s as cardiology training programs in medical schools and many stand alone hospitals resulted in upwards of 800-900 newly trained cardiologists annually around the world, the growth in numbers at the annual meeting ultimately necessitated convention centers that were able to accommodate 25,000 attendees.

When smaller convention facilities sufficed, the ACC met in Houston on two occasions in the 1970s. One of which was in 1974 when Dr. Henry McIntosh was president of the ACC. Serving as the meeting's chairman, Dr. McIntosh asked Drs. Chapman and Winters to serve as the local arrangement chairmen and they agreed, volunteering their wives, Mary Louise Chapman and Barbara Winters, to be in charge of social activities for the spouses in attendance.

To facilitate the accomplishment of their assigned tasks and to be readily available to answer questions and solve problems, the two volunteers were promised a prominent desk in the convention facilities. When they arrived on the first day to arrange trips to NASA, the Astrodome, the Museum of Fine Arts, and Museum of Natural History, as well as tours of Galveston and the well-manicured homes and mansions of River Oaks in Houston, they found their desk not only was front and center but also their first names had been switched and printed incorrectly on the sign. "It read 'Barbara Chapman' and 'Mary Lou Winters,'" Dr. Winters recalled, noting that the printed misnomers remained unchanged for the duration of the meeting. "To this day, 40 years later, a few still recall that misstep and merrily refer to them by their adopted name. So much for the best laid plans by good intentioned people."

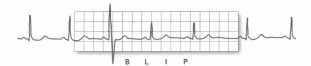

THE ART OF
HOSPITAL MANAGEMENT

*I*n the late 1970s, Dr. Peter Kellaway, a noted neuroelectrophysiologist at Baylor College of Medicine and The Methodist Hospital, spearheaded a plan to have a portrait of Ted Bowen produced, and the services of Everett Raymond Kinstler were procured. At the time, Mr. Kinstler was a young but very talented portrait artist whose reputation was to grow exponentially. In the intervening four decades he has become world famous for his portraits, including those of presidents Gerald Ford, Ronald Reagan, and George W. Bush that hang in the White House. He has painted a total of seven presidents and several of their wives, more than 50 Cabinet members, numerous congressmen, and a multitude of well-known personalities. Prior to the delivery of the painting of Mr. Bowen to The Methodist Hospital, a contingency of couples from Houston trekked to New York City to view the portrait and visit the artist in his studio. "Accompanying Mr. Bowen and wife June for the trip were Dr. Kellaway and wife JoAnn, and my wife Barbara and I, who all found Mr. Kinstler to be a most gentlemanly and proper host," Dr. Winters said. "Shortly thereafter, the large, full-figure portrait of Mr. Bowen was delivered to Houston and hung next to the main elevator in what was then the entrance to the main hospital building off of Bertner Avenue. It remains there to this day."[1]

---

1. On September 29, 1999, Ted Bowen died at the age of 78, and June Bowen died on December 2012 at the age of 91.

IMAGES

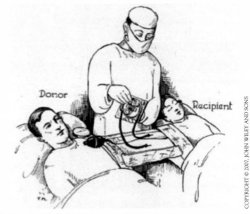

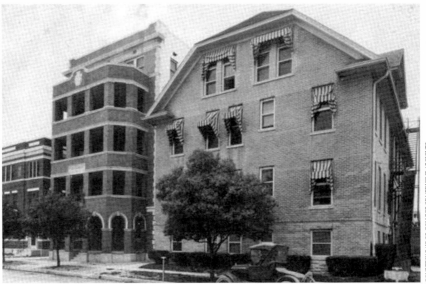

Originally invented and patented by Dr. Michael E. DeBakey and Charles Ernest Schmidt in 1935, the DeBakey Roller Pump with a ratchet to prevent backflow was used for direct donor-to-patient transfusion. When citrated stored blood became available in blood banks, this manual roller pump was obsolesced for transfusion. A motorized version in 1953 enabled the first successful open-heart surgery.

When The Methodist Hospital in Houston opened its doors to the public on June 12, 1924, it was located at the corner of San Jacinto Street and Rosalie Avenue in downtown Houston and comprised two adjacent buildings with a total capacity of 90 beds and 10 bassinettes.

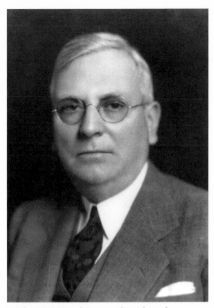

Walter W. Fondren, co-founder of Humble Oil and a major benefactor of The Methodist Hospital, was one of the hospital's original trustees in 1924.

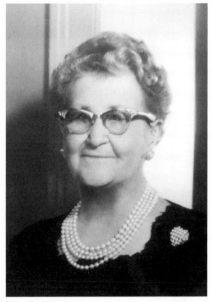

Ella Cochrum Fondren, widow of Walter W. Fondren, became a trustee of The Methodist Hospital after the death of her husband in 1939 and was one of its major benefactresses.

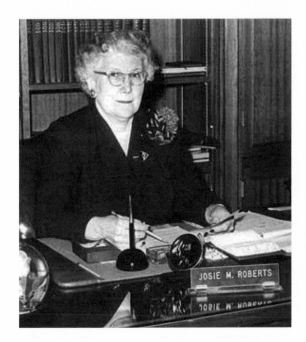

Josie Mooring Roberts, hired to be business manager in 1923, was named administrator of The Methodist Hospital in 1931. On the 29th anniversary of her employment in 1953, she resigned and Ted Bowen succeeded her.

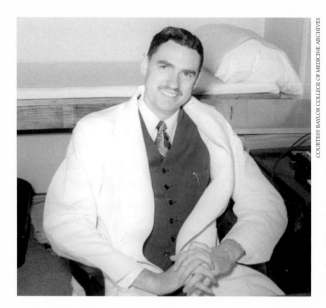

Dr. Don W. Chapman, recognized as the first cardiologist in Houston, joined the faculty at Baylor University College of Medicine in 1944 as an instructor in medicine.

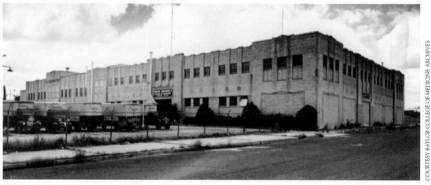

When Baylor University College of Medicine moved to Houston in 1943, while its new campus was under construction in the Texas Medical Center the first classes were held in a converted Sears, Roebuck and Co. warehouse on Houston's Buffalo Drive.

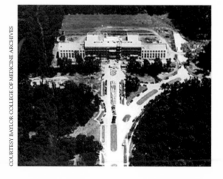

The Roy and Lillie Cullen Building of the new Baylor University College of Medicine in the Texas Medical Center opened in 1947.

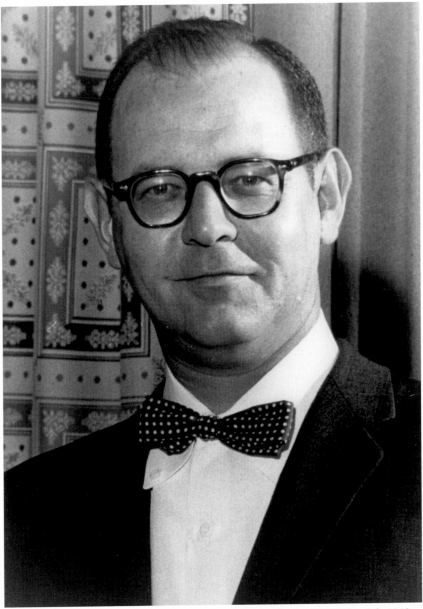

Ted Bowen became the assistant administrator of The Methodist Hospital in July 1948. He became president and chief executive officer at age 32 in 1953, a position he held until retiring in 1983.

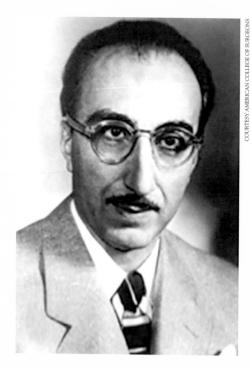

COURTESY AMERICAN COLLEGE OF SURGEONS

Dr. Michael E. DeBakey came to Houston in 1948 to become the chairman of the Department of Surgery at Baylor University College of Medicine.

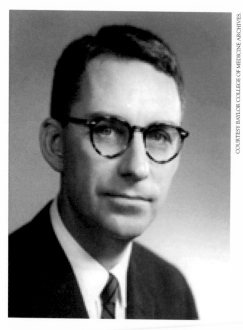

COURTESY BAYLOR COLLEGE OF MEDICINE ARCHIVES.

Dr. Oscar Creech Jr. joined Dr. DeBakey in 1949 and served as head of the peripheral vascular unit at Baylor University College of Medicine until his departure in 1956 to become Chairman of the Department of Surgery at Tulane University.

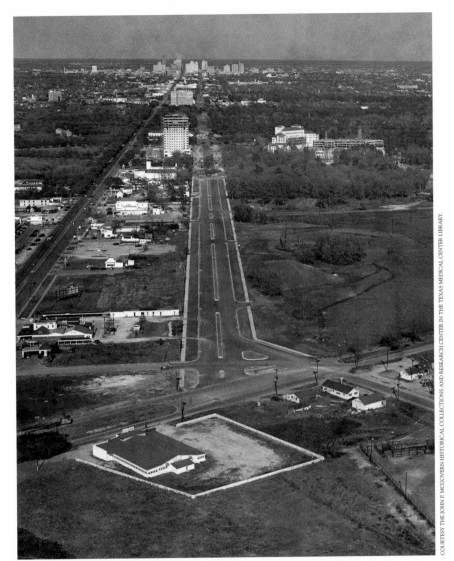

Before construction began in The Texas Medical Center in the late 1940s, there were only vacant lots at the corner of Fannin Street and Holcombe Boulevard. The large white structure visible to the right of Fannin was Hermann Hospital, constructed in 1925.

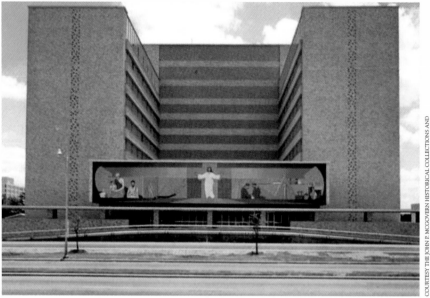

After its 1963 renovation and expansion The Methodist Hospital included an additional 375 beds and artist Bruce Hayes' colorful, 98-foot-long, 16-foot-high mosaic mural, *The Extending Arms of Christ*, installed above the hospital's new, primary entrance on Fannin Street.

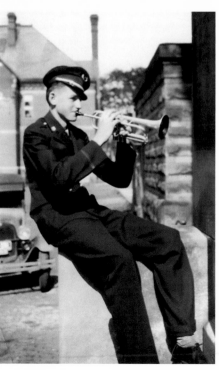

Called to service in the U.S. Army Medical Corps during the Korean War in the 1950s, Dr. Don Chapman was assigned to the 5th General Hospital in Stuttgart Bad-Cannstatt, where he also practiced his skills with a coronet. A decade later, when the all-physician band "The Heartbeats" was created in 1965 in Houston, he became one of the charter members.

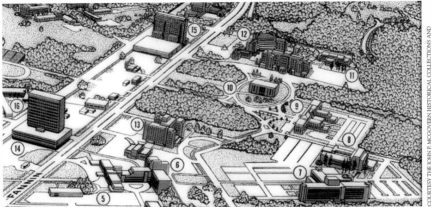

Map of the Texas Medical Center in the mid 1950s illustrates its rapid growth. Adjacent to The Methodist Hospital (13) are the new Texas Children's Hospital (5) and St. Luke's Episcopal Hospital (6), both opened in 1954. The Texas Medical Center Library (10), opened in 1953, is adjacent to Baylor University College of Medicine (9). Also illustrated is new M.D. Anderson Hospital (7), adjacent to the University of Texas Dental Branch (8).

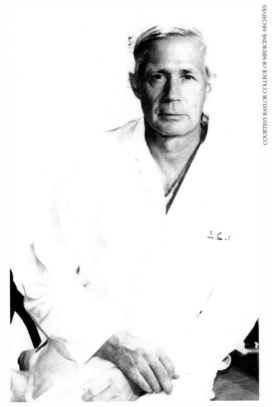

Dr. George C. Morris, Jr. served as the first surgical resident under Dr. Michael E. DeBakey in 1950 when he began residencies in general and thoracic surgery at Baylor University College of Medicine.

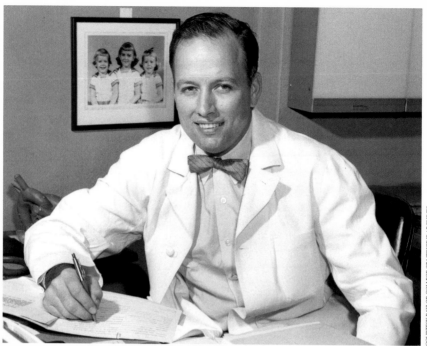

Dr. Denton A. Cooley joined Baylor University College of Medicine in 1951, the year The Methodist Hospital opened in the Texas Medical Center.

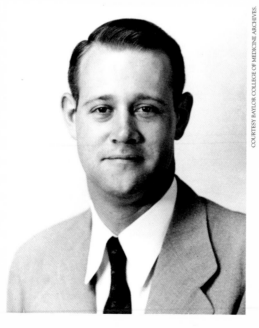

Dr. James K. Alexander was named chief of the cardiology section of the Department of Medicine at Baylor University College of Medicine in 1954 and began working at Jefferson Davis Hospital and The Methodist Hospital, eventually moving to Ben Taub.

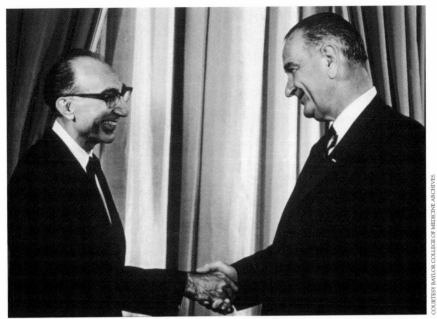

Dr. Michael DeBakey was awarded the Presidential Medal of Freedom by President Lyndon Johnson on January 20, 1969.

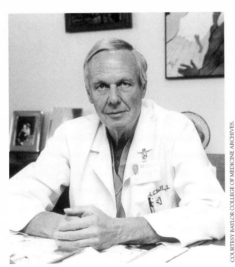

Dr. Arthur C. Beall joined Baylor University College of Medicine in 1954 as a first-year resident rotating through the surgical services at The Methodist Hospital, Jefferson Davis Hospital and the Veteran's Administration Hospital.

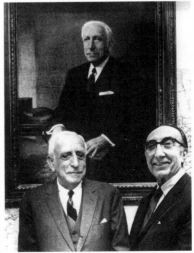

Houston businessman and philanthropist Ben Taub and Dr. Michael DeBakey first met in 1949 and became lifelong friends, having breakfast together every Sunday until his death at the age of ninety-two in 1982.

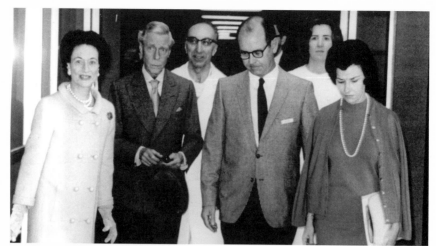

The Duke of Windsor leaves The Methodist Hospital after his 1964 operation with the
Duchess of Windsor, Dr. Michael DeBakey, Ted Bowen and Betty Hahneman.

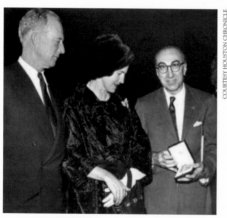

COURTESY HOUSTON CHRONICLE

Abdicated King Leopold and Princess
Liliane of Belgium presented Dr.
Michael DeBakey with the Grand Cross
Order of Leopold in 1962.

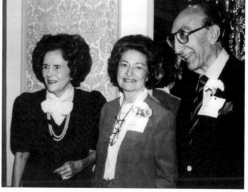

COURTESY THE MARY LASKER PAPERS, NATIONAL LIBRARY OF MEDICINE

Mary Lasker and Lady Bird
Johnson visited with Dr. Michael
DeBakey after the 1963 Lasker
Foundation Awards luncheon
in New York.

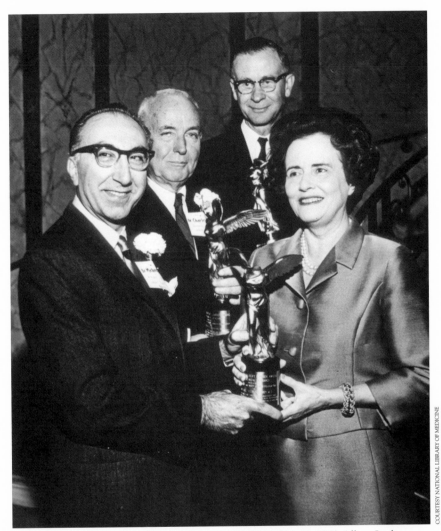

On October 30, 1963, the Albert and Mary Lasker Foundation's 1963 Albert Lasker Award for Clinical Research was presented to Dr. Michael E. DeBakey and Dr. Charles B. Huggins. Receiving the Albert Lasker Basic Medical Research Award was Lyman C. Craig. The three recipients posed with Mary Lasker for pictures after the awards ceremony in New York.

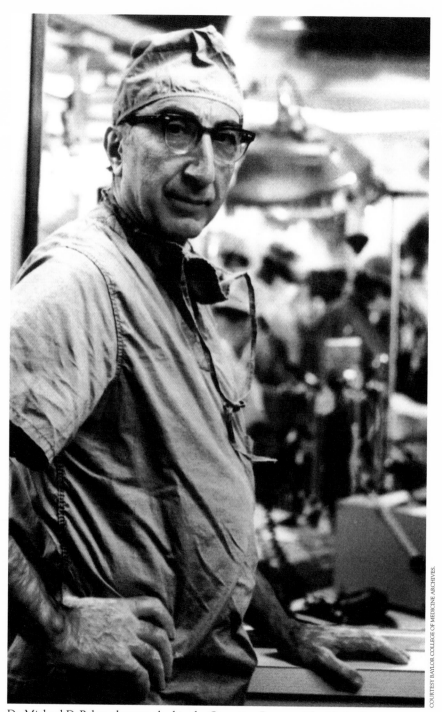

Dr. Michael DeBakey photographed in the Operating Room at The Methodist Hospital in 1964.

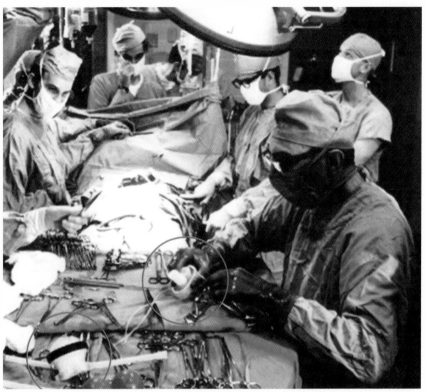

Dr. Michael DeBakey (right) and Dr. Jimmy Howell (left) implant one of the first
Baylor/Rice ventricular assist devices (circled in red) at The Methodist Hospital in 1966.

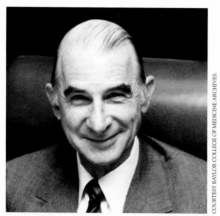

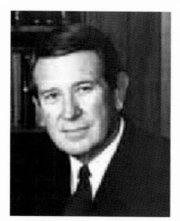

COURTESY BAYLOR COLLEGE OF MEDICINE ARCHIVES.

Dr. Jimmy F. Howell joined the Baylor University College of Medicine faculty in 1964 and has been a full professor of surgery since 1975.

Dr. W. Sam Henly, a former surgical resident at Baylor College of Medicine, joined Dr. Michael DeBakey's surgical team and in 1965 he became one of the founding members of the Surgical Associates, the third professional medical association formed in the city of Houston.

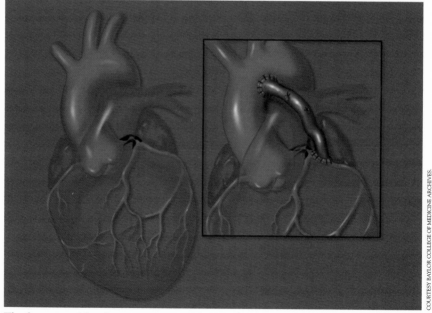

COURTESY BAYLOR COLLEGE OF MEDICINE ARCHIVES.

The first successful saphenous vein-coronary artery bypass operation was performed at The Methodist Hospital in 1964. Since the breakthrough was not published at the time, but seven years later, it became known as the first successful case with longest follow-up of a functioning coronary bypass graft.

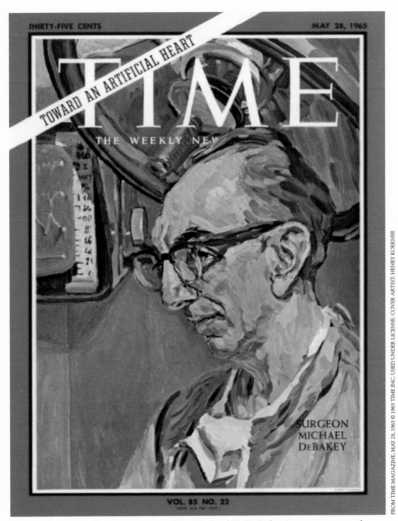

The in-depth article accompanying Dr. Michael E. DeBakey's appearing on the cover of the May 28, 1965, issue of *Time* was titled "The Texas Tornado," in which the magazine described "the incredible drive for perfection, the unending concern for his patients, and the utter domination of his life by his profession."

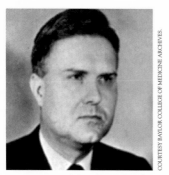

Dr. H. Edward Garrett joined
Baylor University College of
Medicine in 1961 and directed
Dr. DeBakey's clinical service
for six years. He left Houston
in 1967 to serve as chairman of
the Section of Cardiothoracic
Surgery at the University of
Tennessee.

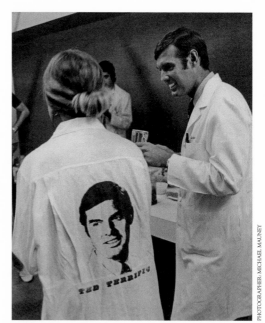

Dr. Edward B. Diethrich, a member of Dr. DeBakey's
surgical team from 1966 to 1970, earned the
nickname "Ted Terrific," as illustrated by this
tribute on a technician's gown at the Arizona Heart
Institute, founded by Dr. Diethrich in 1971.

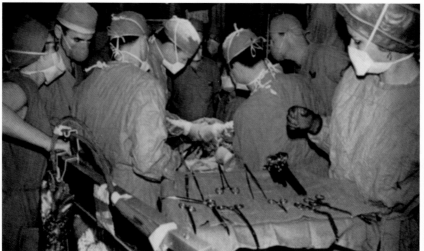

Dr. Denton Cooley performed the first successful heart transplant in the United States
and the ninth worldwide on May 2, 1968. The recipient, Everett C. Thomas, was a
patient referred by Dr. Don W. Chapman, who scrubbed in for the historic operation at
Texas Heart Institute.

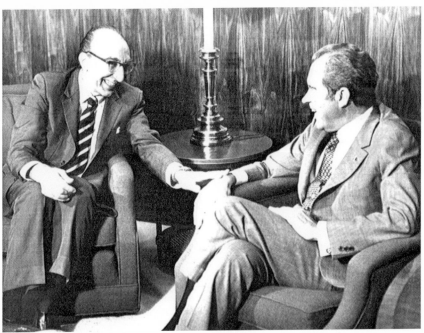

At the Western White House in San Clemente, California, in July 1973, Dr. Michael DeBakey and President Richard Nixon met to discuss the surgeon's recent trip to the Soviet Union.

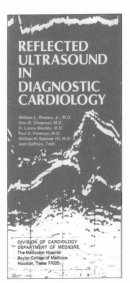

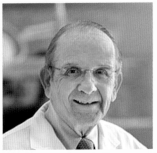

Dr. Charles H. McCollum trained with Dr. DeBakey and joined his surgical team in 1966 before leaving to join Surgical Associates in the late 1960s. He returned to Baylor College of Medicine and The Methodist Hospital in early 1970s, where he and Dr. George P. Noon created the first vascular laboratory.

When Dr. William L. Winters Jr. and The Chapman Group established the echocardiography laboratory in the basement of The Methodist Hospital in 1970 it was the only such laboratory in the southwest at that time. A second echocardiography laboratory was established by Baylor College of Medicine at the hospital in the early 1970s and both laboratories operated independently until 1977

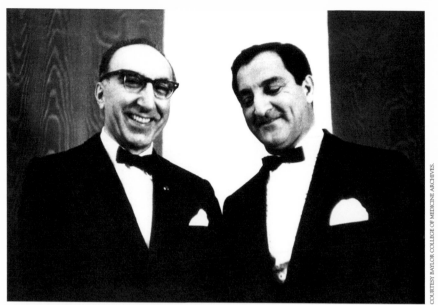

Photographed together at a fund-raising event in the 1970s, Dr. Michael DeBakey and Danny Thomas, noted entertainer and founder of St. Jude's Children's Research Center, were longtime friends.

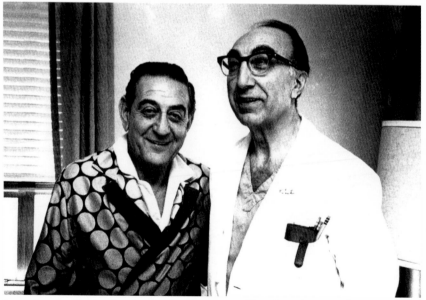

Legendary bandleader Guy Lombardo, whose annual broadcast for more than five decades with his Royal Canadians orchestra on New Year's Eve in New York City was synonymous with the ball drop in Times Square, visited with Dr. Michael DeBakey after the bandleader's September 1977 open-heart surgery at The Methodist Hospital.

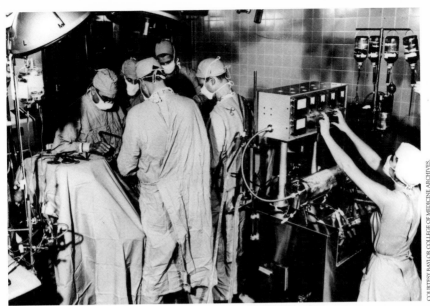

As a technician adjusts the heart-lung machine, Dr. DeBakey and his surgical team perform an open-heart operation at The Methodist Hospital in the early 1970s.

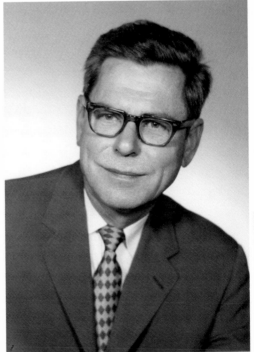

Dr. Henry D. McIntosh became the first occupant of the Bob and Vivian Smith Professor and Chair of Internal Medicine at Baylor College of Medicine and chief of internal medicine at The Methodist Hospital in June 1970.

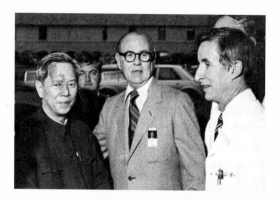

Vice Premier Fang Li of China is welcomed to The Methodist Hospital by Ted Bowen and Dr. Antonio M. Gotto Jr., Chief of the Internal Medicine Service on February 2, 1979.

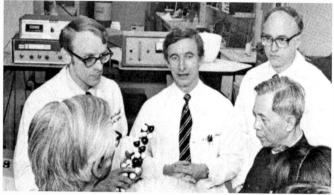

Dr. Joel Morrisett, Dr. Antonio Gotto Jr., and Dr. William T. Butler with Vice Premier Fang Li of China in the National Heart and Blood Vessel Research and Demonstration Center at The Methodist Hospital.

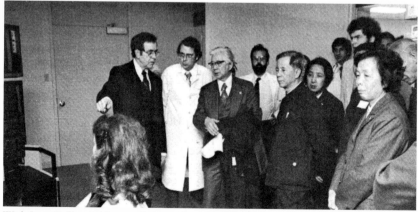

With Jean Gaffney Nelson at the console in the Echocardiography Laboratory at The Methodist Hospital, Dr. William L. Winters Jr. and Dr. Miguel Quiñones describe ultrasound imaging of the inner heart to Vice Premier Fang Li of China in February 1979.

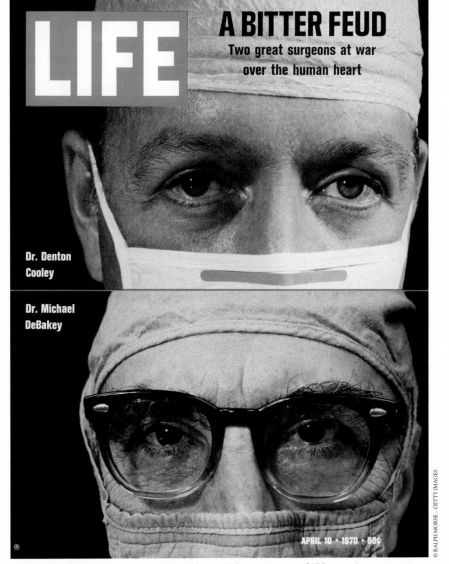

The 1970 *Life* magazine cover story by Thomas Thompson stated "Houston's two master heart surgeons are locked in a feud," identified as "The Texas Tornado Vs. Dr. Wonderful."

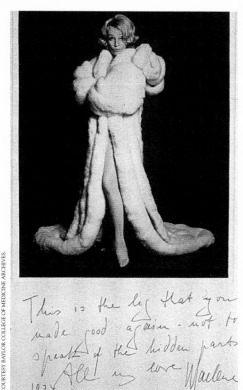

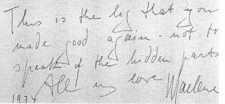

The 1974 autographed thank-you photo to Dr. DeBakey from Marlene Dietrich: "This is the leg that you made good again—not to speak of the hidden parts. All my love, Marlene."

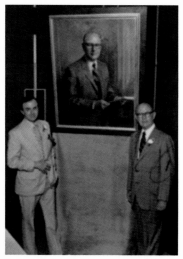

Renowned portrait artist Everett Raymond Kinstler with his subject Ted Bowen at his painting's dedication at The Methodist Hospital in the late 1970s.

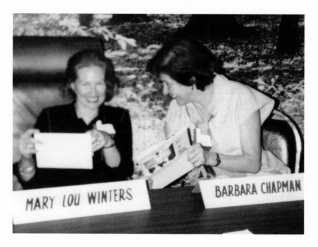

For Barbara Winters and Mary Lou Chapman, commandeering the social activities for spouses at the 1974 American College of Cardiology annual March meeting in Houston included their unexpectedly assuming new identities when the sign maker switched their first names.

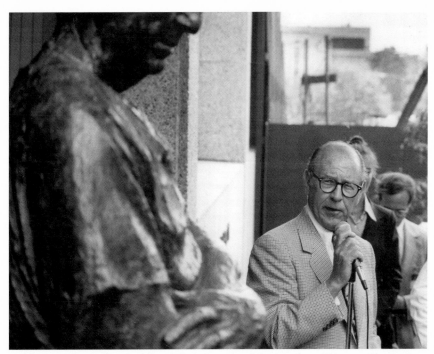

Ted Bowen officiated at the May 1978 dedication of the four-foot, 300-pound bronze bust by French artist Georges Muguet of Dr. Michael DeBakey. Commissioned and donated by the abdicated King Leopold and Princess Liliane of Belgium, it was placed in the lobby of Dunn Tower at The Methodist Hospital.

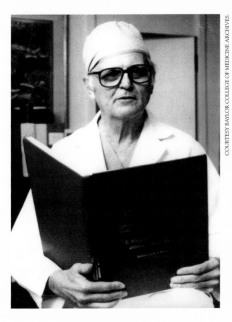

COURTESY BAYLOR COLLEGE OF MEDICINE ARCHIVES.

Recognized as one of the leading authorities in thoracoabdominal aneurysms and aortic disease, Dr. E. Stanley Crawford, who joined Baylor University College of Medicine in 1954, and his son, Dr. John L. Crawford II, published *Diseases of the Aorta: An Atlas of Angiographic Pathology and Surgical Technique* in 1985 to critical acclaim.

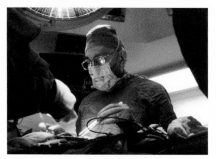

At the age of 77 in 1985, Dr. Michael DeBakey had performed heart surgery more than 60,000 times, traveled an average of 200,000 miles a year, and showed no signs of slowing down.

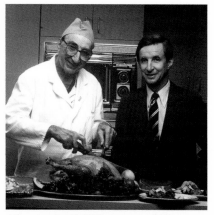

After the April 1981 opening of Chez Eddy, a gourmet restaurant in The Methodist Hospital's Scurlock Tower, Dr. Michael DeBakey and Dr. Tony Gotto advocated a hands-on approach to that eatery's heart-healthy cuisine.

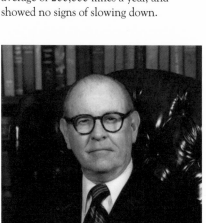

Ted Bowen unexpectedly stepped down as president of The Methodist Hospital at the age of 63 in October 1982. Unable to continue his duties due to poor health, he had been the hospital's administrator for 30 years.

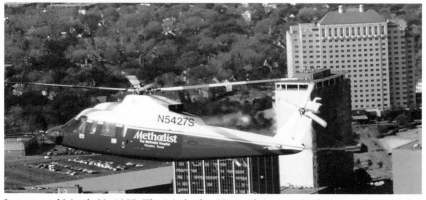

Inaugurated March 23, 1987, The Methodist Hospital Aeromedical Services became the first such service to focus exclusively on the cardiovascular patient in Texas.

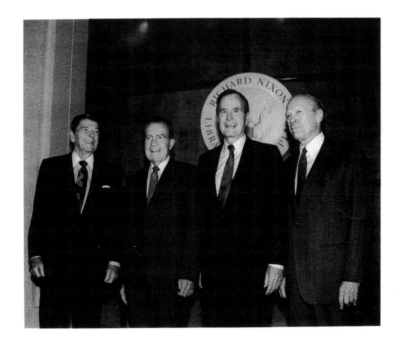

Dr. De Bakey,

With Best Wishes and Appreciation,

The four living Republican presidents of the United States, Ronald Reagan, Richard Nixon, George Bush and Gerald Ford, expressed their best wishes and appreciation to Dr. Michael DeBakey in this autographed memento from the July 1990 dedication of the Richard Nixon Library and Birthplace in Yorba Linda, California.

196

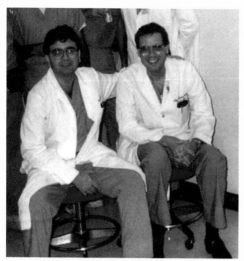

Dr. William A. Zoghbi (left), who joined the
Baylor College of Medicine faculty in 1985,
and Dr. Miguel Quiñones (right), a faculty
member since 1977, pictured together in the
echocardiography laboratory at The Methodist
Hospital in the late 1980s.

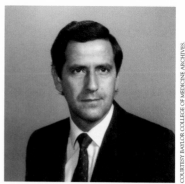

Cardiologist Dr. Mario S. Verani
became intrigued with the
diagnostic possibilities evident
in the evolving field of nuclear
cardiology in the late 1970s.
With Dr. Richard Cashion, he
established the nuclear cardiology
laboratory in 1978, introduced four
types of cardiac scanning at The
Methodist Hospital, and became
one of the recognized pioneers in
nuclear cardiology.

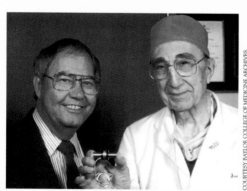

David Saucier, a NASA engineer who underwent
a heart transplant in 1984, arranged for his
surgeon Dr. Michael DeBakey to meet with other
space agency engineers to collaborate on the
design of a battery operated heart pump based
on the space shuttle's rocket engine pump. A
decade later, they presented the result of this
collaboration: the three-inch long, one-inch
diameter, implantable ventricular-assist device to
strengthen the beat of a weakened heart known
as the MicroMed-DeBakey VAD.

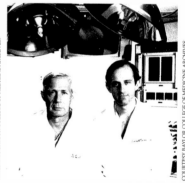

Surgeons Dr. George C. Morris
(left), Dr. DeBakey's first surgical
resident in 1950 who became
one of the recognized pioneer
in cardiovascular and peripheral
surgery, and Dr. Gerald M. Lawrie
(right), who joined the surgical
team in 1974 and subsequently
confirmed the feasibility of surgical
intervention on a variety of serious
arrhythmias in 1985.

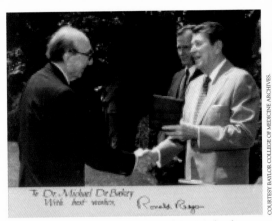

President Ronald Reagan presented Dr. Michael DeBakey the Presidential Medal of Science in the Rose Garden of The White House in June 1987.

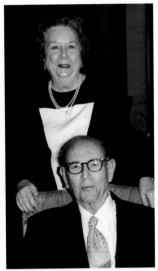

COURTESY BAYLOR COLLEGE OF MEDICINE ARCHIVES.

June and Ted Bowen, who retired in 1982 because of poor health, continued his avid interest in The Methodist Hospital for more than a decade.

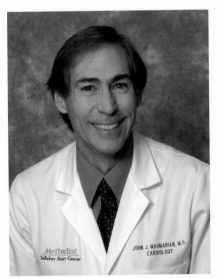

Joining Baylor College of Medicine in 1987, Dr. John J. Mahmarian became chief of nuclear cardiology in 2001. With a clinical focus on preventing heart disease, acute coronary syndromes, and myocardial infarction, he has published extensively on myocardial perfusion imaging and CT angiography. He was named president of American Nuclear Cardiology Society in 2011.

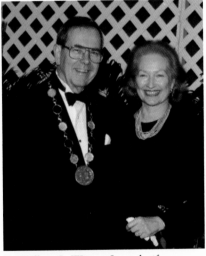

Dr. William L. Winters Jr., and wife Barbara celebrated his induction as President of the American College of Cardiology (ACC) at its 1990 annual scientific session in New Orleans.

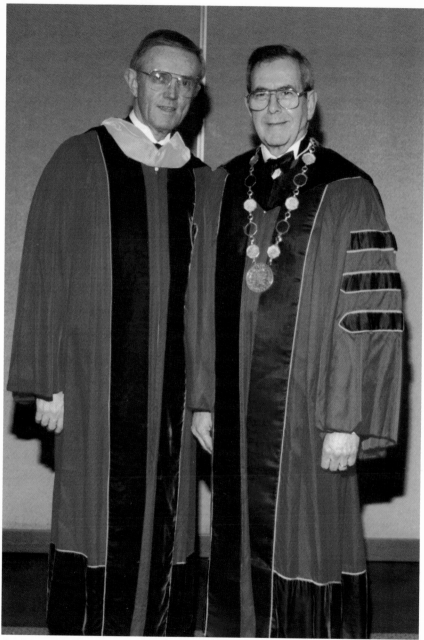

ACC Executive Vice President William D. Nelligan with Dr. William L. Winters Jr. after his presidential investiture of at the 1990 ACC Annual Scientific Session in New Orleans.

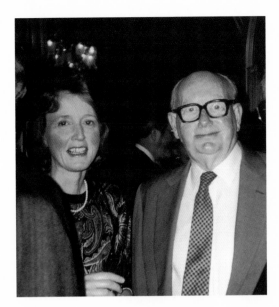

London's Dr. David Brooks and wife Leslie Brooks attended the presidential investiture ceremonies for Dr. William L. Winters Jr. at the 1990 ACC Annual Scientific Session in New Orleans.

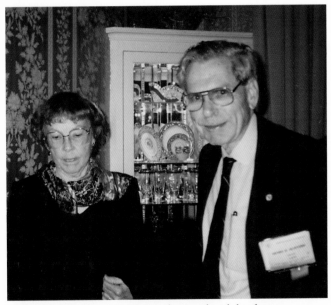

Harriet and Dr. Henry D. McIntosh visited with his former colleagues while attending the 1990 ACC Annual Scientific Session in New Orleans.

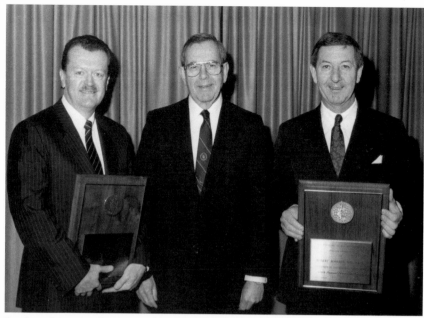

Dr. Craig Pratt, Dr. William L. Winters Jr., and Dr. Robert Roberts with plaques for serving as co-chairmen of the 1991 ACC Annual Scientific Session in Atlanta.

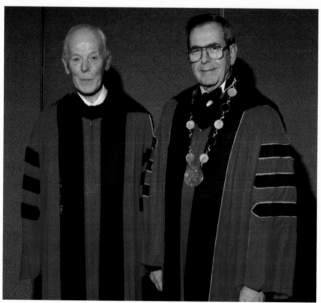

Dr. Inge Edler, known as the "Father of Echocardiography," received the ACC Distinguished Fellowship Award from ACC President William L. Winters Jr. at the 1991 ACC Annual Scientific Session in Atlanta.

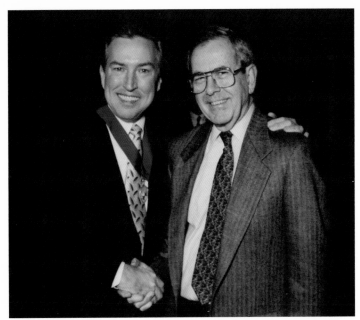

Dr. William L. Winters Jr. congratulated Larry Mathis after his January 1993 investiture as Chairman of the Board of Trustees of the American Hospital Association in Washington, D.C.

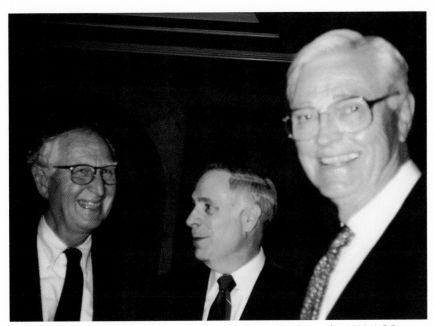

Dr. Richard Judge, Dr. Francis Klocke, and Dr. H. Liston Beazley at the 1999 ACC Annual Scientific Session in New Orleans.

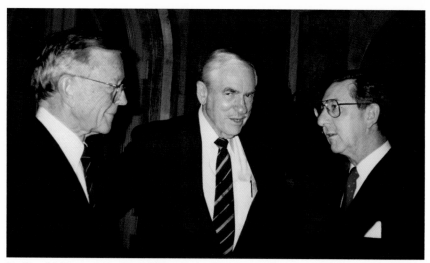

Dr. Dan McNamara, Dr. Don Chapman, and Dr. Robert Roberts together at the 1990 ACC Annual Scientific Session in New Orleans.

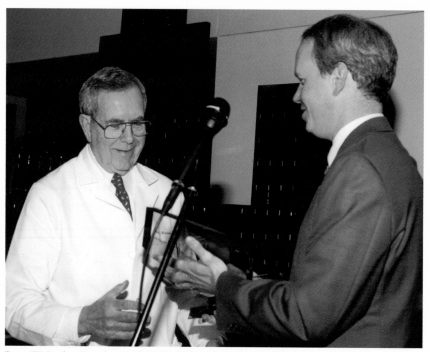

Peter W. Butler, President and CEO of The Methodist Health Care System, presented the 1998 John Overstreet Award to Dr. William L. Winters Jr. at The Methodist Hospital.

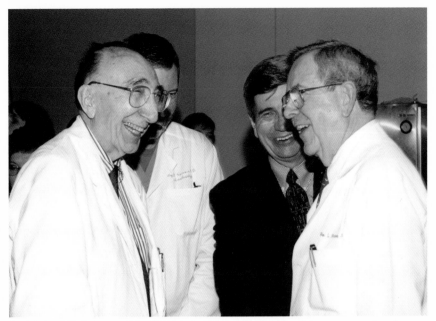

Dr. Michael DeBakey and Dr. William L. Winters Jr. shared a light moment after the 1998 presentation of the John Overstreet Award at The Methodist Hospital.

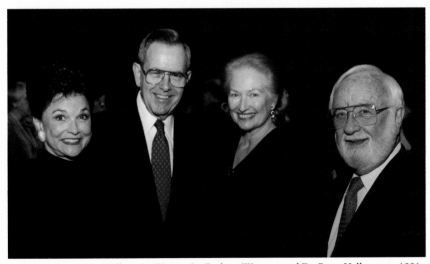

Joanne Kellaway, Dr. William L. Winters Jr., Barbara Winters, and Dr. Peter Kellaway in 1991.

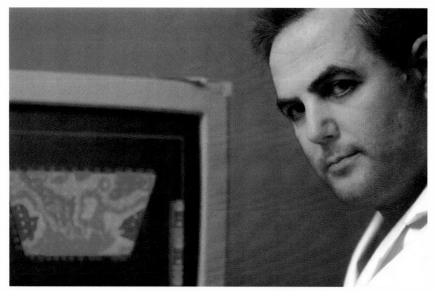

In addition to his flourishing electrophysiology program at Baylor College of Medicine and The Methodist Hospital in 1994, Dr. Antonio Pacifico established and directed The Texas Arrhythmia Institute.

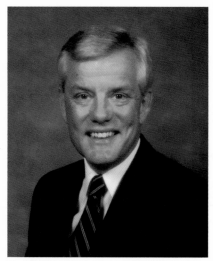

Dr. William H. Spencer III left The Chapman Group in September 1994 with Dr. William L. Winters Jr. to join the faculty at Baylor College of Medicine at The Methodist Hospital.

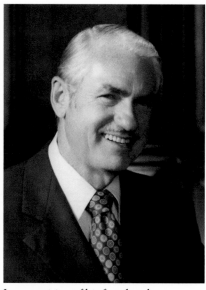

In recognition of his five-decade, legendary career as a cardiologist in 1996, Dr. Don W. Chapman received the Harris County Medical Society's highest award — the John P. McGovern Compleat Physician Award.

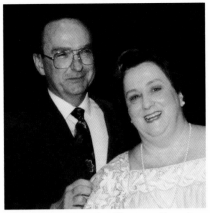

In the early 1990s, The Chapman Group's Dr. Richard Cashion and his wife Pamela Cashion left Houston to live and work in College Station, Texas.

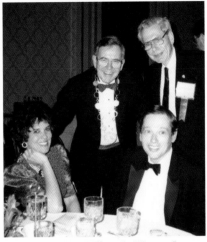

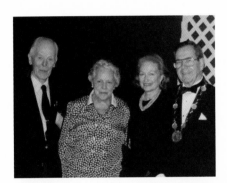

Judy Girotto, Dr. William L. Winters Jr., Ron Girotto, and Dr. Henry D. McIntosh together at the 1990 ACC Annual Scientific Session in New Orleans.

Dr. Inge Edler and wife Karen Edler visited with Barbara Winters and Dr. William L. Winters Jr. at the 1991 ACC Annual Scientific Session in Atlanta.

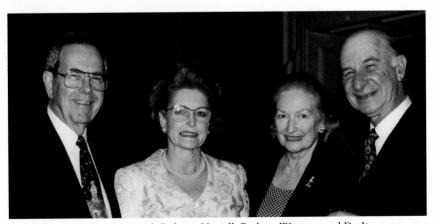

Dr. William L. Winters Jr., with Roberta Howell, Barbara Winters, and Dr. Jimmy Howell in 1998.

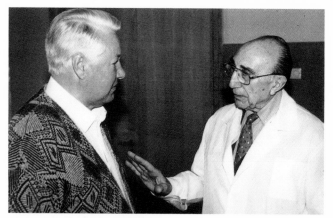

Russian President Boris N. Yeltsin conferred with "magician of the heart" Dr. Michael DeBakey after "the man with a gift for performing miracles" served as a consultant on his successful 1996 coronary bypass operation in Moscow.

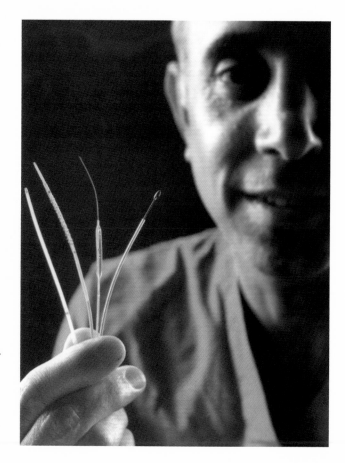

Dr. Albert Raizner and the four plaque-busting catheters used in the Cardiac Catheterization Laboratory at The Methodist Hospital in the 1990s.

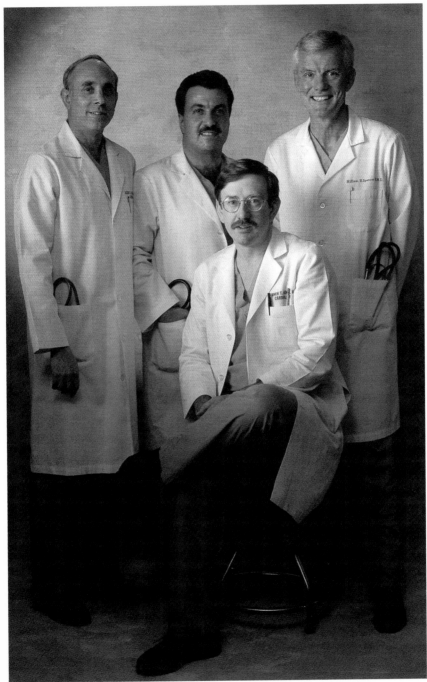

Dr. Albert Raizner, Dr. Nadim Zacca, Dr. William Spencer, and Dr. Steve Minor photographed in the Cardiac Catheterization Laboratory at The Methodist Hospital in the 1990s.

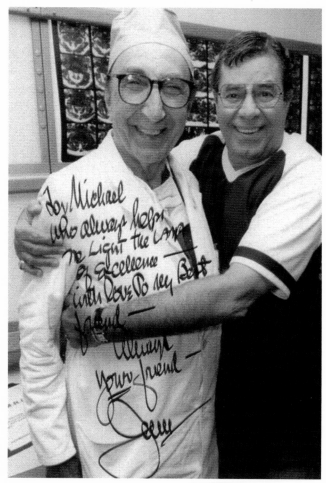

Dr. Michael DeBakey became the personal physician and close friend of Jerry Lewis in 1978 when he diagnosed his almost fatal abdominal ulcer. He not only supervised the comedian's subsequent double bypass operation, he served 20 years on Muscular Dystrophy Association Board of Directors, 17 as its vice president, and appeared on the comedian's Labor Day MDA telethons whenever he was asked.

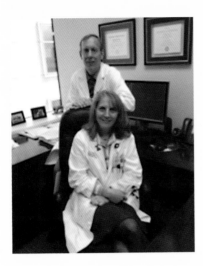

The first husband/wife team of cardiologists at Methodist DeBakey Heart & Vascular Center were Drs. Karla M. Kurrelmeyer and John M. Buergler, who joined the cardiology faculty at Baylor College of Medicine in 1999.

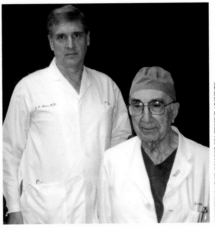

COURTESY BAYLOR COLLEGE OF MEDICINE ARCHIVES.

After Dr. Michael E. DeBakey stopped performing operations at the age of 90 in 1998 he was known to accompany his long-time colleague Dr. George P. Noon in the operating room just to observe.

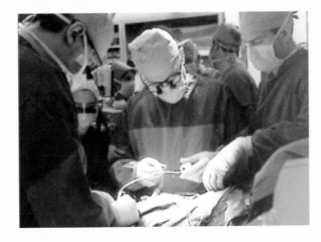

With assistance from surgeons from Berlin and Vienna in 1998, Dr. Noon had implanted the first MicroMed DeBakey VAD® into European patients. Two years later he implanted the first MicroMed DeBakey VAD in the United States into a patient at The Methodist Hospital in June 2000.

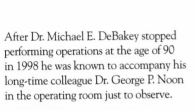

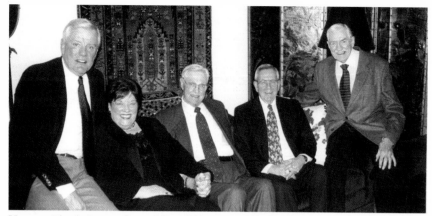

Honoree Glenda Sawyer, (second from left) retiring secretary of Dr. Don W. Chapman in 2003, reminisced with Dr. William H. Spencer III, Dr. H. Liston Beazley, Dr. William L. Winters Jr., and Dr. Don W. Chapman.

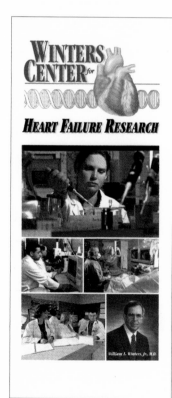

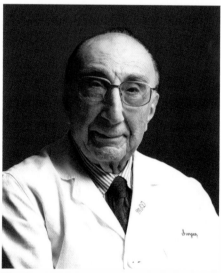

The 92-year-old Dr. Michael E. DeBakey was honored by the Library of Congress in 2000 as one of the 84 individuals the library recognized as a "Living Legend" who embodied the American ideal of individual creativity, conviction, dedication and exuberance.

The Winters Center for Heart Failure Research was established at The Methodist Hospital and Baylor College of Medicine in 2000 to develop, design, and conduct basic and clinical research studies.

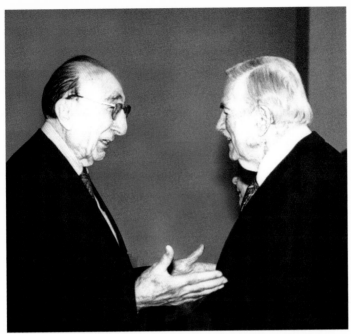

Dr. Michael E. DeBakey and Dr. Don W. Chapman, colleagues for more than 50 years, recalled the past while predicting the limitless future of the Methodist DeBakey Heart Center at its 2001 dedication.

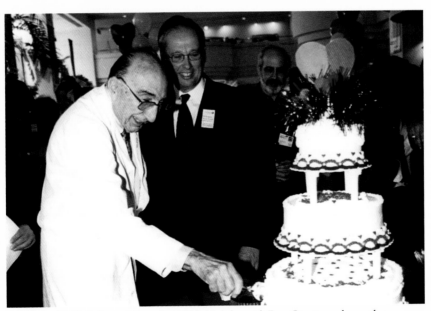

Dr. Michael E. DeBakey celebrated his 95th birthday with Ron Girotto and countless colleagues and admirers at The Methodist Hospital in 2003.

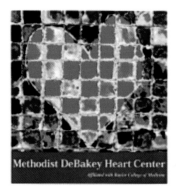

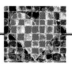

Methodist DeBakey Heart Center
Dedication
Monday, February 19, 2001
The Methodist Hospital
3:00 p.m.

Invocation	The Reverend Theodore M. Smith
Welcoming Remarks	Peter W. Butler
Proclamation Presentation	Martha Engel, D.D.S. Assistant Director of Community and Personal Health Services
Employee Recognition Presentation of Gifts	Albert E. Raizner, M.D. Debra F. Sukin
Recognition of Michael E. DeBakey, M.D.	Joseph S. Coselli, M.D.
Unveiling	Lynn Schroth, DrPH
Closing Remarks	Peter W. Butler

Methodist
DeBakey Heart Center

Dedication of the Methodist
DeBakey Heart Center at
The Methodist Hospital was
February 19, 2001.

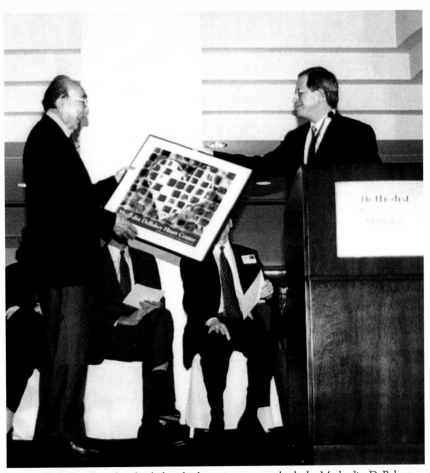

Dr. Joseph S. Coselli, right, chief of cardiothoracic surgery at both the Methodist DeBakey Heart Center and Baylor College of Medicine, presented Dr. Michael E. DeBakey a commemorative poster during the 2001 dedication ceremonies of the Methodist DeBakey Heart Center at The Methodist Hospital.

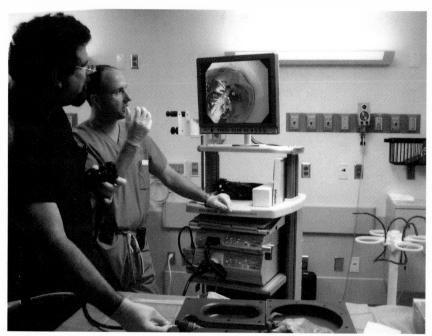

Dr. Brian Dunkin and learner in a laboratory of the Methodist Institute for Technology, Innovation, and Education (MITIE).

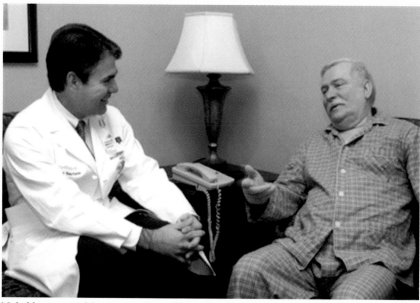

Nobel laureate and former president of Poland Lech Walesa, implanted with a biventricular pacemaker-defibrillator in February 2008 at the Methodist DeBakey Heart & Vascular Center, visited with his cardiologist Dr. Guillermo Torre after the procedure.

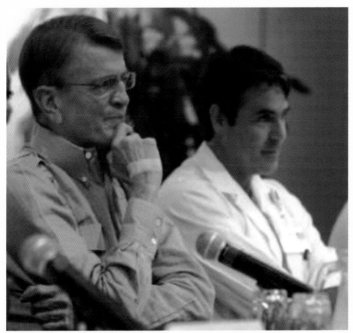

After receiving a heart transplant at the Methodist DeBakey Heart &
Vascular Center in September 2007, Texas Congressman Charlie Wilson
and his cardiologist Dr. Guillermo Torre appeared together at a press
conference at the hospital.

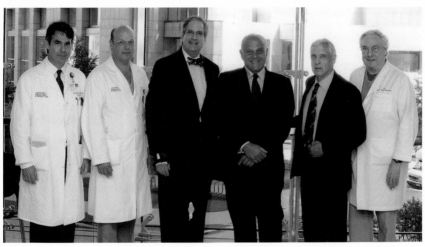

The world-renown Egyptian-born cardiothoracic surgeon Sir Magdi Habib Yacoub from
London's Imperial College was the honored speaker at the second annual Michael E.
DeBakey Lecture in 2010 at The Methodist Hospital where he (third from right) was
welcomed by (left to right) Dr. Guillermo Torre, Dr. Matthias Loebe, Dr. Robert Jackson, Dr.
George P. Noon, and Dr. O. H. "Bud" Frazier.

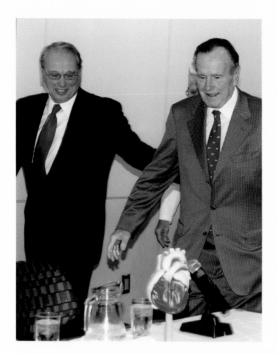

Ron Girotto escorted former President George H. W. Bush to the press conference to announce the successful outcome of former First Lady Barbara Bush's 2009 aortic valve replacement operation at The Methodist DeBakey Heart & Vascular Center.

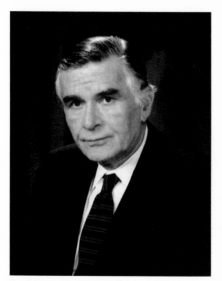

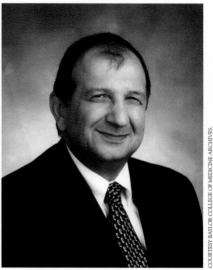

Dr. Manus F. O'Donnell, a trained cardiologist and graduate of the Medical School of Queens University in Ireland, joined the full-time Baylor College of Medicine cardiology faculty at The Methodist Hospital in 1965 and practiced there for more than 35 years.

Trained for four years by Dr. Michael E. DeBakey, surgeon Dr. Hazim Safi became his chief resident in the early 1980s, joining Dr. E. Stanley Crawford as an associate in 1983 to concentrate his clinical focus on aortic aneurysm surgery.

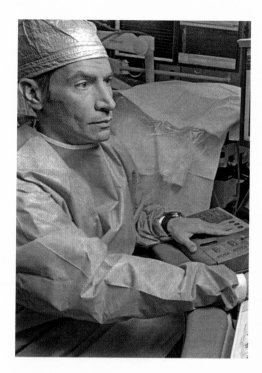

One of the national training leaders for Hansen Robotics in the early 2000s was Dr. Miguel Valderrábano, chief of cardiac electrophysiology at the Methodist DeBakey Heart & Vascular Center.

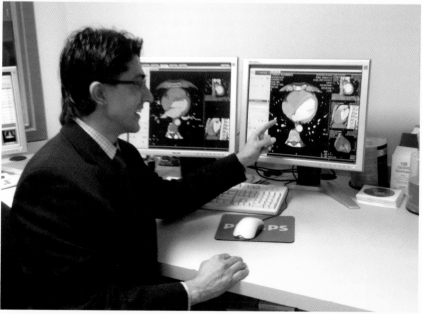

Joining the Methodist DeBakey Heart & Vascular Center in 2010 in multi-modality imaging was Dr. Faisal Nabi, a board-certified cardiologist with Level III training in echocardiography, nuclear cardiology, cardiac CT, and cardiac MRI.

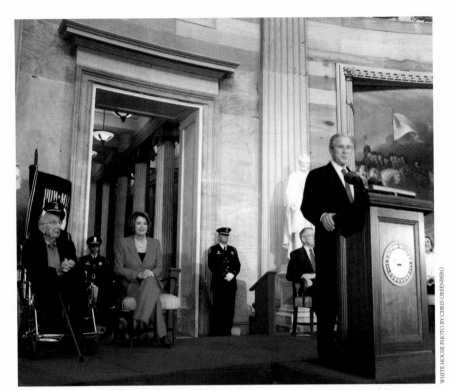

President George W. Bush speaking at the April 2008 ceremonial presentation of the
Congressional Gold Medal to Dr. Michael E. DeBakey in the rotunda of the U.S. Capitol.

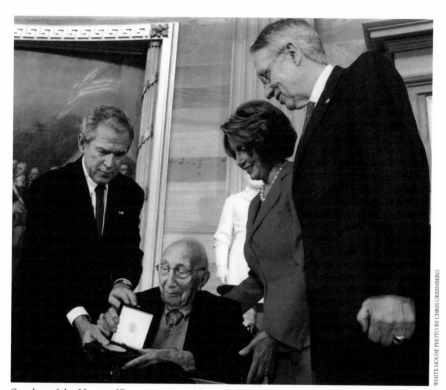

Speaker of the House of Representatives Nancy Pelosi and Senate Majority Leader Harry Reid joined President George W. Bush for the April 2008 ceremonial presentation of the Congressional Gold Medal to Dr. Michael E. DeBakey in the rotunda of the U.S. Capitol.

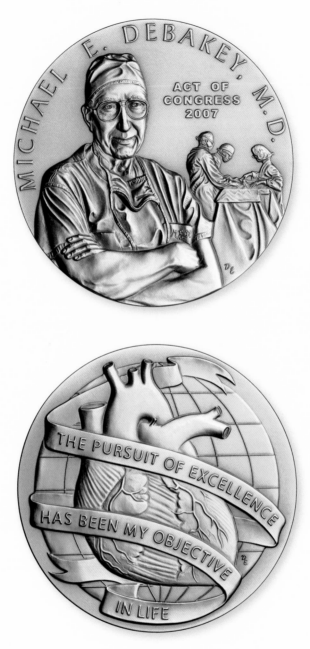

MEDAL DESIGNED BY UNITED STATES MINT SCULPTOR-ENGRAVER DON EVERHART.

The front and back of the Congressional Gold Medal presented to Dr. Michael E. DeBakey by President George W. Bush at the U.S. Capitol on April 23, 2008.

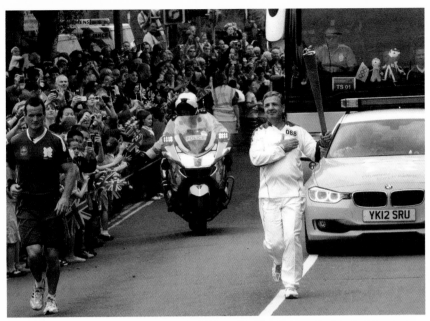

2112 Olympic Torch Relay participant Dr. William Zoghbi photographed in the historical town of Bicester, Oxfordshire, England, as he patriotically fulfilled his duty.

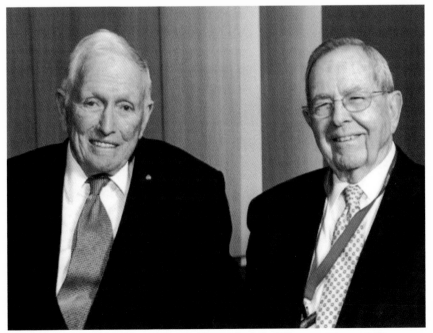

Dr. Denton A. Cooley and Dr. William L. Winters Jr. at the fifth annual Pumps & Pipes conference in December 2011.

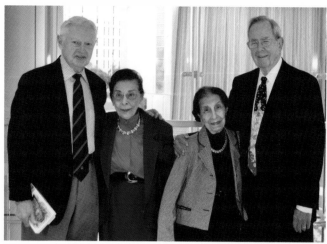

While visiting Houston in 2007, Yale University School of Medicine surgeon, educator, and acclaimed author Dr. Sherwin B. Nuland visited with Dr. Lois DeBakey, Selma DeBakey, and Dr. William L. Winters Jr.

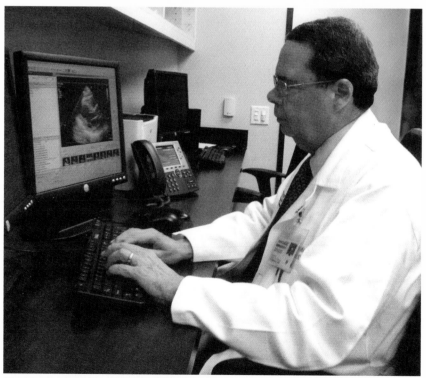

Shown at work in the echocardiography laboratory in 2007, Dr. Miguel A. Quiñones, chairman of the Department of Cardiology at The Methodist Hospital and medical director of the Methodist DeBakey Heart & Vascular Center.

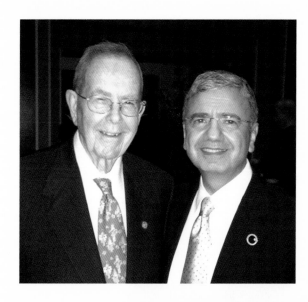

Former ACC President
William L. Winters Jr.
(1990) congratulated 2012
ACC President William
Zoghbi after his investiture
in Chicago.

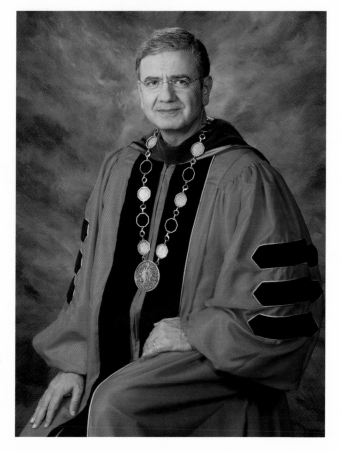

Dr. William Zoghbi
was installed in 2012
as President of the
American College
of Cardiology at its
annual convocation
in Chicago.

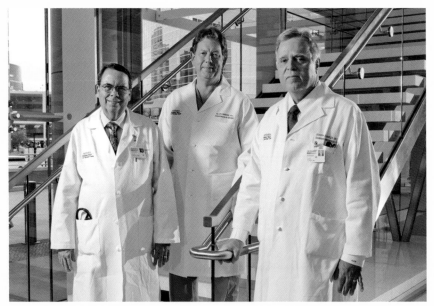

Photographed at the Methodist Hospital Research Institute in 2011, Dr. Miguel Quiñones, chairman of the Department of Cardiology, Dr. Alan Lumsden, chairman of the Department of Vascular Surgery, and Dr. Joseph J. Naples, chairman of the Department of Anesthesiology.

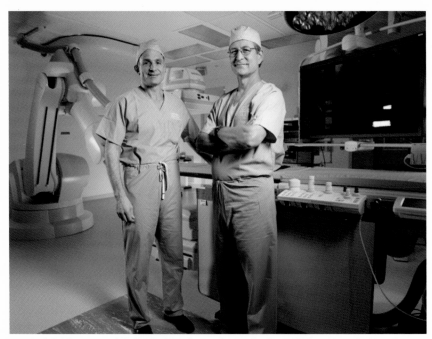

Dr. Neal S. Kleiman and Dr. Mike Reardon in the Methodist DeBakey Heart & Vascular Center hybrid catheterization laboratory in 2011.

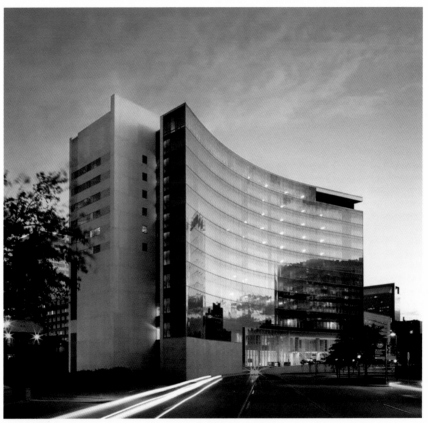

The Methodist Hospital Research Institute, founded in 2004 for the sole purpose of supporting, managing, and conducting clinical and translational research for the advancement of patient care, opened in 2010. The new building is located on Bertner Avenue at the site of the hospital's original entrance.

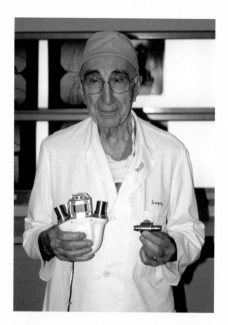

Dr. Michael E. DeBakey demonstrated
the difference between the miniaturized
MicroMed DeBakey VAD in his left hand
and first-generation device in his right hand.

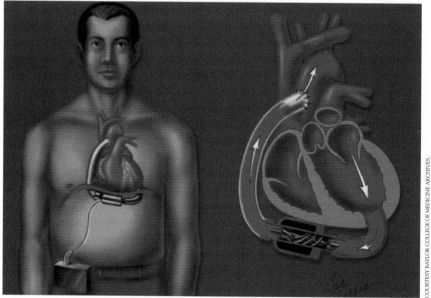

The first implants of the DeBakey VAD, the miniature continuous-flow device co-designed
with NASA engineers, were performed in November 1998 in Germany at the German
Heart Institute Berlin, where the chair and head of surgery Dr. Roland Hetzer performed
the implant with the assistance of Dr. DeBakey and Dr. Noon. These landmark cases were
the first ever of implantable rotary blood pumps to support long-term bridge to transplant
patients. In 1999, the DeBakey VAD was inducted into the U.S. Space Foundation's Space
Technology Hall of Fame.

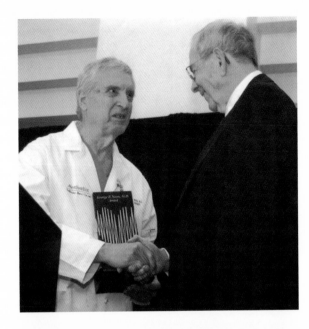

Dr. George P. Noon presented the first George P. Noon M.D. Award in March 2011 to Dr. William L. Winters Jr. in recognition of his leadership, service, and lifelong commitment to excellence in treating cardiovascular disease.

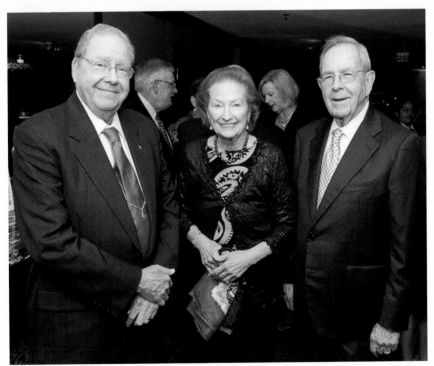

At a celebration held in his honor, Dr. Richard Wainerdi, who served as president and CEO of the Texas Medical Center for more than 28 years before stepping down in December 2012, reminisced with Barbara and Dr. William L. Winters Jr.

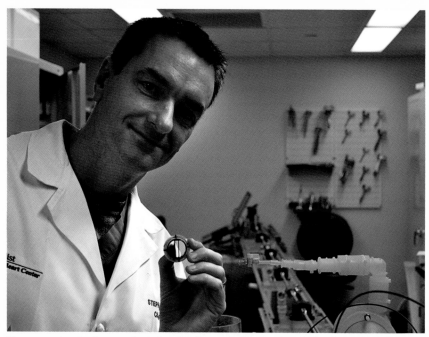

Demonstrating the latest technical tools of his trade, Dr. Stephen H. Little, medical director of the Valve Clinic and director of heart valve research at the Methodist DeBakey Heart & Vascular Center in 2013.

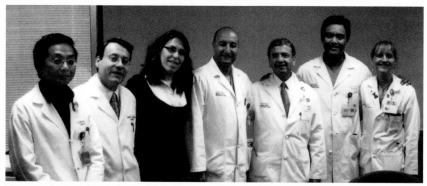

Photographed in the Methodist DeBakey Heart & Vascular Center Echocardiography Department in 2013 were (left to right) Dr. Su Min Chang, Dr. Sherif Nagueh, Dr. Sagit Ben Zekry, Dr. Selim R. Krim, Dr. William Zoghbi, Dr. Rey Percival Vivo, Dr. Karla Kurrelmeyer.

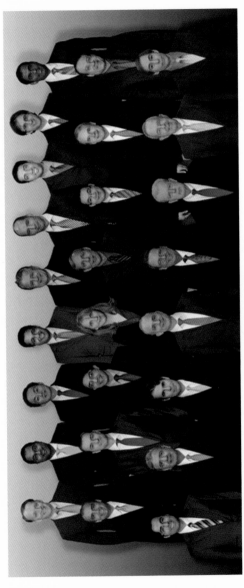

Methodist DeBakey Cardiology Associates in 2013 included (*left to right*):

Back row: Drs. Colin M. Barker, Sanjay Kunapuli, Su Min Chang, Amish S. Dave, George Schroth*, Miguel Valderrábano, Guha Ashrith, Barry H. Trachtenberg, Arvind Bhimaraj

Second row: Drs. Dipan J. Shah, Stephen H. Little, Faisal Nabi, Karla M. Kurrelmeyer, John M. Buergler, C. Huie Lin, Anton Nielsen, Sherif F. Nagueh

First row: Drs. Jerry D. Estep, William A. Zoghbi*, Guillermo Torre-Amione, Neal S. Kleiman*, Miguel A. Quiñones*, Craig M. Pratt*, William L. Winters Jr.*, John J. Mahmarian*

*25 years or more at *The Methodist DeBakey Heart & Vascular Center*

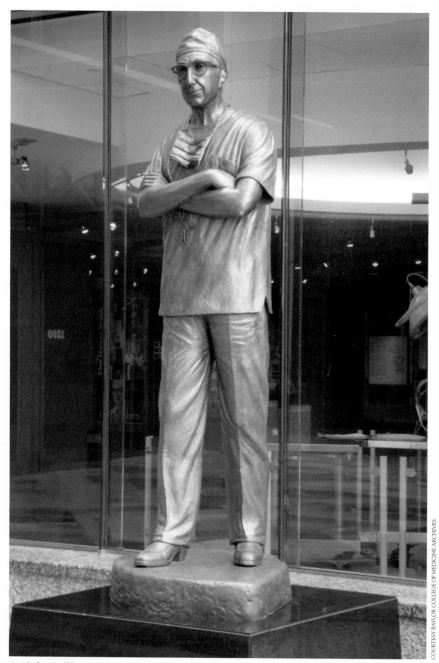

A 12-foot tall bronze figurative portrait of Dr. Michael E. DeBakey, by Texas sculptor Edd Hayes, was unveiled in May 2010 in front of the newly opened DeBakey Library and Museum at Baylor College of Medicine. Housed on the ground floor of the DeBakey Center for Biomedical Education and Research and open to the public, the resource center is a tangible tribute to the genius of Dr. DeBakey.

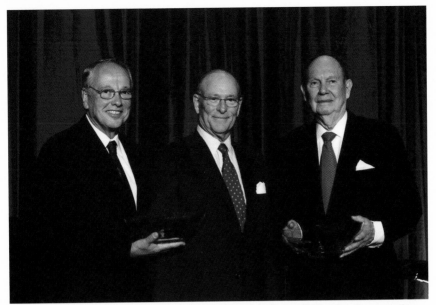

Ron Girotto (left) and John Bookout (right) receive the Ella and Walter Fondren award in November 2011 for their work as CEO and Board Chairman at Houston Methodist from David Underwood (center), grandson of the Fondrens.

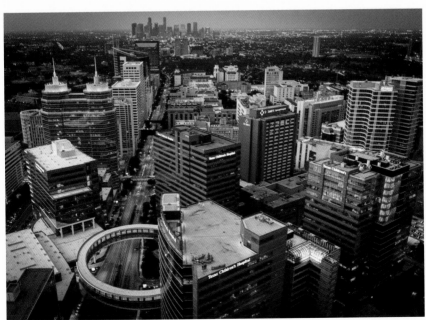

With downtown Houston in the distance, the 2013 Texas Medical Center was the largest medical complex in the world with 54 institutional members, eight hospitals, two medical schools, and Rice University.

COURTESY HOUSTON CHRONICLE

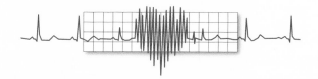

CHAPTER ELEVEN

THE ACADEMIC BUILDING BLOCKS
1969 - 1979

"Building blocks focus on making things better, not bigger."
H. JACKSON BROWN JR.

I n an ideal interdisciplinary center for cardiovascular research and training, as envisioned by Dr. DeBakey in the 1950s and presented to Congress in 1960, there was to be a capability of advancing knowledge and developing the most effective techniques and methods for the clinical management and prevention of cardiovascular disease through research, teaching, and patient care.[1]

The first embodiment of this concept was the Cardiovascular Research and Training Center at The Methodist Hospital, established by a $5 million, 10-year program project grant in 1960 from the National Heart Institute. In its first decade, the Cardiovascular Research and Training Center had become Baylor College of Medicine's financial lifeblood.[2]

The renewal of the National Heart Institute grant was to become one of Dr. DeBakey's top priorities as the first president of the newly independent Baylor College of Medicine. Beginning in 1969 and continuing through 1979, he and the medical school's board of trustees were to create an era of unprecedented growth, one that effectively laid the foundation for its future preeminence as a health science center.

Necessary for major federal and private funding for research efforts such as the Cardiovascular Research and Training Center was the recruitment of renowned physicians and research scientists to bolster the medical school's scientific credibility. Also of strategic importance to the future clinical management and prevention of cardiovascular disease at The Methodist Hospital was the strengthening of the medical school's Department of

Internal Medicine, in which cardiology was a subspecialty. Without a chairman since the departure of Dr. Pruitt in 1968, the department initially was under the administration of a committee of three senior faculty members, Drs. Harold Brown, Robert Hettig, and Daniel Jenkins. Eventually named "acting chairman" was Dr. Brown, who was to continue to serve in that position until the arrival of the new chairman.

To enhance recruitment efforts for a new chairman of the Department of Internal Medicine and the multiple other vacant chairs in 1970 was a revision in the medical school's new affiliation agreement with The Methodist Hospital. Approved by the boards of both institutions in January, a provision stated that newly selected chairs of clinical departments at Baylor College of Medicine also would become chiefs of clinical services at The Methodist Hospital.[3] In addition, anyone appointed a medical staff member at The Methodist Hospital must agree to become a member of the school's clinical faculty and assist in the teaching, research, and other services.

Though the full-time faculty welcomed these administrative changes mandated in the affiliation agreement, many among the clinical staff of private practitioners at The Methodist Hospital were reticent to approve it, expressing their fears of the loss of control of important professional decisions to the medical school.[4] Apprehensive that their "open staff" privileges were in jeopardy, more than 80 active staff members formed a coalition to seek an improved balance of power between the hospital and school. In an effort to thwart the immediate implementation of the new agreement, this coalition formed a committee to meet with the hospital's executive committee. To reach a compromise, their discussions were to continue for six months.

One notable exception to the skeptics among the private practitioners was Dr. Cummings, the Houston internist who not only served as the hospital's clinical chief of internal medicine since 1946 but had also been one of the persuasive advocates of the original affiliation with the medical school in the early 1950s. He was to seize an opportunity to demonstrate his enduring advocacy for maintaining close ties between the two institutions in 1970.

The opportune moment arose when the foundation of one of Dr. Cummings' patients pledged to endow a chair in internal medicine at Baylor College of Medicine. "For a long time I had been working on trying to get the medicine service, in some way, endowed so that we could really attract people of prominence and people who could relate better to other medical schools and hospitals across the country," Dr. Cummings said. "I was successful in getting Mr. R. E. 'Bob' Smith to make a contribution. He offered to give a million dollars to set up the chief of service, but, when the time came, he decided to make it two million, so, it came out all right."[5]

Reflecting Dr. Cummings' convictions, the resulting endowment from the Bob and Vivian Smith Foundation reiterated the institutions' new affiliation agreement. Included in its wording was the stipulation that the person occupying the Bob and Vivian Smith chair would serve both as chairman of the Department of Internal Medicine at the medical school and chief of the corresponding service at The Methodist Hospital.[6] "That's when we looked at various people from all over the country, had four or five of them visit down here," Dr. Cummings recalled.[5]

Offering to step down from his position at The Methodist Hospital once the ideal candidate to fill the chairmanship was selected, Dr. Cummings personified his support for both institutions' cohesive relationship. Such selfless efforts facilitated the successful recruitment of Dr. Henry Deane McIntosh, a distinguished academic cardiologist who served as chief of the cardiovascular division at Duke University School of Medicine.

In preliminary discussions of his taking over the chairmanship, Dr. McIntosh had advised the school's trustees that his acceptance was contingent on the implementation of the new affiliation agreement.[6] After the eventual approval of the compromise agreement by the hospital's clinical staff in June 1970, Dr. McIntosh became the first occupant of the Bob and Vivian Smith Professor and Chair of Internal Medicine at Baylor College of Medicine and chief of internal medicine at The Methodist Hospital.

In a gracious tribute to his predecessor at The Methodist Hospital, Dr. McIntosh said upon his July 1970 arrival, "It is a rare privilege and a tremendous opportunity to join Hatch W. Cummings and his colleagues in their untiring efforts to maintain quality undergraduate and graduate education and patient care at The Methodist Hospital." Noting how he planned to lean on Dr. Cummings for advice and guidance, Dr. McIntosh continued, "I am confident that the staffs of The Methodist Hospital and Baylor College of Medicine, and the citizens of Houston appreciate the quality and quantity of service that Dr. Cummings has rendered."[7]

Thus began a seven-year period at the Baylor College of Medicine in which the contributions made by Dr. McIntosh were to become legendary. As one colleague remembered, he was able to successfully recruit the best candidates to fill the vacant chairs in the department, create new sections, implement advanced training for residents, fellows, and post graduates, and thrust the internal medicine department into national prominence by "going through the Texas Medical Center as the 'Texas Tornado' others there claimed to be."[8]

Though his whirlwind of accomplishments began in his first few weeks on the job and was evident throughout his tenure, Dr. McIntosh's dogged determination to accomplish his mission was to have a polarizing effect. Seemingly impervious to others' opposing opinions of some of his contrarian ideas, he often was involved in heated discussions with his fellow faculty members as well as numerous private practitioners. Recalled Dr. Joseph M. Merrill, the medical school's executive vice president at the time, "He and I fought over many things, but there was never any question in my mind but that Henry intended building the strongest possible department of medicine for Baylor."[9]

Universally accepted by all parties was Dr. McIntosh's immediate establishment of a cardiology section in the Department of Medicine in June 1970. Having pledged to bring a "more meaningful arrangement" between The Methodist Hospital and Baylor College of Medicine, Dr. McIntosh began to augment the hospital's slender academic clinical cardiology staff during his first month as chairman.[6]

With the 1970 departure of Dr. Kinard, who accompanied cardiovascular surgeon Dr. Diethrich when he departed to establish the Arizona Heart Institute, there were only two remaining academic faculty members in clinical cardiology, Drs. Edward Dennis and Manus O'Donnell. Both Drs. Ben McCall and John Fitzgerald had departed for St. Joseph Hospital in downtown Houston. Recalling Dr. McIntosh's July arrival at The Methodist Hospital, Dr. O'Donnell said, "He arrived on the scene and proceeded to antagonize everyone in sight, but he didn't interfere with Dr. Dennis and me."[10]

As director of three catheterization laboratories, two on the ninth floor of the main building of The Methodist Hospital, Dr. Dennis was responsible for managing the increasing number of diagnostic cardiac catheterizations performed in the late 1960s and early 1970s. Coronary angiography was becoming a very important aspect of cardiac catheterization, so that hemodynamic studies were less emphasized and angiography was more emphasized. This was because the vast number of coronary bypass procedures being performed at that time by surgeons at The Methodist Hospital required more anatomic detail than the basic hemodynamic information.

In addition to performing angiograms on the coronary artery bypass patients in the catheterization laboratories, the cardiologists were responsible for whatever further testing was required for an accurate diagnostic evaluation. Should surgery be indicated, the cardiologists then became responsible for the patients' postoperative recovery and medical care. "In other words, we were the ones ultimately responsible for the outcomes," Dr.

O'Donnell explained. "That was DeBakey's philosophy, 'I got 'em out of the operating room alive and it's up to you to keep them alive.'"[10]

Since more than 10,000 coronary bypass procedures had been performed at The Methodist Hospital between 1964 and 1975, the cardiologists on staff, those in The Chapman Group, and other private practitioners often found themselves working around the clock. The high volume of coronary bypass surgeries was a testimony to Dr. DeBakey's widely published philosophy about this revascularization procedure's benefits. Following his 12th heart transplant in January 1970, Dr. DeBakey declared a moratorium on that procedure. Comparing his experience with 12 heart transplant patients, of which only two survived more than a year, to "the overwhelming success of the coronary bypass operation" in which patients "are free of discomfort and pain and able to go about their business," Dr. DeBakey concluded the new method of fixing hearts was preferable. Directly influencing that conclusion, he said, was his surgical team's successfully fixing the hearts of patients at The Methodist Hospital "who would have been candidates for heart transplants" a few years ago.[11]

A contrary point of view concerning the benefits of coronary bypass surgery already existed among a select group of cardiologists in the early 1970s. Prominent among them was Dr. McIntosh, who also began to question the increasing number of arteriograms performed in conjunction with the bypass procedures. He was not to speak publicly about his viewpoint until the late 1970s, but his colleagues were to become fully aware of his stance on both subjects much earlier.

Instead of immediately confronting those issues upon his arrival, Dr. McIntosh chose to concentrate his efforts elsewhere by creating a new laboratory for noninvasive diagnostic techniques. Named the Cardiology Diagnostic Laboratory and located on the fourth floor of the conjoined Fondren and Brown Buildings, known thereafter as the Fondren-Brown Building, it was designed to accommodate the performance of vectorcardiograms, electrocardiograms, treadmill exercise tests, cardioversions, and hydrogen electrode studies and echocardiography.

Serving as that laboratory's first director was one of Dr. McIntosh's first recruits, Dr. Kinsman E. "Ted" Wright Jr. A former colleague of Dr. McIntosh at Duke University Medical Center, where he had served his postdoctoral fellowship, Dr. Wright joined Drs. Dennis and O'Donnell on The Methodist Hospital clinical cardiology staff in July 1970. Clarifying his mission as director of the newly established Cardiology Diagnostic Laboratory, Dr. Wright stated: "The concept of noninvasive techniques has several hidden meanings. Since the procedures are done without insertion of catheters and take little time, they are relatively inexpensive and are available to large numbers of individuals. We plan to utilize the available techniques, develop new techniques, and apply them to the care of the hospital's inpatient and outpatient population."[12]

Because of an increasing demand at The Methodist Hospital for echocardiographic studies of valvular heart disease and artificial heart valves, and the function of the heart, an echocardiograph unit was included in Dr. Wright's laboratory. Even though it was a duplicate of the hospital's first echocardiography laboratory established the previous year in the basement by The Chapman Group, both laboratories were to operate independently throughout the early 1970s, eventually merging in 1977 with the arrival of Dr. Miguel Quiñones.

The next area of expertise in cardiology to be enhanced by Dr. McIntosh's recruitment efforts was cardiovascular research. Arriving with Dr. McIntosh from Duke in 1970 were two more cardiologists to join the Department of Internal Medicine at Baylor College of Medicine. The most senior, recruited to become chief of the new computer sciences section of the department created by Dr. McIntosh, was Dr. Howard K. Thompson. The other was Dr. Mark L. Entman, who joined the Cardiovascular Research Center as an investigator. Named chief of the cardiovascular sciences section of the Department of Medicine in 1977, Dr. Entman was to develop a highly productive laboratory research program in myocardial biology throughout the following three decades.[13]

Another of Dr. McIntosh's recruitments was to have a dramatic impact on the future of cardiology as well as all areas of medicine. Recruited to establish the genetics section at Baylor College of Medicine and to serve as its chief was Duke University School of Medicine graduate Dr. C. Thomas Caskey, who previously had served as senior investigator in the laboratory of biochemical genetics and head of the section of medical genetics at the National Heart and Lung Institute at the National Institutes of Health (NIH). Noting that the molecular and human genetics program initiated by Dr. Caskey was to become recognized as one of the most outstanding in the world, Dr. Merrill said, "Henry McIntosh, by recruiting Tom Caskey was responsible for introducing Baylor to the new genetics, one of the 'hot' areas of biological science at that time."[14]

From the NIH came another recruitment destined to have a major impact on the Cardiovascular Research Center. Culminating a two-year effort was the 1971 recruiting of Dr. Antonio M. Gotto Jr., who had been pursuing research related to cholesterol and lipoproteins at the NIH. A former Rhodes Scholar in biochemistry at Oxford University, where he earned his doctorate degree, Dr. Gotto subsequently had graduated Alpha Omega Alpha at Vanderbilt University School of Medicine and trained in internal medicine at Massachusetts General Hospital before joining the NIH.

The initial efforts to recruit Dr. Gotto to Houston had begun in 1968 with an invitation issued by a former colleague, Dr. Joseph Merrill. "When I was a medical student at Vanderbilt and rotating, making rounds, and a clerkship at the VA Hospital, I met Dr. Joseph Merrill, who subsequently left Vanderbilt, went to the National Institutes of Health (NIH), and then came to Baylor," Dr. Gotto said. "While I was at the NIH in 1968, he called me to see whether or not I would have any potential interest in coming to Baylor. I told him I had looked at a number of medical schools and that I was probably not going to leave NIH for at least another two years or more, but if he wanted to invite me down, I would be willing to come."[15]

His subsequent visit to Houston occurred in 1969 when there was no chief of medicine at Baylor College of Medicine and Dr. DeBakey had just become president. "The Department of Medicine was not structured enough at that time, I felt, for me to start out in," Dr. Gotto said afterward. "I felt I probably needed a more structured situation to begin my career. And so, it seemed to me that it would be better to wait until the department recruited a chairman and things got better organized."[15]

Upon Dr. McIntosh's acceptance of the chairmanship in 1970, Dr. Merrill once again contacted Dr. Gotto to invite him for a return visit to discuss the various departmental chairmanships available in the newly organized Department of Medicine. Determined to succeed in his efforts, Dr. Merrill recalled the motivating factor of his relentless pursuit: "To compete nationally, the Cardiovascular Research Center needed science, so Dr. McIntosh and I went after Dr. Gotto."[16]

Such enthusiastic interest was reciprocated during Dr. Gotto's second visit to The Methodist Hospital and Baylor College of Medicine. In discussions with Drs. Merrill, McIntosh, and DeBakey, Dr. Gotto defined his aspirations to develop both a basic research laboratory and clinical activities. With the clear intent of using basic biochemistry as a way of understating and treating disease, he stated his desire to have a section or division in the Department of Medicine in which he could carry out basic and clinical research on lipoproteins, lipoprotein structure, and metabolism and their relationship to cardiovascular disease.

When Dr. Gotto also expressed interest in having a clinical consultation service for patients with lipid disorders, "that brought me into direct negotiations and discussions with Mr. Bowen and others in The Methodist Hospital's administration," Dr. Gotto said. "My wife and I met with Dr. DeBakey in Washington and in repeat visits to Houston I met with Mr. Bowen and talked with him about setting up a lipid laboratory and lipid service. I had been impressed since my first visit in 1968 with the efficiency of the administration of The Methodist Hospital."[15]

In addition to persuasive conversations with Dr. DeBakey and Mr. Bowen, ultimately influencing Dr. Gotto's decision to accept the offer were the opportunities presented by the large population of patients with cardiovascular disease at The Methodist Hospital; the apparent limited activity in cardiology and preventative cardiology; the absence of concentrated areas in his chosen field; the efficient administration of the hospital; and the strong support and interest in the cardiovascular area expressed by the Houston community. "It's civic pride," Dr. Gotto said. "They think that the medical center is something that deserves their pride. They see people coming from all over the world for treatment and see recognition for the research that is done here and they take pride in it."[15]

Appointed a professor of medicine and biochemistry in 1971, Dr. Gotto was named chief of the newly created section on arteriosclerosis and lipoprotein research at Baylor College of Medicine and The Methodist Hospital and scientific director of the Cardiovascular Research Center, a position previously held by Dr. Merrill.

Within months of his 1971 arrival in Houston, Dr. Gotto applied for three new program grants. Competing with other medical centers for two new programs of the National Heart and Lung Institute, Dr. Gotto succeeded in obtaining grants for a Specialized Center of Research in Arteriosclerosis and a Lipid Research Clinic. His third application for a grant from the John Hartford Foundation also was successful. "This support, along with institutional support, helped us develop and build the program," Dr. Gotto said.[15] "Under Mr. Bowen's leadership, The Methodist Hospital provided the facilities and resources to house and support the Specialized Center of Research in Arteriosclerosis and the Lipid Research Center."[17]

In the provided facilities of the Fondren-Brown Building, sophisticated laboratories were developed for studying the structure and metabolism of the plasma lipoproteins. Dr. Gotto recruited Drs. O. David Taunton, Joel D. Morrisett, and Ellison Wittels to begin studies to determine the role of plasma lipoproteins in the development of arteriosclerosis and cardiovascular disease, determine how they are bound together, and investigate ways to prevent the accumulation of cholesterol in arterial walls. [18] Beginning in 1975, research activities in these laboratories were to include more than 15,000 laboratory tests, eventually growing to more than 25,000 in 1980.

As originally envisioned by Dr. Merrill, the contributions of Dr. Gotto were to significantly enhance the medical school and hospital's standing in the scientific community. Within three years of his arrival, the necessary resources were available for Baylor College of Medicine and The Methodist Hospital to respond to a new congressional mandate calling for the establishment of a National Heart and Blood Vessel Research and Demonstration Center.

Spearheaded by Drs. DeBakey and Gotto and enthusiastically supported by Mr. Bowen and the two institutions' boards, a proposal for the $13.3-million grant was submitted in 1973. "After a fierce competition among 25 leading academic centers, the National Heart and Lung Institute selected The Methodist Hospital and Baylor College of Medicine as the site for the nation's first National Heart and Blood Vessel Research Center," Dr. Gotto said, noting how the new center reflected Dr. DeBakey's 1960 vision of a multidisciplinary approach to combating cardiovascular disease. [17]

With plans to incorporate the Specialized Center of Research in Arteriosclerosis and the Lipid Research Center into the new research center, Dr. Gotto said, "This center differs from earlier ones in that it combines within one organization clinical and basic research, education programs for the general public, schools, health professionals, and finally, demonstration programs to test methods for rapid translation of medical advances into community practice. The establishment of the center has made it possible to coordinate cardiovascular activities from basic laboratory research to the bedside and to the community." [17]

During the formal dedication ceremonies of the nation's first National Heart and Blood Vessel Research and Demonstration Center in March 1975, its co-principal investigators, Drs. DeBakey and Gotto, who also served as its scientific director, announced plans for the imminent $5.5-million expansion of the Brown Building. Through the generosity of Albert Alkek, Mr. and Mrs. Don McMillan, and the DeBakey Medical Foundation, five floors were to be added within the coming year to house the center's expanding programs. Expressing his gratitude for the generous community support, Dr. DeBakey said. "One of the most important aspects of this center is that it has attracted more and more scientists to work with us in our efforts to combat cardiovascular disease." [19]

As the number of cardiovascular scientists at the center increased throughout the 1970s, Dr. McIntosh continued to recruit additional cardiologists to join the clinical staff at The Methodist Hospital. Serving as president of the American College of Cardiology in 1974, he traveled extensively to perform his duties, enabling his search for cardiology section candidates throughout the country. Included among those he recruited were research cardiologists Drs. James S. Cole and Henry G. Hanley and clinical cardiologist Dr. Assad Rizk.[20]

An abrupt alteration of the clinical cardiology staff occurred with the sudden August 1975 death of senior attending cardiologist Dr. Dennis. Since joining the faculty in the 1950s, the 52-year-old workaholic, known to begin work at 5:30 AM and continue until late in the night each day, successfully had created the foundation necessary for clinical cardiology's future substantial growth, one in which he was certain to play an integral role. While on a rare holiday away from the hospital, Dr. Dennis tragically succumbed to a cerebral hemorrhage.

His unexpected death stunned his colleagues, particularly Dr. O'Donnell. "He had just built a summer house in Maine, of all places, and he and his wife were taking their first vacation there," he recalled. "He went yachting with friends and was hit in the head by the boom. He wasn't knocked out, but it must have been quite a hit. He told his wife he was going to take a couple of aspirin and go to bed and in the middle of the night he had a massive cerebral hemorrhage and died. Having undergone heart valve surgery several years before, he was on Coumadin, the blood thinner, and after his post mortem in Houston, the pathologist confirmed the cause of death was a cerebral hemorrhage exacerbated by the Coumadin."[21]

Named immediately thereafter by Dr. McIntosh to assume Dr. Dennis's duties was Dr. O'Donnell. As interim director of the three catheterization laboratories at The Methodist Hospital, Dr. O'Donnell became responsible for some of the hospital's most trafficked diagnostic laboratories, ones in which the volume was to continue to escalate exponentially. As a harbinger of this phenomenon, following the 3,500 cardiac catheterizations performed in 1974, there were to be more than 7,000 performed in 1975.

The correlating escalation in diagnostic angiography in the hospital's catheterization laboratories during the mid-1970s mirrored that of coronary bypass surgeries. "At The Methodist Hospital, coronary bypass surgery was five years ahead of the rest of the country, maybe more, and the catheterization laboratories were the epitome of efficiency in cardiology," said Dr. Albert E. Raizner, recruited from Emory University School of Medicine by Dr. McIntosh in 1972. "The importance of coronary bypass surgery was well ingrained, sophisticated and well developed at The Methodist Hospital and in Houston in general. In fact, that was one of the major reasons I came here. It seemed to be light years ahead of what I had experienced—even at a very fine place like Emory in the early '70's."[22]

Rather than becoming a member of the clinical cardiology staff at The Methodist Hospital, Dr. Raizner began his Houston career at the Veterans Administration Hospital (VA). Working in the catheterization laboratory with "a great, great staff" that included Drs. Alfredo Montero, Robert Chahine, and Virendra Mathur, he patiently awaited his promised move to the clinical cardiology staff at The Methodist Hospital. "When I had taken the job originally, the initial plan was to spend several years at the VA and then move to The Methodist Hospital," Dr. Raizner said. "But Dr. McIntosh began a crusade at that time, thinking that there were too many cardiologists at The Methodist Hospital, so two years became three, three years became four, four years became five."[22]

Also affected by Dr. McIntosh's efforts to limit the number of cardiologists at The Methodist Hospital was a newly recruited member of The Chapman Group, Dr. William H. Spencer III, a former cardiology fellow at Duke University School of Medicine where he had graduated as valedictorian of his 1965 medical school class. While a fellow at Duke University Hospital, Dr. Spencer had spent one year in its catheterization laboratory where "we just did diagnostic coronary arteriograms and we thought if we did 18 a week that was the maximum workload." Recalling his amazement upon learning that many and more were done on a daily basis at The Methodist Hospital, he said, "Lord, it was all the difference of night and day."[23]

To Dr. Spencer's dismay, "When I first came here in 1972, Henry McIntosh had determined that he wanted The Methodist Hospital to have a closed staff and he was not going to grant 'cath' privileges to just anybody," he recalled. "And Henry had also tried to entice me to work for him and Baylor College of Medicine instead of The Chapman Group, and I think that also played into it. So Henry made me catheterize with one of my partners in the room or in the vicinity for a full year."[23]

Constrained by the inability to do catheterizations at will, Dr. Spencer sought the advice of Drs. Chapman and Winters as to what he should do. They suggested that he get involved with the implantation of artificial pacemakers, a surgical procedure that took place in the operating room in the early 1970s. More often than not, because of the surgeons' busy operating schedules at The Methodist Hospital, these procedures usually occurred at the end of the day. This predicament was much to the chagrin of the cardiologists, who often had to "wait until 7 or 8 or 9 o'clock at night to have a surgeon help us put in a pacemaker" and proved to be a strong incentive to change the process.[23]

In offering his assistance to the surgeons in the operating room, Dr. Spencer learned the intricacies of the pacemaker implantation procedure by both observation and hands-on participation. "The surgeon would isolate the brachial vein and put the pacemaker leads just a little bit in it, and then I would advance the lead down and position it in the apex of the right ventricle and make sure that the thresholds and sensing characteristics were satisfactory and then turn it back over to the surgeon, who would make the pocket and attach the generator and sew everything up," he said. "So that's what I did a lot of."[23]

These experiences with surgical pacemaker implantations in the operating room throughout the 1970s were to serve as the necessary foundation for Dr. Spencer's future endeavors in cardiac pacing, an emerging field that was to become known for rapid shifts in hardware and techniques.[24] Introduced in the 1950s, implantable pacemakers able to sense electrical activity in the heart as well as pace were to undergo myriad technological improvements in the following two decades. In tandem with the advances made in understanding the spectrum of arrhythmias arising from atrial disease, pacemakers were to become a major aspect of the broader transformation of cardiovascular medicine.

With the advent of a peel-away sheath, the cardiologist was able to provide percutaneous access to the subclavian vein. This development, plus the increasing complexity of pacemakers, led to the change of site for pacemaker implantation from the operating room to the catheterization laboratory. This effort, led by Dr. Spencer, revolutionized the practice of cardiac pacemaking at The Methodist Hospital.

The contributions made by Dr. Spencer were substantive and included: atrial ventricular (AV) sequential pacing, a method that never became mainstream[25]; subclavian vein angiogram to enable a safer means for correctly introducing the pacing catheters[26]; early investigator for the Cordis dual chamber pacemaker; and early investigator for dual chamber rate adaptive pacing and biventricular pacing for patients in heart failure.[27]

As the demand for more sophisticated devices to meet the evolving indications for artificial pacemaking began to increase in the late 1960s, the number of manufacturers multiplied. Soon each manufacturer began to offer unique technological innovations to differentiate its complex device from others in the market. However, a recurring problem with all devices was the short life of the pulse generator, a mercury-zinc battery with a 20- to 30-month lifespan. The inevitability of battery failure necessitated replacing all pacemakers every two years to preclude any catastrophic difficulties.

Even though the number of pacemakers implanted at The Methodist Hospital totaled less than 250 during a five-year period during the early 1970s, Drs. Wright and McIntosh expressed great enthusiasm about the device's benefits and guarded caution about its shortcomings. "The development of artificial pacemakers for the electrical control of the cardiac rhythm has greatly enhanced the physician's ability to treat cardiac dysrhythmias," they stated in a 1973 report. "The long-term management of patients in whom pacemakers have been implanted becomes progressively more complex. Any malfunction of the pacemaking system or deterioration of the pulse generator has the potential for serious consequences."[28]

To monitor the functional integrity of the various implanted devices and greatly expand the useful lifespan of each, Dr. Wright created the pacemaker evaluation laboratory, an extension of the cardiology diagnostic laboratory at The Methodist Hospital. When the laboratory's fully equipped clinic designed exclusively for pacemaker follow-up opened in November 1974, it was one of the first such clinics in Texas and was accessible to all Houston-area physicians' referred patients. Describing its services, Dr. Wright said: "The objectives are threefold: to keep the referring physician advised on the current status of his patient's generator; to be a source of information to the patient on matters regarding his pacemaker; and to gather data on the performance characteristics of each different pacemaker model."[29]

Rapidly improving the performance characteristics of pacemakers nationally was an innovation introduced in 1973, a long-lived pacemaker battery based on lithium chemistry. The lithium battery rapidly became the standard of every pacemaking device manufactured thereafter, a development that was to impact the field of cardiac pacing immeasurably in the late 1970s.

In the 30 years since the invention of the totally implantable artificial pacemaker, the number of patients implanted nationally was to rise from half a dozen in the 1950s to an estimated half-million in 1980.[30] Indicative of that trend, more than 480 pacemakers were to be implanted at The Methodist Hospital in 1975, twice the number implanted during the previous five years. When Dr. Wright left for Chattanooga, Tennessee in 1977, Dr. Spencer became director of the hospital's pacemaker clinic. Subsequently, the volume of pacemaker implantations was to increase substantially on an annual basis.

Also experiencing unbridled growth was the number of electrocardiograms processed in Dr. Wright's noninvasive diagnostic laboratory at The Methodist Hospital. In the laboratory's first decade, the number of electrocardiograms administered was to accelerate from 28,000 in 1970 to more than 57,000 in 1980. Another reflection of the average daily census of 200 cardiovascular patients during each year of that decade was the annual increases in the total number of noninvasive diagnostic cardiology tests performed, growing from 6,865 in 1975 to more than 11,000 in 1980.

As was the case in the catheterization laboratories, capacity levels had been reached in all other areas of service in the cardiology section at The Methodist Hospital in the mid-1970s. Even though there was an immediate need for additional physical space to house each area adequately, none was available in 1975. Having grown from 300 beds to 1,040 in its first two decades in the Texas Medical Center, The Methodist Hospital was using all existing space in its physical plant.

While future expansion plans for the hospital existed, none included the additional space required by the rapidly expanding cardiology section. Already in progress in 1975 was the construction of three major projects: the Neurosensory Center, a three-towered structure built adjacent to the Fondren-Brown Building to house the institutes of ophthalmology, neurology, and otorhinolaryngology and communicative disorders; the Total Health Care Center, a 21-story facility across the street from the hospital designed to meet the needs of outpatients; and the four-story Alkek Tower addition to the Brown Building to house the cardiovascular research programs of the National Heart and Blood Vessel Research and Demonstration Center.

The solution to the problem of overcrowding in the cardiology section of The Methodist Hospital presented itself in spring 1976. Announced by the board of trustees of the Fondren Foundation was a $7.4-million grant for the addition of six floors to the Fondren building. Including subsequent contributions from other major donors, the Catherine Fondren Underwood Trust and Houston Endowment, funding for the project was to total more than $10 million. Another major gift received from the Fondren Trusts enabled the furnishing of the new addition's twelfth-floor luxury suites in memory of Sue Fondren Trammel. Upon completion in 1979, at the request of the Fondren Foundation trustees, the 12-story building was to be rededicated to honor not only Mrs. Fondren, as before, but also her late husband, Walter W. Fondren.

At the time of the Fondren Foundation's announced grant in spring

1976, Mrs. Fondren had become a permanent resident of The Methodist Hospital. Ensconced in one of her favorite, corner rooms furnished with her belongings, the 95-year-old benefactress had around-the-clock nurses as well as the devoted attention of Mr. Bowen and members of his administration. Twice a week, one of the assistant administrators would escort Mrs. Fondren out of the hospital to one of her favorite restaurants for lunch. Because she was hard of hearing, one young administrator recalled how all others dining in the restaurant were able to eavesdrop effortlessly.

Many of those loud conversations centered on Mrs. Fondren's continuing, avid interest in the day-to-day operations of The Methodist Hospital. As to whether she was made aware of the overcrowded conditions in the cardiology section was not documented but entirely possible. As the guiding force behind her foundation's grant for the 1960 construction of the original building to house Dr. DeBakey's envisioned Cardiovascular Research Center, she undoubtedly played a major role in the Fondren Foundation's 1976 grant for its expansion as well.

Having been an active participant in the ribbon-cutting ceremonies for each new facility opened at The Methodist Hospital during its previous two decades, Mrs. Fondren planned to bring the sterling silver scissors she had purchased for such occasions to the 1979 rededication of the building bearing both her and her late husband's names.

Also making definitive plans for that building's completion were Dr. McIntosh and all the cardiologists at The Methodist Hospital. Embracing the "Fondren expansion" as their opportunity to create a centralized location for the cardiology section, they began to configure the plans accordingly. In the allotted space on the ninth floor shared with the pulmonary section, Dr. McIntosh carved out an area for cardiology offices. The ample additional space on that floor was allocated for Dr. Wright's greatly enlarged noninvasive diagnostic laboratory.

Planned for a major portion of the space allocated to the cardiology section on the tenth floor plans were three spacious heart catheterization laboratories and a recovery room. Nearby was to be an expanded medical intensive care unit (ICU) and coronary care unit boasting 24 beds and improved monitoring capabilities. In additional space provided on the 11th floor, there were to be patient beds for the exclusive use of the cardiology and pulmonary sections.

With construction projected for completion in 1979, these new areas in the Fondren expansion were to become tangible evidence of Dr. McIntosh's successful efforts to create, enhance, and expand the cardiology section at

The Methodist Hospital.

Having been equally involved in building and enlarging all the other sections in the Department of Medicine during his nearly seven years as chairman, Dr. McIntosh had succeeded in advancing academic development in the training of residents, expanding the program to include not only The Methodist Hospital and the other Baylor-affiliated facilities, Ben Taub General Hospital and the Veterans Administration Hospital (VA) but also St. Luke's Episcopal Hospital. Integrating the assignments of residents across the four hospitals, he also greatly expanded the teaching responsibilities of the voluntary faculty at each facility.

Enhancing the housestaff training program was a priority established by Dr. McIntosh upon his arrival in 1970. To stress the growing importance of caring for the critically ill, he implemented training programs in the newly created ICUs. Residents also began to receive essential training in the care of patients with cardiac crises from cardiologists in the coronary care unit and began to make rounds with pulmonary specialists in the medical ICU. In addition, in an area deemed insufficiently covered in the past by Dr. McIntosh, concentrated attention was given to "Code Blue," emergency care for acute cardiac patients.[31]

Integrated into Dr. McIntosh's academic development plan was an expanded education program in the study of lipid disorders inaugurated by Dr. Gotto at The Methodist Hospital in 1971. These efforts, coupled with his new team's ongoing scientific discoveries, were to effectively increase awareness of the importance of determining levels of blood lipids and the use of drugs and dietary management for treatment among residents and students.

By the fall of 1976, Dr. McIntosh's dedicated efforts had elevated the Department of Medicine's graduate-level training program for interns, residents, and subspecialty fellows to a position of national rank, where it was to remain for decades. With his constant input, participation, guidance, and support of the faculty, the quality of both the program and the trainees was to escalate in tandem. Having originally attracted 86 trainees in 1971, it was to grow to more than 185 in six years.

Immediately afforded national recognition when instigated in 1970 was the two-year, postgraduate training program in cardiovascular disease. Divided into four areas, the program was designed to address acquisition of clinical skills used in diagnosis, mastery of laboratory techniques, instruction and management of various types of heart disease, and opportunity for research.

Although the emphasis on research opportunities in a clinical training program was unusual, Dr. McIntosh believed its inclusion was essential. "The experience of identifying a problem worthy of study, going through the literature to see what is already known, working out a protocol, studying the protocol under skillful supervision, executing the necessary studies, evaluating the results and writing up the whole study for presentation to colleagues in verbal or written form is an important and instructive exercise," he said, noting he fully was aware it would either positively impact a trainee's future career in academic medicine or have no impact at all. "Some trainees have no interest in research and it is quite possible that their forced immersion in on-going investigative programs will be tedious and time-wasting for all concerned."[32]

Squandered time was anathema to Dr. McIntosh. "He was strongly motivated to develop and lead a successful program," said Dr. Edward C. Lynch, one of his colleagues in the Department of Medicine. "In pursuing his objective, he made a very high commitment of his personal time. In his more than six years as chairman, he may well have put in 10 years of chairman's work. He was an activist, with a direct approach to problems. Perhaps, at times, he should have walked around the wall rather than climb over it. But his approach usually worked."[33]

However, to those in the hospital's administration, Dr. McIntosh's propensity to confront problems head-on proved to be an annoying trait. "Keeping a good working balance between the full time faculty and the town physicians was always a challenge, and Dr. McIntosh tended to make decisions that disrupted that balance," recalled Michael Williamson, a hospital administrator. "Eventually, Dr. DeBakey and Mr. Bowen became disenchanted with him."[34]

Tactfulness notwithstanding, Dr. McIntosh's many accomplishments had become second nature to him. "I have met few men as well organized, persevering, and hard working as Henry McIntosh," Dr. Manuel Martinez Maldonado said, recalling the time he worked with him in Houston. "His loyalty and devotion to his faculty are difficult to match. His enthusiasm for the projects he felt were novel and exciting and those he wasn't so sure about that were carefully probed were responsible for his frequent successes."[8]

Also true to character was Dr. McIntosh's spontaneous decision to step down as chairman of the Department of Medicine in October 1976 "to get back to patients and teaching." Vowing to remain on staff as a professor of cardiology, he planned to work more closely with community programs that emphasized prevention of heart diseases. "The administration duties keep me from doing many of those things I think I do best," he explained. "Our department now is one of the strongest in the nation with a very large and strong house staff that serves in five affiliated hospitals, so I feel like I can think about turning over the administration to someone else."[35]

Primary among the multiple off-campus activities of Dr. McIntosh was an organization he founded, Heart Beat International, whose purpose was to provide new pacemakers to indigent people in developing countries. The program flourished and was endorsed and supported by Rotary International and InterMedics Corporation.

In recognition of his effort, Dr. McIntosh received a citation from President Ronald Reagan in a Rose Garden ceremony in 1986. He also was honored for his effort by receiving the North American Society of Pacing and Electrophysiology (NASPE) Distinguished Service Award in 1991. Also heavily invested in Dr. McIntosh's program was Dr. Spencer, who was actively involved until retiring in 2011.

Another crusade of Dr. McIntosh was directed to the tobacco industry, which he proclaimed as "The Seven Merchants of Death." It was a crusade he pursued until his dying day. He also remained active in activities of the American College of Cardiology as an Emeritus on the board of trustees. He would engage all who would participate in early morning jogs at each annual meeting—a ritual of his lasting many years.

Upon accepting Dr. McIntosh's resignation in 1976, Dr. DeBakey announced that a search committee would be formed to find his replacement. In the meantime, unburdened from the constraints of his chairmanship, Dr. McIntosh began to publicly participate in one of the medical community's most fierce debates. The catalyst for the controversy was the surgical procedure that had been known by many names since its inception in the 1960s: direct myocardial revascularization, distal coronary bypass, saphenous vein autograph replacement, coronary bypass surgery, to name a few. Eventually to become known as coronary artery bypass grafting and referred to by its initials, CABG, the operation was becoming a major bone of contention in the early 1970s, particularly between cardiologists and surgeons.

The basic quarrel was concerning the lack of scientific evidence to show that CABG was life prolonging or capable of preventing heart attacks. Studies to assess the long-term benefits of CABG were in progress, but they were not to be completed until the latter part of the 1970s. Consequently, those in the field of cardiology who were skeptical about the benefits of CABG began advocating a more conservative medical treatment of blocked arteries rather than surgery. By 1976, when more than 80,000 CABG surgeries were being performed nationally, these skeptics had become more vociferous in their avocation for a more cautious approach.

For more than six years at The Methodist Hospital, Dr. McIntosh discreetly had questioned the efficacy of CABG as well as the necessity for the volume performed. His discretion was understandable. Even though several nationally prominent cardiologists shared his opinions at the time, they starkly contrasted with Dr. DeBakey's oft-quoted praise of the successful results experienced with CABG at The Methodist Hospital.[36]

Such discretionary tactics were abandoned at a November 1976 American Heart Association symposium in Miami, as the resulting front-page story in *The New York Times* was to attest. "The evidence to date suggests, but does not prove life may be prolonged by bypass surgery," Dr. McIntosh reportedly said. Furthermore, the newspaper reported, he said bypass surgery should be limited to only those patients with crippling angina who did not respond to more conservative treatment because "I do not believe that in 1976 surgery is indicated for the asymptomatic patient."[37]

For Dr. McIntosh, this publicly stated opposition to the status quo was indicative of his tempestuous tenure at Baylor College of Medicine and The Methodist Hospital. Well known by his colleagues for imparting "the quote of the day," he had become the personification of one attributed to Theodore Roosevelt that was prominently displayed on his desk: "It is not the critic who counts; not the man who points out how the strong man stumbled, or where the doer of deeds could have done them better. The credit belongs to the man who is actually in the arena, whose face is marred by dust and sweat and blood; who strives valiantly; who errs and comes short again and again; who knows the great enthusiasms, the great devotions; who spends himself in a worthy cause; who at the best knows in the end the triumph of high achievement, and who at the worst, if he fails, at least fails while daring greatly, so that his place shall never be with those timid souls who know neither victory nor defeat."[38]

Because Dr. McIntosh was to continue to dare greatly without timidity, his career as a cardiologist at The Methodist Hospital was to be short-lived. Its conclusion followed his coauthorship of a comprehensive review of the first decade of CABG. Culled from more than 450 articles and scientific studies, the detailed manuscript was submitted for publication in 1977 but not published until March 1978.

Acknowledging that more than 300,000 CABG operations had been performed in the United States despite the ongoing controversy about the indications for its use, Dr. McIntosh and coauthor Dr. Jorge A. Garcia presented their manuscript in hopes "that the physician could better make intelligent decisions about the use of this procedure as a 'remedy' in the management of his patients."[39]

Stated in the manuscript's overview was the authors' summary, an affirmation of the skeptics' greatest concerns about CABG: "Despite a low operative mortality and rate of graft closure, available data in the literature do not indicate that initial symptomatic improvement necessarily persists, or that myocardial infarctions, arrhythmias, or congestive heart failure will be prevented, or that life will be prolonged in the vast majority of operated patients."[39]

This conclusion did not represent the consensus at The Methodist Hospital or Baylor College of Medicine, nor did a July 1977 nationally published editorial in which he announced the necessity for "state of the art" guidelines for the "accelerating use" of arteriograms. As the immediate past chairman of the American Heart Association's council on clinical cardiology, Dr. McIntosh reported that a committee of "carefully chosen" cardiologists had been deliberating such guidelines since 1975. This committee's recently submitted recommendations had, when possible, been based on published data rather than personal opinion because of the "divergent points of view by competent cardiologists as to the indications for coronary arteriography."[40]

Before either of these potentially controversial articles was published, Dr. McIntosh announced his plans to retire from academia, move back to his home state of Florida, and enjoy "the relative academic obscurity" of "practicing medicine at the grass roots of 'middle America' in Watson Clinic, Lakeland, Florida."[38] On June 10, 1977, his last day at Baylor College of Medicine, the chief residents honored his many contributions to residency training by establishing the Henry D. McIntosh Award to be presented annually to the outstanding resident in internal medicine.

Also to continue was the impact of Dr. McIntosh's creating and expanding the section of cardiology at The Methodist Hospital. In the decades to come, the programs he initiated were to flourish, ultimately becoming one of the key components of a cornerstone of the Methodist DeBakey Heart & Vascular Center.

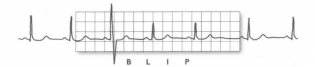

THE USSR ACADEMY OF SCIENCE

*I*n January 1973, Drs. DeBakey and Noon, along with Ellen Morris, Bonnie Noon, and June and Ted Bowen, traveled to Moscow to care for the president of the USSR Academy of Science, Mstislav Keldysh, the Soviet Union's highest ranking scientist. "The request for Dr. DeBakey came from President Leonid Brezhnev, the Minister of Health Dr. Boris Petrovsky, and Professor Eugene Chazow," Dr. Noon explained. "On January 10, 1973, we performed a bypass from the abdominal aorta to both external iliac arteries with a DeBakey Dacron bifurcation graft; bilateral femoral popliteal bypass above the knee with autogenous saphenous vein; bilateral lumbar sympathectomies and cholecystectomy. He had a satisfactory complete recovery."[1]

---

1. Winters, William L. Jr. (Methodist DeBakey Heart & Vascular Center, The Methodist Hospital, Houston, Texas). Personal correspondence with: Dr. George P. Noon (Methodist DeBakey Heart & Vascular Center, The Methodist Hospital, Houston, Texas). 2013 Apr

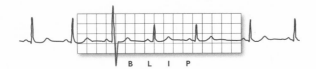

THE PACER CAR
ON THE INFORMATION FREEWAY

*W*hen the information superhighway became a freeway to biomedical information, Dr. DeBakey, as chairman of the National Library of Medicine
(NLM), was steering the pacer car along with Vice President Al Gore. At a
June 26, 1997, Capitol Hill press conference, the two of them announced free
public access to "Medline," the library's extensive database service introduced in
1971. Created at the recommendation of the President's Commission on Heart
Disease, Cancer and Stroke, chaired by Dr. DeBakey, the heretofore fee-based
service originally provided instantaneous, online bibliographic searching capabilities for medical schools, medical libraries, hospitals, and research institutions
around the country.

After the 1991 inception of the World Wide Web, Dr. DeBakey had be-
come an activist for the seemingly endless possibilities this advance presented to the
NLM. By 1993, the NLM had become one of the first federal web sites on the
World Wide Web. After President Bill Clinton and Vice President Gore's 1996
announcement about their commitment to the Next Generation Internet (NGI)
Initiative, based on research and development programs across federal agencies,
Dr. DeBakey advocated the library's inclusion.

To garner the national funding required to expand the library's Internet presence, Dr. DeBakey testified to Congress in early 1997: "I believe that it is absolutely essential that the Library be included in the so-called Next Generation
Internet program. I think there is no aspect of today's society that is more worthy
of reaping the benefits of the expanding national information infrastructure than
medical research and health care today. I believe that the health care professionals
and consumers should be able to tap into the most recent medical information, for
that is a public service, not a commodity. Even with all our modern advances in
health care, I still consider good information to be the best medicine. Mr. Chairman, I realize you must consider many worthy competing claims for the resources.
Nevertheless, I would suggest that a 9 to 10 percent increase in the National Library of Medicine over the fiscal year 1997 to support a health component in the

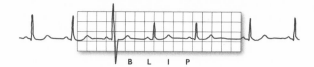

Next Generation Internet initiative and to improve access to health information would be in the Nation's best interest."[1]

As Dr. DeBakey predicted, the nation rapidly recognized its value in 1997. In the first month of free public access to the NLM "experimental" database, which later became known as PubMed, there were approximately two million searches. Today, the current daily average of searches on PubMed exceeds three million.[2]

1. Departments of Labor, Health and Human Services, Education, and Related Agencies: Appropriations for 1998. U.S. Government Printing Office website. http://www.gpo.gov/fdsys/pkg/CHRG-105hhrg41305/html/CHRG-105hhrg41305.htm. Accessed October 1, 2013.

2. PubMed turns 10. NLM In Focus: National Library of Medicine website. http://infocus.nlm.nih.gov/2006/01/pubmed-turns-ten.html. Created January 1, 2006. Accessed September 29, 2013

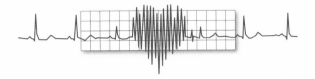

CHAPTER TWELVE

BEYOND THE STETHOSCOPE
1970 - 1980

"Whatever you can do or dream you can do, do it.
Boldness has genius, power, and magic in it. Begin it now."
GOETHE

In the early 1970s, although there had been significant progress achieved in surgical operations of the heart by Dr. DeBakey and other cardiovascular pioneers, disease of the heart and blood vessels was still responsible for the majority of all deaths in the United States.

Advances made during the previous two decades in terms of understanding cardiovascular disorders and improving medical care had produced the favorable developments of a reduced death rate in acute myocardial infarction, a decreased incidence of rheumatic heart disease, an increase in the survival in congenital heart disease, and extended longevity for patients with severe hypertension. However, even with the resulting reduction in death rates, overall mortality and morbidity due to heart disease remained the nation's leading health problem.

When one anticipated panacea, heart transplant surgery, proved to be impracticable due to the insurmountable problems of rejection and the chronic shortage of suitable donors, Dr. DeBakey concentrated his efforts in another direction. While continuing to perform the escalating number of CABG and myriad other cardiovascular operations, he announced in 1973 that finding the cause of heart disease would be a solution to the heart health problem, in terms of prevention, and was to be "the most significant factor for future research."[1]

Beginning in the early 1970s and fully endorsed by the American Heart Association, the prevention of atherosclerosis, or coronary artery disease, became the primary emphasis of cardiovascular research. One already-known method of preventing heart attacks and strokes had been advocated by Dr. DeBakey since the early 1960s but was relatively unknown by the public. In an effort to increase awareness, Dr. DeBakey had included a recommendation for a nationwide effort to increase the screening and treatment of high blood pressure in the 1965 Report of the Commission on Heart Disease, Cancer, and Stroke. This initiative had yet to be acted upon in 1972, and Dr. DeBakey once again capitalized on his previous lobbying experience by joining forces with fellow noble conspirator Mary Lasker to achieve this elusive goal.

Serving as chairman of the Lasker Foundation's newly formed Citizens for the Treatment of High Blood Pressure, one of the first health advocacy organizations to be formed around a specific chronic disease, Dr. DeBakey headed "a group of distinguished individuals who will marshal private and voluntary resources for professional and public education on the importance of early detection and treatment of high blood pressure."[2] Informally referring to themselves as "Citizens," this lobbying organization was successful in its mission, later recognized as being instrumental in the 1972 establishment of the National High Blood Pressure Education Program at the National Heart and Lung Institute (NHLI).[3]

With a collaboration of federal agencies, professional organizations, and voluntary resources, the Citizens also were responsible for the launch of a nationwide advertising and public awareness program to alert both consumers and physicians to the dangers of high blood pressure, a leading cause of heart attacks and strokes. Describing hypertension as a "silent killer" with virtually no symptoms and warning that "half the people who have it don't know it," the campaign urged individuals to have their blood pressure checked and, if required, controlled by medication and diet.[4]

The Citizens also successfully urged Congress to enact legislation to establish the National Heart, Blood Vessel, Lung, and Blood Act of 1972, the legislation that authorized the 1974 creation of the nation's first National Heart and Blood Vessel Research and Demonstration Center at the Baylor College of Medicine and The Methodist Hospital.[5]

As the co-principal investigators of that multidisciplinary center in Houston since its 1974 creation, Drs. DeBakey and Gotto had endeavored to bring together heart disease research with a broad-based community effort aimed at prevention. Embracing the philosophy "that prevention is the only way to significantly reduce death and sickness from heart disease and that prevention requires an informed and motivated public," Drs. DeBakey and Gotto coauthored a book that was critically praised as providing the layman "with a concise, authoritative guide to the cardiovascular system, how it functions, and what can go wrong and why."[2]

Published in 1977 and detailing what had been learned in the previous 25 years about the diagnosis and treatment of heart disease, *The Living Heart* was one of the first books to address in layman terms what could be done to prevent, contain, or repair damage to the heart or blood vessels.[6] Exposure of the book and its message was greatly enhanced when newspapers throughout the country published a serialization of its contents and syndicated columnist Ann Landers described the "superb book" which "will help you understand the function and value of your heart and may well add years to your life."[4]

It was these two heart specialists' collaborative efforts to increase public awareness of heart disease prevention, in tandem with the established national and international reputation of the cardiovascular center at The Methodist Hospital, that served as a catalyst in bringing together 210 physicians, scientists, educators, communicators, and support staff to the multidisciplinary research and demonstration center at The Methodist Hospital and Baylor College of Medicine.

The influx of skilled scientists who had the ability, training, and background to do cardiovascular research was indicative of one of Dr. DeBakey's many successful missions as president of Baylor College of Medicine. Upon taking office in 1968, he had realized "the only way we were going to improve the standards of the college was to bring in some new people."[7]

Throughout Dr. DeBakey's tenure as president of Baylor College of Medicine in the 1970s, he concentrated on recruiting the most outstanding candidates to help build the college. "I think you should put your money where the track record shows that it works best—in people who pursue excellence in the field, can innovate, and do good research," he said. "Concentrate on excellence. Concentrate on innovation. Concentrate on making advances, and you will get recognition, and you will get patients, no matter what."[7]

The embodiment of Dr. DeBakey's recruitment philosophy had been Dr. Gotto, who consistently had undertaken breakthrough studies since the 1971 establishment of the Specialized Center of Research in Arteriosclerosis and the Lipid Research Center at The Methodist Hospital. Recognized nationally and internationally for his laboratory's research on the structure and function of plasma lipoproteins and for accomplishing the first total synthesis of apolipoprotein C-1 in 1975, Dr. Gotto and his associates also had developed the theory of the amphipathic helix to explain the mechanism by which the blood fats are bound and transported.[8]

These noteworthy contributions to scientific research were the first of many to be made by Dr. Gotto and his associates during the following two decades, during which he would become internationally recognized as an authority on atherosclerosis and abnormalities of cholesterol metabolism. Although Dr. Gotto had been on staff for only six years in 1977, many of his colleagues had anticipated he would be selected to assume the leadership role unexpectedly vacated by Dr. McIntosh. "He had developed excellent relationships at Baylor College of Medicine," said Dr. Edward Lynch, recalling Dr. Gotto's collaborative efforts with Dr. DeBakey and various department chairmen. Also obvious to his colleagues was the fact Dr. Gotto "was highly regarded by the leaders of The Methodist Hospital, in particular by the president, Mr. Ted Bowen."[9]

The subsequent appointment of Dr. Gotto as chief of internal medicine at The Methodist Hospital and chairman of the Department of Medicine at Baylor College of Medicine was effective in February 1977, four months after Dr. McIntosh stepped down to become a member of the cardiology staff at The Methodist Hospital. After announcing he was going to continue in his capacity as a professor of atherosclerosis and lipoprotein research, Dr. Gotto appointed Dr. Lynch to serve as associate chairman of the Department of Medicine and associate chief of the medical service at The Methodist Hospital.

After assuming his new responsibilities, Dr. Gotto immediately began to recruit candidates to become the newest leaders of many of the subspecialty sections of the department. To those already recruited by Dr. McIntosh, Dr. Gotto sent reconfirmation letters to advise of the transition in leadership. One of the recipients was Dr. Miguel A. Quiñones, a former cardiology fellow at Baylor College of Medicine who had been recruited the previous December by Dr. McIntosh to become the new director of the cardiology noninvasive laboratory at The Methodist Hospital. "He had already stepped down as chairman at that time, so I had no illusions," Dr. Quiñones said. "I heard from Dr. Gotto the following April or May informing me he was taking over as chairman and he was looking forward to my coming back."[10]

It was a sentiment shared by Dr. Quiñones. After spending 90 percent of his fellowship at Ben Taub Hospital with Dr. James Alexander and an additional six months in the catheterization laboratory at the Texas Heart Institute at St. Luke s Episcopal Hospital between 1971 and 1974, he enthusiastically looked forward to becoming a member of the cardiology staff at The Methodist Hospital.

Since each of Baylor College of Medicine's affiliated hospitals had an independently structured fellowship program until 1977, Dr. Quiñones had spent little or no time at The Methodist Hospital during his training, a circumstance that appealed to him at the time. "If you were a cardiology fellow at The Methodist Hospital, you got to see a lot of different cases, but because of the volume, there were a lot of things missing academically," he said, recalling how taking care of all of Dr. DeBakey's cases had monopolized the cardiologists' time. "Back then, the best track for an academic interested in a research career was at Ben Taub."[10]

Whether to continue that academic career path was the question Dr. Quiñones faced at the completion of his military commitment in 1977. "I was not completely sure I wanted to spend my life in academics," he said, recalling his initial conversations with Dr. McIntosh about his possible return to Houston. "I had been very successful in my training years in academics, but I also loved taking care of patients. I knew that at any point I could decide to convert and go into private practice. There was no question that if I was going to give academics a try, I had to be at The Methodist Hospital, where the action was. Actually, it was the only way I would have come back."[10]

In addition to securing the return of Dr. Quiñones, the previous efforts of Dr. McIntosh to build an academic-oriented Department of Cardiology at The Methodist Hospital and Baylor College of Medicine had included the recruitment by Dr. Antonio Gotto of its first chief of cardiology, Dr. Richard Miller. A senior faculty member at the University of California at Davis, one of the powerhouses in cardiology at the time, Dr. Miller was scheduled to assume his position in August 1977.

The simultaneous arrival of Drs. Miller and Quiñones during the first week of August marked the beginning of the transformation of the cardiology area at The Methodist Hospital into an academic center of excellence. Eager to establish their new positions, both cardiologists were surprised to find themselves immediately immersed in the day-to-day activities of one of the largest cardiovascular centers in the world. "On day one we both had consults from Dr. DeBakey," Dr. Quiñones said, recalling his initial excitement of interacting with the legendary surgeon. "So, for me, being 33, to be a consultant to Dr. DeBakey was like being a kid in a candy store. It was fantastic."[10]

At the age of 69, Dr. DeBakey still traveled all over the world, still testified in Washington and the state capitol of Austin, and still performed multiple operations at The Methodist Hospital. While maintaining a hospital patient population that often exceeded 100 on a daily basis, Dr. DeBakey followed an established pattern for a majority of his cardiology consultations in 1977. "He mostly used the Baylor academic group, in particular, Manus O'Donnell," Dr. Quiñones said. "Following the death of Dr. DeBakey's number one cardiologist, Ed Dennis, Manus inherited Dr. DeBakey's patients. Manus was a very, very experienced, astute clinical cardiologist. He could take care of the sickest of the sickest. He would take care of the richest and the poorest."[10]

After becoming known as "one of Dr. DeBakey's favorite cardiologists," Dr. O'Donnell was to be involved in the medical management of such well-known patients as bandleader Guy Lombardo, movie star Marlene Dietrich, comedian Jerry Lewis, prizefighter Joe Lewis, baseball legend Leo Durocher, and abdicated King Leopold of Belgium, who, with Princess Liliane, commissioned a four-foot bronze bust of Dr. DeBakey. Dedicated in 1978 and depicting the surgeon in surgical hat and gown with his hands folded across his chest, the statue subsequently was placed in the atrium lobby of the Dunn Tower of The Methodist Hospital.

As for another type of monumental occasion that occurred in the 1970s with one of Dr. DeBakey's patients, Chicago mob leader Sam Giancana, Dr. O'Donnell was not involved. "Ed Dennis took care of him," Dr. Quiñones explained, recalling the newsworthy events that followed that surgery during the summer of 1975. "He had a very simple gall bladder or something similar done and was discharged. The nurses loved him because he gave them presents, but about a week later he was murdered in his home. Somebody let him in and they shot him in the back of the head and that was the end of Sam."[11]

Regardless of his patients' fame or lack thereof Dr. DeBakey treated all "with the same dedication to the relief of human pain and suffering," Dr. Gotto said. "He and I traveled together often, and whether we were in Turkey, China, or Russia, he would be approached by people who thanked him for saving or extending the life of a spouse, child, or loved one. He treated the rich, the famous, and the powerful, and he treated the poor and humble, too."[12]

Included in Dr. DeBakey's vast number of cardiovascular operations performed in the 1970s was a steadily increasing number of CABG operations, the efficacy of which remained an ongoing debate in the medical and surgical fields. The controversy centered on the conflicting answers to two questions: does it prolong life and does it improve quality of life? When the results of the 1977 Veterans Administration (VA) Cooperative Study of 1,000 patients at 13 hospitals were published, stating it found no benefit of surgery for patients whose disease was not extensive, Dr. DeBakey vociferously questioned the validity of its findings.[13] The published report's finding that the mortality rate in bypass surgery was two or three times higher than had been reported by major heart centers was particularly objectionable to not only Dr. DeBakey but also to many other cardiovascular surgeons who found such a conclusion to be distorted.

When the lay media highly publicized the VA study's results, it "not only created considerable controversy within the medical community, but also caused confusion and concern among patients," Dr. DeBakey said. Challenging the study, Dr. DeBakey published his own 13-year assessment of CABG in the February 27, 1978, issue of the *Journal of the American Medical Association*. "That the preliminary study of a small, highly selective group of patients operated on by surgeons with variable experience and observed for a mean interval of only 21 months should have received such enormous attention indicates the passion and partisanship that have enveloped this subject," he stated. "In most major medical centers such as ours, with more than a decade of extensive experience with both medical and surgical treatment of coronary-artery disease, careful analysis with good follow-up evaluation has provided sound criteria for determining the appropriate method of therapy for individual patients."[14]

In Dr. DeBakey's opinion, the limited number of surgical patients included in the VA Cooperative Study further compromised the validity of its conclusions. "Remember that there were seven patients per year in the 13 hospitals contributing to that study," he stated in a speech made to the American Society of Contemporary Medicine and Surgery in 1978. "We are doing seven bypass operations every day."[15]

Among this decidedly larger number of cases at The Methodist Hospital, Dr. DeBakey pointed out that fewer than 2 percent of his CABG patients died in the hospital, and 92 percent were "living as long as their counterparts in the general population of the same sex and age." Without corrective surgery, in his opinion, these patients would be unable to earn wages or pay taxes. "In other words," he said, "They have been restored to a normal life span."[15]

Since the life expectancy estimates in the United States had been revised in 1977 by the U.S. Census Bureau to add four years to the projected life span of females and almost three years more for males, the beneficial results of CABG encompassed an ever-aging population.[16] Although the projected increase in life span reflected a 10 percent drop in the mortality rate for heart disease in the previous seven years, cardiovascular disease still remained the leading cause of death in the United States with more than one in every three deaths attributable to heart attacks, amounting to more than one million annually.[17]

Nationally, there was increased awareness of the ability of individuals to control their own lives intelligently to prevent heart disease. When medical studies in 1977 also indicated that the rate of treatment for hypertension was twice the number reported five years earlier, Dr. DeBakey credited this achievement to the public awareness increased by the education campaign mounted in the early 1970s. "We know that hypertension or high blood pressure is a very important risk factor that contributes significantly to heart disease," he stated, urging the public to accept medical advice to take measures about the other known factors and to quit smoking, reduce weight, and exercise more to fight heart disease. "This is one factor we are beginning to control with the proper education of the public about hypertension, with much better drugs to control high blood pressure."[18]

With more than one in every three deaths in the United States attributed to heart attacks, extensive research into methods of prevention, diagnosis, and treatment of cardiovascular disease remained a priority at The Methodist Hospital. In order to fulfill the mandate of Drs. DeBakey and Gotto to substantially strengthen the hospital's cardiology clinical research program, Drs. Miller and Quiñones had to assemble a new team of clinicians and research scientists. "When we arrived, the only other cardiologist on the faculty besides Dr. O'Donnell was Dr. Mohammed Attar, who had completed his fellowship training at The Methodist Hospital and remained on staff as junior faculty," Dr. Quiñones said. "Mohammed had no interest in research, but he was terrific clinically. Basically, the three of us worked for Dr. DeBakey clinically and Rich and I started doing whatever research we could do while we gradually began to recruit new faculty."[10]

One source of future cardiology staff members was to be the greatly enhanced training program previously implemented by Dr. McIntosh at Baylor College of Medicine. Instead of training only in one hospital, as Drs. Quiñones and Attar had in the past, a growing number of fellows rotated between all of the college's affiliated hospitals for two years. Also new to the enhanced training program was an additional, mandatory year of research.

Even though a majority of the fellows was expected to go into private practice, the ability to conduct meaningful research was considered a necessary skill in the practice of cardiology, both privately and academically.

"We believed that during your formative years, if you spend some time in research it would pay off because you would become a different kind of doctor in the community because you have learned to be more scholarly; you have learned to appreciate science; you also have learned how to interpret science; and you were not just going to be persuaded by anything that somebody just writes or tells you about," Dr. Quiñones said, echoing a mindset promulgated by Dr. McIntosh nearly a decade earlier. "So you will become a thinker; you will become a better physician."[10]

To meet the immediate need to increase the clinical research capabilities at The Methodist Hospital, Dr. Miller recruited a former colleague who had been a junior faculty member at the University of California at Davis, Dr. Craig Pratt. Subsequently named director of the hospital's coronary care unit (CCU) in 1978, Dr. Pratt became responsible for the newly expanded 24-bed unit on the tenth floor of the Fondren-Brown Building. First established in 1970 as a five-bed area located in the medical intensive care unit, the new CCU provided specialized, immediate care for patients during the first three to four days following an acute myocardial infarction, the critical time period in which 75 percent of the deaths in such hospitalized patients occurred.

Also admitted directly to the CCU were patients with cardiac syncope, cardiac pacemaker failure, acute hypertensive crisis, shock related to heart failure, cardiac arrhythmias, possible dissecting aneurysms, and other possible, catastrophic situations involving the cardiovascular system. High nurse-patient ratio and sophisticated monitoring equipment provided an opportunity for the optimal recovery of each patient. When the risk of mortality was reduced, the CCU transferred the patient elsewhere

While there had been ongoing investigations into the unresolved medical problems experienced in the CCU since its inception, there had been a paucity of structured research undertaken. In February 1978, Dr. Miller began to aggressively pursue an opportunity to participate in a clinical trial sponsored by the National Heart, Lung, and Blood Institute (NHLBI). Announcing that it was accepting applications, the NHLBI described the first clinical trial as one designed to determine whether the regular administration of the beta-blocker drug propranolol to people who had had at least one documented acute myocardial infarction would result in a significant reduction of mortality from all causes over the follow-up period.[19]

Approved in September 1978 by the NHLBI as one of the 37 principal investigators in the national double-blind clinical trial known as the

Beta-Blocker Heart Attack Trial (BHAT), Dr. Miller effectively paved the path to countless future clinical trials as well.[19] The enormity of his accomplishment did not go unrecognized by his colleagues, particularly Dr. Quiñones. "That clinical trial was a big thing, because it had never happened before in cardiology at The Methodist Hospital," he said. "There was a lot of basic research going on, but very little clinical. Craig Pratt was the person who got directly involved with it and actually we ended up being one of the centers that enrolled the most number of patients in that trial. We had a very successful participation in that trial."[10]

Participants in Dr. Pratt's study had been recruited while in the hospital for acute myocardial infarction. That the number of volunteer patients at The Methodist Hospital far outnumbered those in the 36 other study centers was indicative of the established volume of cardiovascular cases treated therein. Once the availability of this patient population was established, the BHAT was to be followed by many pioneering studies conducted by Dr. Pratt in The Methodist Hospital's CCU..

In the coming three decades, Dr. Pratt was to publish more than 200 scientific journal articles, books, and book chapters, garnering an international reputation for being a "cardiologist with a proven background in advancing ECG applications and investigating the cardiac impact of pharmaceuticals."[20] As an appointee, at the recommendation of Senator Lloyd Bentsen of Texas, Dr. Pratt was a member of the Food and Drug Administration Committee on Cardiovascular and Renal Drug Advisory Committee from 1986 to 1987, serving as chairman between 1987 and 1993. At The Methodist Hospital and Baylor College of Medicine, Dr. Pratt focused his research on the development of new drug and device therapy for the treatment of arrhythmias, heart failure, ischemia, and hypertension. He frequently received awards for excellence in teaching.[21]

In tandem with the introduction of new drug and device therapies in the cardiology section at The Methodist Hospital, numerous advances were made in noninvasive diagnostic techniques for cardiac disorders in the late 1970s. Of particular interest to Dr. Miller and all the cardiologists at The Methodist Hospital was the potential for clinical information made evident in myocardial perfusion scans that used an intravenous injection of thallium-201 chloride in combination with exercise on a treadmill. This use of technologies such as CT scanning combined with infusions of radioisotope markers, to create highly detailed two-dimensional and three-dimensional views of the heart was to mark the beginning of nuclear cardiology, a term that heretofore did not exist.

Although only introduced in 1976, the thallium stress test already was a familiar diagnostic procedure to Dr. C. James Costin, a new member of The Chapman Group. He had trained with one of the cardiologists credited with the first documented stress myocardial perfusion imaging studies, Dr. Barry L. Zaret at Yale University School of Medicine. Recognized as one of the founders of nuclear cardiology, Dr. Zaret had introduced the use of CT scanning combined with infusions of radioisotope markers to create highly detailed two-dimensional and three-dimensional views of the heart.

Nuclear cardiology was to begin in Houston one year after its national introduction. Required for the testing was a Baird atomic first-pass camera and one of the first in Houston was delivered to the office of The Chapman Group, who began to offer office-based nuclear stress tests in 1977. Such an innovative idea turned out to be prescient, since the concept eventually was implemented throughout the country.

When referrals to The Chapman Group for the nuclear stress tests rapidly multiplied, an alternate location was necessary to accommodate the demand. "Our group became concerned regarding the scheduling of out patients in our office since the schedule became cluttered with so many referrals," said Dr. W. Richard Cashion, who gained clinical experience with Dr. Costin in the tests, handling isotopes and performing and interpreting studies. "A decision was made in our office to move the equipment to The Methodist Hospital. When one looks back on that decision and the current and prior reimbursements for nuclear stress tests, it's interesting that our group gave it to the hospital—we gave up a huge income producer."[22]

Upon receipt of the donated nuclear equipment in 1978, Drs. Miller and Quiñones created space in the plans for the cardiology noninvasive laboratory on the ninth floor of the Fondren Building, naming the new area the Radioisotope-Cardiac Laboratory. "There was a huge controversy with radiology and nuclear medicine at The Methodist Hospital regarding that laboratory," Dr. Cashion said. "I was low man on the totem pole and did not participate in those discussions, but Tony Gotto was instrumental in accomplishing the establishment of nuclear cardiology at The Methodist Hospital."[22]

Recalling those initial discussions, Dr. Quiñones attributed the desired outcome to both Dr. Gotto and Dr. Miller: "We were one of the first places in the country to do nuclear cardiology. From day one, it was in the noninvasive cardiology laboratory and belonged to cardiology; everywhere else in the country it belonged to either radiology or nuclear medicine. Rich Miller recruited the first nuclear cardiologist on the Baylor College of Medicine staff at The Methodist Hospital in 1978, Dr. Lawrence A. Reduto."[10]

A former American Heart Association fellow at Yale-New Haven Hospital, Dr. Reduto had trained with Dr. Zaret and the pioneering cardiologists credited with the first stress myocardial perfusion imaging studies documented in the early 1970s. Named co-director of the CCU with Dr. Pratt in 1978, Dr. Reduto also became the director of the new Radioisotope-Cardiac Laboratory at The Methodist Hospital.[23] Although he was expected to spearhead the development of nuclear cardiology at the hospital, his tenure was brief, less than two years, and other cardiologists were to become instrumental in accomplishing that mission. Prominent among them was Dr. Cashion, who continued to demonstrate his avid interest in the emerging subspecialty.

Wishing to enhance his more than 600 hours of time invested in performing nuclear stress tests with Dr. Costin in The Chapman Group office, Dr. Cashion sought further training and enrolled in a six-week, basic science course in nuclear medicine at Bethesda U.S. Naval Hospital in 1979. "I took a course of intensive training handling radioisotopes and radiation safety that concluded with a certifying examination," he recalled. "I returned to Houston and then spent several months with Dr. John Burdine, director of nuclear cardiology in nuclear medicine at St. Luke's Episcopal Hospital."[22]

The emerging concept of nuclear cardiology also had garnered the rapt attention of Dr. Mario S. Verani, director of the Hemodynamics Laboratory at the VA Medical Center in 1978. The cardiologist was to become so intrigued with the limitless possibilities of nuclear cardiology that he decided to devote the rest of his career to this new field. "Among the recently developed diagnostic techniques in cardiology, cardiac scanning procedures play a major role," he said in 1978. "This technique, which has come of age in the last four years, is rapidly being incorporated as a routine test in the evaluation of cardiac patients throughout the nation's major medical centers."[24]

Together with Dr. Cashion, Dr. Verani began to develop nuclear cardiology in the newly established laboratory at The Methodist Hospital. After the laboratory's inception, four types of cardiac scanning were being performed in 1978. One cardiac scan was available to detect the existence of myocardial infarction; one was for myocardial perfusion; one was for the detection of cardiovascular shunts, the abnormal mixing of arterial and venous blood; and one was for the study of the motion of the heart and its pumping function.

The enhancement of diagnostic capabilities had been evident. "The experience accumulated thus far suggests that the ability to diagnose coronary artery disease before myocardial infarction has occurred is greater using thallium scans than using only exercise electrocardiograms," said Dr. Verani, who was to perform more than 850 such scans in 1981.[25] "Also, the thallium perfusion scans frequently help to identify a relative large number of people who have normal coronary arteries but who had a 'false positive' stress electrocardiogram."[24]

The evaluation of the most common cardiac disorder—coronary artery disease—was enabled by the cardiac scan studies of the motions of the heart by radionuclide angiograms of the left ventricle. "These studies not only uncover unsuspected problems but also give good indications as to how much heart muscle is involved, as well as which coronary arteries are diseased," said Dr. Cashion. "Rapid advances in medical technology have made it possible for physicians to obtain information valuable in the diagnosis and treatment of cardiac disorders using noninvasive studies such as radionuclide angiograms."[26]

Although it was impossible to foresee the exponential growth of nuclear cardiology in the coming decade, Dr. Verani nonetheless accurately predicted one aspect when he was recruited by Dr. Miller from the VA to become co-director of the laboratory in 1982: "It is anticipated that the cardiac scans will become an essential part of the diagnostic evaluation of cardiac patients. In certain cases, replacing the cardiac catheterization and in others complementing the information obtained through the catheterization."[24]

Diagnostic cardiac catheterizations at The Methodist Hospital averaged more than 20 per day in the late 1970s, a volume that showed no indication of decreasing. Dr. Miller began searching for a new medical director for the three new cardiac catheterization laboratories opening in 1979 on the tenth floor of the Fondren-Brown Building. Having served as the interim director of the laboratories since the death of Dr. Dennis in 1975, Dr. O'Donnell planned to step down whenever asked to do so. That request came when Dr. Miller successfully convinced Dr. Albert E. Raizner at the VA Hospital to join the staff at The Methodist Hospital and to assume the position as medical director of the cardiac catheterization laboratories in 1979.

The efficiency of the newly opened catheterization laboratories at The Methodist Hospital was evident to Dr. Raizner upon his arrival. "The staff was fabulous," he said, recalling the volume of procedures performed daily.

"They told you the case would be ready in fifteen minutes, and in fifteen minutes things were ready. The equipment was, to say the least, archaic. We would take pictures and then everybody would move over to the monitor and squint and say, 'I think I see a blockage there.' But we did very well and it was a very, very rapid moving laboratory. In my training, every catheterization was a project. Even at the VA Hospital there were long cases. We did a lot of hemodynamics and lot of other things. The lab here was different. It was functional. It was quick. You got your information. You didn't shortchange a thing, but you got the information that was needed and the case was completed."[27]

There also was increased volume experienced by Dr. Quiñones in the new noninvasive cardiology diagnostic laboratory on the ninth floor of the Fondren-Brown Building in 1979. Designed by its original director Dr. Wright, who had since returned to his home state of Tennessee to practice, the spaciousness of this laboratory enabled Dr. Quiñones to include Dr. Reduto s Radioisotope-Cardiac Laboratory and to expand the area designated for echocardiography, the diagnostic procedure in which he had excelled.

When the diagnostic technique of echocardiography first gained recognition in the early 1970s, Dr. Quiñones was in his fellowship with Dr. Alexander at Ben Taub Hospital. Intrigued with the possibility of incorporating the new technique into the catheterization laboratory to combine it with pressures and do some continuous measurements of cardiac dilations, he had discussed his ideas with Dr. Alexander. "I am a first year fellow who had been in fellowship for three months," Dr. Quiñones said, remembering how he had brought along various articles from medical journals and photos of echocardiographic equipment to illustrate his request. After agreeing to purchase a $7,000. Smith Kline Echo Machine and set it up at Ben Taub, Dr. Alexander also granted Dr. Quiñones' request to be trained by an expert, Dr. Dick Popp, for two weeks at Stanford. "I learned a little bit and came back and started doing it," Dr. Quiñones said. "I worked with Bill Gaasch, who was a natural born researcher, and in two years we had written probably six or seven papers that to this day are very well respected."[28]

To enhance future clinical research in echocardiography, Dr. Quiñones conceived a personal plan. Since his 1977 arrival at The Methodist Hospital, Dr. Quiñones had become fully aware of how Dr. McIntosh often had conflicted with the non-Baylor physicians in the past. To ameliorate the situation, Dr. Quiñones endeavored to eliminate the residue of any so-called "town and gown" complications in cardiology.

One obvious manifestation of the previous friction at The Methodist Hospital was the existence of two separate echocardiograph laboratories. "Instead of going to Dr. Winters, who was the first person to bring echocardiography to Houston, and having everything together in one lab, Dr. McIntosh recruited Ted Wright to run his own echo lab," Dr. Quiñones discovered. "Obviously, all the private doctors went to Dr. Winter's lab, where they got a better job and quality than the other lab. Everything was fragmented. So the town and gown atmosphere was really bad."[10]

Since its origination in 1969, The Chapman Group's echocardiography lab had existed under the stairs in the back of the basement of the Fondren Building. Its less-than-ideal location was a reflection of the existing relationship between the clinical and academic faculty at the time. Remembers Dr. Winters: "I had an appointment with Baylor College of Medicine and was given a clinical associate professor title when I arrived in 1968 because I wanted to teach. My observation through that period of time was that Baylor really gave short shrift to the clinical faculty. They didn't recognize their contribution; they didn't tout their achievements. They took what they could get, but gave very little in return. The students and residents loved us; we had no problems at all with them, but I was always kind of disappointed in the fact that we could never get Baylor to recognize the value of their clinical faculty."

Because of their mutual interest in echocardiography, Drs. Quiñones and Winters quickly collaborated on research around the emerging diagnostic techniques made possible by ultrasound, publishing multiple papers together in peer-reviewed journals. They also developed a lasting friendship. When Dr. Winters served as program director of a three-day program on echocardiography jointly sponsored by Baylor College of Medicine and the American College of Physicians in October 1978, Dr. Quiñones was one of the lecturers. "Together, after concurring it was ridiculous to have two separate echocardiography laboratories at The Methodist Hospital, we made the decision to create one large combined echocardiography laboratory," Dr. Winters recalls. "Inaugurated in 1979 and located in the noninvasive laboratory on the ninth floor, the laboratory was co-directed by both of us."

Rather than being a fractious merger, as some feared this town-and-gown effort might be, it became a symbiotic one. Since the voluntary faculty members in the cardiology service, such as members of The Chapman Group, consistently had been well regarded by the housestaff at The Methodist Hospital, the combined laboratory was universally accepted from its inception. In addition, the technical staff members harmoniously blended as well. Jean Nelson, who was a young medical tech who worked in the original echo lab, became the main supervisor of the combined lab. She later was to become the director of all diagnostic catheterization laboratories at The Methodist Hospital.

In addition to the new diagnostic techniques available in nuclear cardiology at The Methodist Hospital, those of echocardiography in the noninvasive cardiology laboratory had been enhanced by the introduction of pulsed Doppler echocardiography (PDE) in 1978. Used in combination with M-mode echocardiography, this new technique facilitated the study of the flow of blood inside the heart chambers or in the great arteries. Its clinical applications augmented the unique role played by echocardiography in the noninvasive diagnosis of pericardial effusion and the evaluation of valve abnormalities and left ventricular function. "More than 1,000 studies have been performed at The Methodist Hospital using pulsed Doppler echocardiography," Dr. Quiñones reported in 1978.[29] The lesions detected by PDE included mitral stenosis and mitral regurgitation; tricuspid regurgitation; aortic stenosis, valvular or subvalular; aortic insufficiency, pulmonic stenosis; pulmonic insufficiency; atrial septal defect; secundum defect; ventricular septal defect–membranous; and patent ductus arteriosus. "Results indicate a high degree of sensitivity and specificity in detecting these lesions, particularly valvular ones," Dr. Quiñones said. "In addition PDE complements both conventional and two-dimensional echocardiography in the evaluation of patients with artificial valve replacements."[29]

Before the technologic advances made in the evaluation of patients with heart disease, diagnosis was established based solely on history, palpation, and auscultation. While electrocardiograms were used in the late 1950s to study the electrical activity of the heart and to detect myocardial ischemia and infarction, cardiac catheterization afforded the measurement of the mechanical functions of the heart and paved the way for arteriography in 1958. During the 1960s, the success of a CCU, featuring highly technical electrical equipment for around-the-clock monitoring of patients with myocardial infarctions, was dependent on the availability of specialized care by cardiologists and a trained nursing staff.

Throughout the 1950s and 1960s, the advances made by cardiologists in preoperative diagnosis and postoperative care were critical for the pioneering breakthroughs made in cardiovascular surgery.[30] In tandem with the vascular surgical advances came the rapid succession of new drugs, diagnostic techniques, therapeutic possibilities, and technologic advances in cardiology that made previously untreatable heart conditions controllable. New drugs—beta blockers, angiotensin-converting enzyme (ACE) inhibitors, and statins—were benefiting patients with acute and chronic myocardial ischemia, heart failure, a variety of arrhythmias, and hypertension, prolonging and improving the lives of untold millions of patients worldwide.

Technologic advances in cardiology included several new implantable devices. First introduced in the early 1950s, pacemakers and external defibrillators were combined in 1970, proving in clinical trials to be effective in the secondary and primary prevention of sudden cardiac death.

Also saving lives was the discovery of ways to prevent the recurrence of acute rheumatic fever and thus the development of rheumatic heart disease. While diagnostic capabilities became more sophisticated in echocardiography and nuclear medicine during the 1970s, other concepts and techniques for the understanding, diagnosis, and treatment of heart disease continued to proliferate.

Major advances in the field of cardiology in the 1970s included those made in invasive diagnostic techniques generated by the newly emerging subspecialty of clinical cardiac electrophysiology (EP). For more than a century, cardiologists had used the electrocardiogram (ECG) to record the electrical activities of the heart from the body surface. With the introduction of technologic innovations in the cardiac catheterization laboratory, it became possible to record the internal electrical activities of the heart with intracardiac electrode catheters in the catheterization laboratory and operating room.

The use of intracardiac electrode catheters in these pioneering studies resulted in a better understanding of the mechanisms and management of arrhythmias and the development of cardiac mapping techniques. Just as the initial investigation of the subtleties of cardiac arrhythmias in humans had led to the development of transistorized, implantable cardiac pacemakers in the 1960s, the advanced knowledge gained through intracardiac electrophysiologic studies was to lead to the development of automatic implantable defibrillators in the 1980s.[31-32] Even though the field of EP was in its infancy in 1978, Dr. Miller recognized its potential impact and recruited Dr. Christopher R. C. Wyndham to establish clinical EP at The Methodist Hospital.[10]

By the time both echocardiography and nuclear cardiology had moved into the noninvasive cardiology diagnostic laboratory in the Fondren Building in 1979, Dr. Wyndham joined the section. Recruited following his fellowship at the Abraham Lincoln School of Medicine at the University of Illinois the prior year, Dr. Wyndham was an experienced EP, having trained at one of the most active cardiac electrophysiology laboratories in the country and under the tutelage of one of that field's recognized pioneers, Dr. Kenneth M. Rosen.[33]

With more than 4,000 diagnostic catheterizations performed annually in the three laboratories on the tenth floor of the Fondren Building, Dr. Wyndham began to plan a separate EP laboratory adjacent to the recently renovated catheterization laboratory on the fourth floor of the Brown Building. Equipped with bi-plane fluoroscopy to permit visual imaging of catheterization from two planes simultaneously, this laboratory was to become the site of electrophysiological studies for the diagnosis of electrical disturbances of cardiac rhythm and the implantation of devices to regulate such disturbances.[34]

Although the arrival of Dr. Wyndham marked the formal beginning of EP at The Methodist Hospital, that subspecialty had been prominently represented prior to Dr. Wyndham's arrival. Throughout the previous decade, private practitioner Dr. Spencer had spearheaded most of the EP procedures performed, which included more than 11,000 artificial pacemaker implantations and cardiac pacing procedures. He had become one of the first to join the North American Society of Pacing and Electrophysiology in 1979, the year of its inception. As a member of The Chapman Group, he originally had been only on the periphery of artificial pacemaker implantations, assisting the surgeons during the procedures, but he progressively had assumed the total responsibility.

Recalling how the always-heavy surgical schedule at The Methodist Hospital throughout the 1970s used to dictate the timing of pacemaker implants, Dr. Spencer said: "The surgeons were so busy doing coronary bypass surgery that I finally said 'I'm just going to do it myself,' and only call the surgeons if we got in trouble. The funny thing was that they all said, 'Aw, you can have all those pacemakers.' But after awhile, when we started doing angioplasties and we started taking those bypass surgery patients away from them I became 'the SOB who stole the pacemakers from the surgeons.'"[35]

The advances made in pacemakers were indicative of those made in preoperative diagnosis, treatment, and postoperative care. While diagnosis of heart disease in the early 1950s was established almost solely by history and physical examination, electrocardiograms were used to study the electrical activity of the heart and to detect myocardial ischemia and infarction in the late 1950s. Cardiac catheterization afforded the ability to measure the mechanical functions of the heart and paved the way for arteriography in 1958, a breakthrough with a defined impact on the development of pioneering breakthroughs in cardiovascular surgery, a fact often stated by Dr. DeBakey.[30]

Also directly impacting The Methodist Hospital was the success of the CCU, featuring specialized care delivered by cardiologists, a trained nursing staff, and highly technical electrical equipment for around-the-clock monitoring of patients with myocardial infarctions. The rapid succession of new drugs, diagnostic techniques, therapeutic possibilities, and technologic advances in cardiology in the 1970s had made previously untreatable heart conditions controllable.

The extraordinary progress made in cardiology and cardiovascular science nationally during the previous three decades clearly was evident at The Methodist Hospital in the late 1970s. The combined echocardiography laboratory; the new nuclear cardiology laboratory of Drs. Cashion and Reduto; the invasive diagnostic capabilities available in Dr. Raizner's newly enlarged cardiac catheterization laboratory; the studies conducted in Dr. Wyndham's cardiac electrophysiology laboratory; and the advanced research protocols into medical treatment being conducted by Dr. Pratt in the CCU exemplified the era known as "the golden age of cardiology."[36]

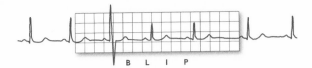

B   L   I   P

SAM "MOMO" GIANCANA

A longtime acquaintance of Frank Sinatra and the reputed leader of the Chicago crime syndicate known as the "Outfit," Sam "Momo" Giancana, known to most as "Mooney," reportedly fell ill "with a pain in his gut that floored him" while in Houston on a business trip in May 1975.[1] He was rushed to The Methodist Hospital and the care of Dr. DeBakey, who promptly performed acute gall bladder surgery. Returning to Chicago to recuperate after his operation, Mr. Giancana developed a blood clot in June and returned to The Methodist Hospital for treatment. When the Senate intelligence committee tried to contact Mr. Giancana for possible testimony about an alleged administration plot against Cuban Premier Fidel Castro, Dr. DeBakey reportedly wrote the committee a letter to advise that Mr. Giancana was his patient and too ill to testify.[2] Although under Dr. DeBakey's strict bed-rest orders, Mr. Giancana decided to leave the hospital and return to Chicago. Dressing himself in white to disguise himself as a physician, Mr. Giancana took the elevator to the basement of the Fondren-Brown Building where he left in his car unnoticed. When the police detectives assigned to tailing him realized he was gone, they raced over to his hotel, The Warwick, where they discovered he had checked out and was waiting outside for a cab. Graciously apologizing for causing any trouble, Mr. Giancana told the detectives he was on his way back to the hospital and would see them there. It was the last they saw of him. Two days later, the 67-year-old Giancana was dead, shot seven times in the basement kitchen of his Chicago home on June 19, 1975.[3]

---

1. William Brashler, The Death of a 'Godfather,' New York, July 28, 1975, page 27-33 [Is this a newspaper article or book? I don't know how to reference it without the full source]

2. Senate group had tried to contact mobster boss. UPI, Star-News. June 21, 1975.

3. Petacque A. Gangland hits take 55 lives since '75. Chicago Sun-Times. January 28, 1986.

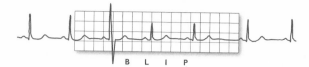

THE LEGS OF MARLENE DIETRICH

*A*fter singing her trademark song, Falling in Love Again, at the end of a November 1973 performance on stage in Maryland, the legendary Marlene Dietrich reached out to shake the hand of her musical conductor, lost her balance, and fell into the orchestra pit. Insisting she was not hurt, but refusing to leave the orchestra pit until the audience had departed the theater, she stood there, smiling and waving goodbye.[1] In December 1973, realizing her right leg was severely bruised and she had torn ligaments and muscles, Miss Dietrich entered a California hospital for a skin graft operation.[2] A month later, concerned her leg was not healing properly, she became a patient of Dr. DeBakey. After being admitted to The Methodist Hospital under an assumed name on January 25, 1974, Ms. Dietrich underwent another skin graft and bypass surgery to the veins in her legs so that sufficient blood would reach the grafts, allowing them to heal.[3] "She was a lovely patient," Dr. DeBakey said decades later. "Her main complaint was that she was having trouble with the circulation in her legs. Fortunately, she had a good result. And she gave me an autographed picture of herself, in a very slinky outfit — sort of an ermine thing, long, but with a slit on the side, showing off her legs — and said, 'This is what you did.'"[4] Among the hundreds of plaques, awards, and photos in Dr. DeBakey's office, the legs of Miss Dietrich always stood out.

1. Dietrich falls in pit. AP, *The Leader-Post*. November 9, 1973.

2. Leg injury hospitalizes Marlene Dietrich. *Knight News Service*. January 27, 1974.

3. Wood E. *Dietrich, A Biography*. London, UK: Sanctuary Publishing Limited; 2002:329.

4. Manier J. On the record, Dr. Michael DeBakey heart surgery pioneer. *Chicago Tribune*. April 23, 2000.

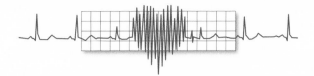

CHAPTER THIRTEEN

NEW PROGRAMS
1978 - 1984

"You lay a firm foundation by laying the bricks that others have thrown at you."
DAVID BRINKLEY

One of the cornerstones for the noteworthy transformation of the cardiology section at The Methodist Hospital was established in the late 1970s with the construction of the new Alkek Tower atop the Fondren-Brown Building.

Completed in late 1978, the addition of 150,000 square feet to the Fondren-Brown Building permitted the expansion of diagnostic, therapeutic, and research capabilities at The Methodist Hospital. As originally planned by Dr. McIntosh, all cardiology clinical services, invasive and noninvasive laboratories, and administrative offices were in one centralized location, the new ninth and tenth floors of the Fondren-Brown Building. Also strategically placed on the tenth floor was the expanded coronary intensive care unit (CCU) with 20 beds, while additional patient beds for cardiology and pulmonology were available on the 11th floor.

The cardiovascular research and clinical services of the federally funded National Heart and Blood Vessel Research and Demonstration Center occupied the 70,000-square-foot, four-floor Alkek Tower. In addition, there were 68 beds for cardiovascular patients and administrative offices for those involved with the national demonstration center, including its director, Dr. DeBakey, who in 1979 was "arguably the most famous doctor in the world" and "the most powerful man" in the Texas Medical Center.[1]

Appointed chancellor of Baylor College of Medicine by the board of trustees the previous year, the 71-year-old cardiovascular surgeon, after serving a decade as the college's first president, had stepped down in November 1979. Even though he maintained his positions as chairman of its Department of Surgery and director of the National Heart and Blood Vessel Research and Demonstration Center at The Methodist Hospital, there was rampant speculation that Dr. DeBakey was contemplating his retirement. To one reporter who asked if this were true, he replied: "I have no plans to change as long as God gives me the ability to keep doing my work. I'm mentally clear. But I don't project. You have to live each day at a time as long as you can. That's one reason I love to get up early. I like to see the day come in every morning."[2]

Having been present at the dawning of open-heart surgery in the 1950s, Dr. DeBakey had become one of the prominent pioneering surgeons responsible for the subsequent proliferation of cardiovascular surgery throughout the 1960s and 1970s. Primarily recognized for his work on the segmental nature of vascular disease[3] and the repair of aortic aneurysms and aortic dissections, as well as his interests in all portions of the arterial tree, he had gained further recognition for his research into the total artificial heart, left ventricular assist devices, and heart transplantations. "It can easily be argued that no other figure in the history of twentieth-century cardiovascular surgery has had such a widespread and permanent impact on advances in the field," said one distinguished medical historian of his contributions.[4]

The public's perception of Dr. DeBakey as a living legend had been fortified by the media's insatiable coverage of his noteworthy contributions to not only cardiovascular surgery but also public health policy and the preservation and extension of medical knowledge. In his tireless, self-directed efforts to export cardiovascular surgical know-how, Dr. DeBakey had traveled the world, receiving more than 82 major awards from such diverse countries as the Soviet Union, Argentina, Belgium, Ecuador, Italy, Lebanon, Peru, Egypt, and Yugoslavia.[5] The recipient of more than 30 honorary degrees from internationally recognized universities, he also collaborated with medical leaders in Saudi Arabia, China, Lebanon, Turkey, and the Soviet Union on the planning and development of cardiovascular centers similar to his at The Methodist Hospital.[6]

While his many trips to other parts of the world were documented in the news, so were those of the countless newsworthy patients who came to see him. Since first gracing the cover of *Time* magazine in 1965 following the Duke of Windsor's aneurysm surgery, Dr. DeBakey had shared the media spotlight with a litany of other such well-known public figures who came to The Methodist Hospital to seek his care. The publicity given to the surgical accomplishments of Dr. DeBakey often overshadowed the significant contributions made by others at The Methodist Hospital. Exemplifying this phenomenon was the "Super Medicine" cover story about the Texas Medical Center in the April 1979 *Texas Monthly*. After devoting the bulk of its multipage article to Dr. DeBakey, the article only listed the names of Drs. Howell, Beall, Crawford, Noon, and Morris in a sidebar under the heading "Some First Rate Heart Surgeons You've Never Heard Of" and the only mention of cardiology was in conjunction to Dr. Gotto's name and his area of expertise in a listing of other "Stars" in the Texas Medical Center.

By the late 1970s, Dr. Gotto had become publicly recognized as a "world famous specialist" in cardiovascular disease and a well-known advocate of heart-healthy diets.[7] In addition to his myriad accomplishments as scientific director of the National Heart and Blood Vessel Research and Demonstration Center, he had coauthored the best-selling *The Living Heart* with Dr. DeBakey,[8] with whom he also had written *The Living Heart Diet*, scheduled for publication in 1984.[9] In a unique effort to promote foods prepared with a minimum of fat and salt, Dr. Gotto collaborated with Mr. Bowen at The Methodist Hospital to create an innovative restaurant.

The location for the gourmet restaurant was to be in the hospital's new Total Health Care Center in the Scurlock Tower, a 560,000-square-foot addition named for a former board member of The Methodist Hospital, Eddy C. Scurlock. Completed in 1981, the new tower comprised outpatient hospital and lab facilities on floors three through six, including the Sid Richardson Institute for Preventive Medicine on the fourth floor, with medical offices and retail space available for lease on other floors as well as multiple floors of indoor parking space. Connecting the new tower to The Methodist Hospital and Smith Tower were pedestrian skywalk bridges.

Months before the official 1981 opening of the Scurlock Tower, physicians and medical-related businesses had leased all the remaining available space. The ability to traverse between the tower and The Methodist Hospital without having to go outside was a major selling point. The Chapman Group was the first to move into the unfinished tower December 30, 1979, choosing the 16th floor because it was the first stop on one of the express elevators.

The location chosen for the gourmet restaurant planned by Dr. Gotto and Mr. Bowen was an area on the fourth floor of the Scurlock Tower adjacent to the skywalk bridge to The Methodist Hospital. One year before its scheduled opening, a French chef trained at the Culinary Institute of Paris was hired to create, test, and perfect the heart-healthy menu. As his creations were being taste-tested by members of the hospital's administration staff, a marketing research team was called in to conduct a research survey as to an appropriate name for the eatery. "The most favorable name was by far 'La Difference,'" recalled one member of the administration staff at that time. "We had a meeting with Mr. Bowen to review the search results and select a name. He rejected all the names submitted and informed us the restaurant would be named Chez Eddy after Eddy Scurlock. So much for market research!"[10]

While newspapers across the country briefly mentioned Dr. Gotto's culinary venture at The Methodist Hospital, the international, front-page headlines in early 1980 were devoted to Dr. DeBakey's ongoing saga with the desperately ill and exiled Shah of Iran, Mohammad Reza Pahlavi. At the request of the Shah's New York physician, Dr. Benjamin H. Kean, Dr. DeBakey accompanied him to Panama for the purpose of removing the Shah's enlarged spleen, a procedure Dr. DeBakey said "would be ticklish technically" because of the Shah's previous operations.[11]

Upon arriving at the Panamanian hospital, the two physicians initially were turned away by security guards and not permitted to perform an examination of the patient, much less an operation. "My first reaction was to withdraw from the situation because I thought that might relieve it," Dr. DeBakey said, recalling the tension between the Panamanian and American doctors at the hospital. "But I made it clear that I would not be an adviser. The only way I could participate was to have control of the operation. There could not be two surgeons."[12]

The tensions eased when the Shah's operation was postponed for a week due to a respiratory infection. On March 23, at the invitation of President Anwar Sadat, the Shah unexpectedly departed Panama for Cairo, Egypt. Five days later, Dr. DeBakey and a surgical team of seven from The Methodist Hospital flew to Cairo, where they successfully removed the Shah's spleen. Although Egypt, like Panama and many other countries, had long prohibited medical practice by foreigners, Egyptian President Sadat made an exception in this case. "In every civilized country," he said, "DeBakey would be welcome to train the doctors."[13]

Such recognition of Dr. DeBakey's vast experience as a general surgeon underscored the starring role he had played in the surgical treatment of heart disease since the 1950s. Conversely, even though what had become routine surgical procedures for heart disease resulted in part from advances by cardiologists in preoperative diagnosis and postoperative care, the integral role of cardiology in cardiovascular surgical accomplishments rarely was credited, much less mentioned, by the lay press.

This seemingly invisible status of cardiology at The Methodist Hospital had begun to change in the 1970s. Because cardiology maintained control of the catheterization laboratories, where arteriography allowed physicians to visualize the site of obstruction to coronary blood flow, the introduction and popularity of coronary bypass surgery (CABG) increased the visibility of cardiologists' diagnostic efforts. By the late 1970s, when cardiac surgeons graduated from single to multiple bypasses with four, five, or even six grafts, the popularity of the procedures continued to increase exponentially.[14] Since all bypass patients were required to undergo preoperative catheterizations for accurate diagnosis for the betterment of the patient, cardiology had begun its transition out of the shadows and into the foreground in the treatment of coronary artery disease by the late 1970s.

The established, collaborative efforts of cardiology and cardiovascular surgery were to gain recognition during the escalating national debate about the efficacy of CABG in the 1970s. Challenging the use of using prospective randomized studies for the evaluation of surgical diagnostic and therapeutic techniques, such as the "scientifically unsound" VA study of CABG, Dr. DeBakey championed a proven, alternative method. In speeches and peer-reviewed publications, he advocated surgical judgment based not on randomized studies but on clinical experience, which he deemed as indispensable in determining whether an operation was worthwhile.[15]

The value of the traditional method of exercising clinical judgment in major medical centers was articulated by Dr. DeBakey in the February 1978 *Journal of the American Medical Association*: "In most centers, the cardiologist first performs the necessary studies and observations and, on the basis of the clinical judgment he has acquired, determines whether surgical treatment should be considered. If, in his opinion, surgical consideration is indicated, the cardiovascular surgeon is consulted, following which the decision regarding the preferred treatment is made on the basis of their combined clinical judgment. Under these circumstances, cardiologists and cardiovascular surgeons do not assume adversarial roles, but rather collaborate in determining appropriate and effective therapy. This traditional method of exercising clinical judgment has proved effective throughout the history of medicine—and remains so today."[15]

In agreement with the optimal results of exercising clinical judgment, Dr. McIntosh nonetheless continued his adversarial opposition to the proliferation of the CABG procedure in the United States. Despite the proven fact that CABG generally lessened the symptoms and functional limitations of patients with angina pectoris, Dr. McIntosh and other adversaries emphasized the lack of evidence as to the procedure's ability to prolong life or prevent myocardial infarction, arrhythmias, and ventricular dysfunction. His resulting conclusions appeared in a 1979 issue of *The American Journal of Medicine*: "Critical assessment of evolving information leads to the conclusion that widespread application of this procedure beyond the alleviation of symptoms refractory to medical therapy is not justified by present data."[16]

As both sides of the CABG debate published reports to substantiate differing points of view in peer-reviewed medical journals and subsequent randomized studies produced additional, conflicting conclusions, the controversy spilled over into the public domain. Even after the popular news media began to identify the ongoing argument as a "major row in the medical fraternity," the result was not a curtailment of the number of CABG surgeries performed nationally. To the contrary, there was a substantial increase to more than 82,000 procedures performed in 1977. Estimating the total cost of each CABG at $10,000, the American Heart Association advised that this cost increased to $20,000 for any patient who underwent extensive drug treatment first, then surgery.[17]

The search for a less expensive method of clearing constricted heart arteries resulted in a possible solution presented by Dr. Andreas Gruentzig at the November 1978 Scientific Session of the American Heart Association in Dallas, Texas. Describing his nonsurgical treatment as "percutaneous transluminal coronary angioplasty," the German physician from the University Hospital in Zurich detailed his technique of guiding a very small balloon-tipped catheter through a coronary stenosis so that the balloon, once positioned within the lesion, was inflated to dilate the stenosis. He reported his experience with this experimental procedure in 80 patients with angina, stating successful dilation in 49.[18]

Many of the cardiologists who witnessed Dr. Gruentzig's presentation in Dallas, including those from The Methodist Hospital, were incredulous about his balloon device as well as his catheterization technique. "I was in the room when it was reported, and several of us looked at each other and said, 'This guy's out of his cotton-pickin' mind. Anybody that is as dumb as putting a catheter in the artery and blowing up a balloon in it – that's just crazy,'" remembers Dr. Winters.

Despite such rampant skepticism, Dr. Gruentzig's innovative technique in vascular intervention already had enticed more than a few cardiologists, heart surgeons, and radiologists to Zurich. Arriving at University Hospital individually and in small groups since word of his first successful procedure in 1977 was published, each physician received one-on-one training from

Dr. Gruentzig in the catheterization laboratory. Insistent on training all who wished to perform the procedure, Dr. Gruentzig, as well as his associates in the laboratory, soon found the constant stream of visitors to be disruptive.

To remedy the situation in August 1978, Dr. Gruentzig grouped all visitors into one three-day live demonstration and training course, the first of its kind in cardiology. Because the size of the group exceeded the limited space in the laboratory, he arranged closed-circuit television coverage to broadcast seven cases to the 28 cardiologists and radiologists from around the world in the nearby basement auditorium. It was to be the first and smallest of five such closed-circuit live demonstrations he would conduct in Switzerland during the following two years.[19]

His second training course, held in August 1979, was decidedly larger, boasting 90 physicians in attendance, with 60 from Europe and 30 from the United States.[20] The dramatic increase was reflective of the worldwide medical community's rapidly evolving awareness of the potentially promising technique. Another contributing factor was the fact that proof of attendance at Dr. Gruentzig's demonstration of percutaneous transluminal coronary angioplasty (PTCA) was a requirement for the purchase of his specially designed balloon catheter. Strictly supervised by its inventor, who originated the initial device at his kitchen table, a small Swiss company, Schneider, was producing the patented double-lumen balloon catheters in limited quantities.[21] By 1978, the five handmade devices produced in the Schneider shop each week rarely met the demand.[22]

Proof of training with Dr. Gruentzig also was required for inclusion in the National Heart, Lung, and Blood Institute's PTCA Registry. Established in June 1979 "to evaluate most completely and expeditiously the promise and limitations of this new technique," the international, voluntary PTCA Registry was to comprise an inventory of investigators to initiate clinical studies of the experimental technique.[23] Its goal was to provide a means of accumulating data promptly for evaluating the safety, efficacy, and long-term effects of PTCA.[24]

Within a year of the PTCA Registry's founding, more than 631 patients had undergone the technique worldwide and the popular media began to shower attention on the technique. After *Time* magazine reported that "a new and highly experimental alternative" to CABG was "a procedure with a tongue-twisting name of 'percutaneous transluminal angioplasty,'" and syndicated newspaper articles identified PTCA as a possible avenue for bypassing the bypass, public interest in the procedure began to intensify.[25]

Among those to express interest in late 1979 was Dr. Gotto. In a conversation with Dr. Walter H. Siegenthaler, the Chief of Medicine at Zurich University Hospital who co-authored many of Dr. Gruentzig's first publications, Dr. Gotto inquired about sending doctors from The Methodist Hospital to learn the technique firsthand. When told those arrangements could be made, Dr. Gotto spoke to Ted Bowen, who also was very supportive and anxious to proceed. As Dr. Winters recalls, "Dr. Gotto proposed that Rich Miller and I go to Zurich, but at the last minute, Rich decided not to go and Al Raizner took his place. Three of us ended up going. Two of us went courtesy of Ted Bowen and The Methodist Hospital and John Lewis, another clinical cardiologist at The Methodist Hospital, went courtesy of himself."

Before attending Dr. Gruentzig's live demonstration and training course in Zurich at the University Hospital in January 1980, the three doctors remained skeptical about PTCA. To their genuine surprise, the week in Zurich with Dr. Gruentzig turned out to be revolutionary, one they later would describe as a seminal event in the course of the diagnosis and treatment of cardiovascular disease at The Methodist Hospital. To this day, Dr. Winters says, "I will never forget that trip to Zurich. It really was a landmark in the evolution of what went on in cardiology in this institution."

The closed-circuit, live demonstration in Zurich they attended in January 1980 was Dr. Gruentzig's third such effort to present his concept of establishing an "audience presence" in the catheterization laboratory so that those observing could see, hear, interact, and experience all aspects of the case as it was performed. Under his direction, the successes, limitations, and complications of PTCA clearly were demonstrated and understood by those in the audience.[26] "Those meetings were astounding to people, to see someone working in a high-risk situation, such as dilating a patient in front of a live audience of peers," said one cardiologist at that 1980 demonstration. "And the astounding thing to me was to see someone applauded probably more for his failures than for his successes. I mean, everybody was in there pulling along with him to get this done. And he saw the teaching value of that, not just to teach the technique, but to teach the potential hazards–he really did control how it went through that meeting."[27]

While Dr. Gruentzig often warned that potential complications are both serious and sudden in PTCA during these demonstrations, he was willing to answer pertinent questions in the midst of performing a procedure. With his outgoing personality, he was a natural showman capable of effectively educating with flair. To illustrate that his patients were fully awake, he would converse on camera with each, often urging them to smile and wave hello to the unseen audience in the auditorium.

The inimitable ability of Dr. Gruentzig to convert skeptics into followers clearly was evidenced by the three cardiologists at The Methodist Hospital in 1980. "After going over there somewhat nonbelievers, but coming back, saying 'this works, and we need to initiate this at The Methodist Hospital,' the three of us started a program of coronary angioplasty," Dr. Raizner said, noting how the entire perspective of the cath lab changed from a purely diagnostic facility to a diagnostic and therapeutic facility.[28]

"The transition was remarkable," Dr. Winters noted. "We started doing our first case in mid-March and the three of us would work together, not knowing what we were doing very much. We managed to struggle through, and then little by little taught the other cardiologists how to do it. It took a year or two to really take hold." In so doing, Dr. Gruentzig's three newly converted disciples effectively had introduced the new subspecialty of interventional cardiology to The Methodist Hospital.

Considered to be in its developmental stages at The Methodist Hospital in the early 1980s, this evolving new mode of therapy was only available to a small minority, approximately five percent, of individuals with significant coronary artery disease. "Further development and modification of the catheters used in the procedure are necessary to apply the procedure to greater numbers of patients," the doctors reported in 1981. "It certainly appears that transluminal coronary angioplasty may be an important adjunct, along with surgical and medical therapy, to the attack on coronary artery disease."[29]

The ability of cardiologists at The Methodist Hospital to offer an alternative mode of therapy for coronary artery disease through PTCA "made the cath lab a treatment lab, not only a diagnostic lab," Dr. Raizner said, recalling the genesis of the eventual transition. "At the same time, since cardiac electrophysiology was coming in to its own, it was no longer just an angiographic laboratory, it was an angiographic and electrophysiologic laboratory. And then ultimately, electrophysiology became therapeutic as well, with the development of ablation procedures. So the whole profile of cardiac catheterization evolved from 100 percent diagnostic to a combination of diagnostic and therapeutic."[28]

The efforts of cardiologists to prevent coronary artery disease were exemplified in the April 1981 opening of Chez Eddy. This innovative approach to promote heart-healthy dining immediately captured the attention of national food critics who were surprised to find the restaurant was occupied in "an unlikely spot between the departments of diagnostic cardiology and ambulatory surgery at The Methodist Hospital."[30] Able to accommodate

120 at linen-covered tables, Chez Eddy was decorated in muted grays and wood tones accented with artwork signed by Frank Stella, the noted American abstract artist. The Belgian recruited by Dr. Gotto to be its manager was Bettina Gerlache, who was known to offer skeptical diners a tally of the consumed calories at the end of a meal "to prove that less can be as satisfying as more."[31]

To the contrary, in Dr. Gotto's thinking, more was better than less when it came to public awareness of preventing cardiovascular disease. As other preventative measures were introduced, as well as various new interventional procedures for treatment, the discipline of cardiology continued its emergence from the shadows of cardiovascular surgery. At the beginning of this transition period in 1981, Dr. Miller decided to step down as chief of cardiology at Baylor College of Medicine and The Methodist Hospital. It took him two or three times to resign before he finally left—having resigned, then unresigned, and then resigned again. At his final resignation, Dr. Gotto and Dr. DeBakey asked Dr. Winters if he would consider being chief, to which he replied, "'Well, I'd like a weekend to think about it.' I had very mixed emotions about that, but in the weekend I was thinking about that, Rich unresigned again."

When Dr. Miller eventually departed in 1982, Drs. Gotto and DeBakey launched a national search for a new chief of cardiology. In the interim, serving as acting chief was Dr. Quiñones, who had agreed to serve on the condition that he was allowed to participate in the interviewing process of potential candidates for the permanent position as chief of cardiology. The reason for this unusual request was clearly articulated by Dr. Quiñones: "We have been developing cardiology over the past five or six years, and this could all be destroyed if you bring in the wrong person."[32]

In the five years Dr. Miller was chief of cardiology, "we went from having almost nothing to a clinical division that had all the bases covered, at least all the bases there were to cover in those days," Dr. Quiñones said, crediting him with the initiation of the development of an academic cardiology department. "Before Dr. Miller came, cardiology had existed primarily to serve Dr. DeBakey and the other cardiovascular surgeons. By the early 1980s we were conducting clinical trials in the CCU; we were publishing in every area; we were beginning to make a name for ourselves. So in the medical community The Methodist Hospital was in the process of going from being the place where Dr. DeBakey does all these wonderful things to suddenly being a place where there also was a respected echocardiography lab, nuclear cardiology lab, cardiac electrophysiology lab, and a diagnostic and therapeutic catheterization lab."[32]

One area in which Dr. Miller had not succeeded was in his unpopular plans to develop an academic clinical program capable of competing with the cardiologists in private practice. Since the number of private practitioners in cardiology at The Methodist Hospital far outnumbered the 10 full-time faculty members at that time in the Department of Cardiology at Baylor College of Medicine, this plan was doomed from the start because, noted Dr. Winters, "the private practitioners said that anything he does we can do better. And basically we did, or so we thought."

Instead of constantly competing, the private practitioners were hoping to work more closely with the full-time faculty to expand the services offered at The Methodist Hospital in the future. Collectively, all agreed that the ideal candidate for the position of chief of cardiology was one in search of an institution where the environment was conducive to limitless growth. One such candidate was Dr. Robert Roberts. "When the call came to look at the job here in Houston, I remembered Gene Braunwald telling me many times, 'When you make your move, go somewhere where the ceiling is not obvious,'" he said, recalling the advice that ultimately influenced his decision. "When I came here, two other things stood out: there was limited research going on in cardiology, yet Baylor College of Medicine and The Methodist Hospital were marvelous institutions that were expanding; secondly, cell biology at Baylor College of Medicine was already one of the top five or six [programs] in the country."[33]

At the time of his interview with Dr. Gotto, Dr. Roberts was an assistant professor of cardiology at Washington School of Medicine and Barnes Hospital in St. Louis, where he served as director of the CCU and head of the cardiovascular research program. For the previous nine years he also had assisted the cardiovascular division chairman, Dr. Burt Sobel, in the creation and development of a cardiology program in which the research base was in biochemistry. "Burt was doing more biochemistry than physiology," Dr. Roberts said. "I became interested in that and I felt at that time that probably might be where the future was as opposed to animal physiology where everybody else was."[34]

Furthermore, having read molecular biologist James D. Watson's 1968 book, *The Double Helix: A Personal Account of the Discovery of the Structure of DNA*, more than 20 times since 1980, Dr. Roberts believed that molecular biology techniques were the key to discovering the alteration of cell growth in cardiomyopathies.[33] In order to pursue this goal, Dr. Roberts wanted to establish the world's first molecular cardiology program. After several trips to Houston and multiple interviews, including one with Dr. Quiñones, Dr. Roberts voiced his desire to establish this one-of-a-kind program at The Methodist Hospital and Baylor College of Medicine.

Upon presenting this concept to Dr. Gotto, he found him to be receptive to the idea, but not totally convinced of its viability. "He said to me, 'Now, Bob, if molecular cardiology does not work out, what will you fall back on?'" Dr. Roberts said. "I am sure I might have been more arrogant than I should have been, but I said, 'Dr. Gotto, I really have to tell you that if it does not work it is not because of the techniques, it will be because of me and you will need to get someone else. These techniques are clearly going to work and I do feel that if I put the effort in and get the right people, it will work."[33]

While no decisions were made during that visit, Dr. Roberts was under the impression that Dr. Gotto thought his proposal to apply the techniques of molecular cardiology and recombinant DNA to cardiology was both plausible and possible. He also felt that Dr. Gotto was in favor of his establishing a molecular cardiology laboratory dedicated to cardiovascular research. However, after returning to St. Louis a few days later, a member of the Baylor College of Medicine search committee phoned him to say there was no research space available for molecular cardiology. This was a seemingly insurmountable problem to Dr. Roberts, who found himself "a little taken aback," convinced he would have to take his vision elsewhere.

To Dr. Roberts' genuine surprise, the inadequate space problem was solved in a matter of days. "Literally, less than 48 hours later, Phil Robinson from The Methodist Hospital came to St. Louis and came to my home on the orders of Ted Bowen, saying, 'I want to show you a plan of the space we have for your lab,'" he said. Unaware of Mr. Bowen's unfailing commitment of space and facilities at The Methodist Hospital over the previous decades to enable the college's development of the cardiovascular center, Dr. Roberts soon learned "that was the way things were done. Ted called my wife and said, 'Don't let him think that there's no space–I have someone coming up to show it to him.' And I have to tell you from that moment on, all I wanted to do was to come here because I felt that kind of enthusiasm and drive. I began to feel right away that I had the opportunity."[34]

As the newly named chief of cardiology, Dr. Roberts arrived in Houston in September 1982 and quickly gained the support of the private practitioners, particularly from those in The Chapman Group, an accomplishment attributed to his disinterest in having academicians compete with the volunteer faculty to become the best clinical cardiologists. "That was not my mission and the fact that people were bringing in patients here and we had an academic mission on top of that was all the better for me," he said. "I thought that was the perfect set up for us. I would certainly develop our clinical programs and would do clinical trials, but my hope was to develop a molecular biology program."[34]

Indebted to Mr. Bowen for his foresight in providing the necessary laboratory space in The Methodist Hospital, Dr. Roberts was stunned when the hospital president and chief administrator suddenly announced his retirement. Having suffered several heart attacks since 1976, Mr. Bowen said he was unable to continue his duties due to poor health and was stepping down in October 1982.

His unexpected announcement caught the entire medical staff at The Methodist Hospital off guard. The sudden departure of Mr. Bowen followed the May 1982 death of Mrs. Fondren, the longtime benefactress who had lived in the hospital the last five years of her life. After a life filled with philanthropic deeds, she died one month short of her 102nd birthday. The combined absence of these two integral members of the hospital family marked the end of an era at The Methodist Hospital. Under Mr. Bowen's guidance and Mrs. Fondren's approval and support, the hospital had doubled in size since its move to the Texas Medical Center in 1950. His administration had overseen the design and construction of the Fondren-Brown, Brown, and Neurosensory Buildings and Scurlock Tower; helped establish and nurture the cardiovascular research center; purchased and managed the Annex; developed Chez Eddy and the Total Health Care Center in Scurlock Tower; organized The Methodist Hospital Health Care System; and helped maintain a close working relationship between The Methodist Hospital and Baylor College of Medicine.

Capitalizing on that established relationship was one of the major thrusts behind Dr. Roberts' planned academic mission to develop the post-graduate cardiovascular training into a nationally recognized fellowship program. Shortly after his arrival he found The Methodist Hospital to be "the centerpiece" to attracting good fellows in search of clinical training with diverse patient care and multiple procedures. "I realized this almost immediately, literally, I think, my third day in the office," he said, recalling his first impressions. "I was looking at what are the positive things I could see around to develop the training program. And I realized when I looked at that time they were doing 20 or 30 caths a day. I thought this is the Cleveland Clinic in the middle of everything else. And I thought this is phenomenal! And immediately we made up brochures. We stressed the fact that at that time there were only two or three places that had anything in common with us in terms of numbers and quality – The Mass General, The Cleveland Clinic and the Mayo Clinic."[34]

Singular to Baylor College of Medicine and The Methodist Hospital in 1982 was the collaborative molecular cardiology laboratory established by Dr. Roberts, Dr. Burt O'Malley, head of cell biology, and Dr. Tom Caskey, head of molecular genetics. Recruited to the laboratory by Dr. Roberts was a former colleague at Washington University, Dr. Ben Perryman, with whom he continued his research focused on enzymology and the assessment and treatment of ischemic heart disease. Another recruit was from the NIH, Dr. Michael Schneider, who initiated research on cardiac cell growth and hypertrophy at Baylor College of Medicine and The Methodist Hospital.[35]

The newly created laboratory was to become the hub of a unique, five-year cardiology training program introduced by Dr. Roberts in 1982. During the first three years fellows trained in the techniques of molecular biology, integrated across cardiology, cell biology, genetics, and physiology, and were exposed to research applying these various techniques to cardiovascular disorders. The following two years of the fellowship concentrated on clinical cardiology. "It became a successful program very early in the game," Dr. Roberts said.[33]

Because both Drs. Gotto and Roberts did not micromanage, there was to be unbridled growth in each of the emerging subspecialty areas in cardiology at The Methodist Hospital. While Dr. Roberts concentrated a majority of his efforts to growing and developing molecular cardiology, he encouraged Drs. Quiñones, Verani, Wyndham, and Raizner to continue building their individual areas of expertise—echocardiography, nuclear cardiology, cardiology electrophysiology, and interventional and diagnostic catheterization. "He was smart enough to leave smart people alone," Dr. Quiñones said, recalling how he and the other subspecialists were given space to do their own thing by both Drs. Roberts and Gotto. "Bob really put us nationally on the map as a serious cardiology division. I do not think we would have had the national recognition as a cardiology division without him on board."[32]

Already recognized by his peers in the early 1980s as one of the country s rising stars in the field of echocardiography was Dr. Quiñones. When two prominent echocardiography groups, one headed by recognized expert Dr. Pravin Shaw and the other by Drs. Jamil Tajik and James B. Seward of the Mayo Clinic, established educational courses at the American College of Cardiology's Heart House in 1983, each invited Dr. Quiñones to participate. "Once I was there as a faculty member, I began to know the staff of the Heart House real well," he said. "Those were the days when Heart House would have four to six echo courses a year because echocardiography became a very, very popular topic for courses because a lot of physicians wanted to train and re-train or update on it. So the Mayo Clinic had one or two courses a year, Pravin had at least one, Cleveland Clinic also started having one. Within a couple of years I applied for our own course and then we started having our own course there."[36]

At The Methodist Hospital, because of the growing interest among the cardiology fellows in echocardiography, an additional year of elective training in that subspecialty was established in 1983. One of the first to follow that fellowship track was Dr. Marian Limacher, "who subsequently went to the University of Gainesville in Florida and had a very successful career there," Dr. Quiñones said. "She later was to become the first trainee from here to serve as a trustee of the American College of Cardiology."[32]

Another extended fellowship track was established in 1983. Its creation was in response to a request made by cardiology fellow Dr. Richard Van Reet, who completed his fellowship and expressed an interest in training an additional year with Drs. Raizner, Winters, and Lewis in the catheterization laboratory. "That was soon after they began doing angioplasties here," said Dr. Quiñones. "In granting his request, we became one of the first places in the country to initiate a full year in interventional cardiology training."[32]

At the time of Dr. Van Reet's interventional cardiology training in 1983, angioplasties were performed in the fourth-floor catheterization laboratory shared with electrophysiology, and the three 10th-floor laboratories were devoted exclusively to diagnostic procedures. Because of the rapid and exponential growth in both areas, many on the nursing staff were new to the job and undergoing on-the-job training as well. "We were lucky at times to get a trained cath lab nurse, but that was far and in between," recalled Patty Chesnick, the registered nurse named director of the catheterization laboratory in 1983. "We had a requirement at that time that they be critical care nurses because we had to be very responsive in code emergencies before a code team would respond. So their training was for three months in diagnostic cath labs, and then they went on for another three more months to get into angioplasties."[37]

As far as Drs. Raizner, Lewis, and Winters were concerned, the beginning years of angioplasties became their own on-the-job training learned from that procedure they first observed in Switzerland with Dr. Gruentzig. "We worked together on all the cases," Dr. Raizner said. "This was the way that we gained experience from each of us. John Lewis was a very talented catheter person. He could do things with the catheter at a time when we were all learning techniques. To John, it was intuitive. He could do a procedure in less time than it took to prep the patient."[28]

Also known to be one of the "most colorful" cardiologists at that time, Dr. Lewis acquired a reputation for being very demanding in the catheterization laboratories. "He was tough," Ms. Chesnick recalled. "He was tough on me, as the director of the lab. He was tough on the staff and he was tough on those fellows. I think the final test of orientation for the nurses was to do a Dr. Lewis case and survive. But let me tell you, we all have John Lewis stories."[37]

Even though that colorful cardiologist became well known for his skills in the diagnostic catheterization laboratories, he and his colleagues were remarkably slower during the beginning months of angioplasties. The time-consuming procedure was exacerbated by the apprehensive caution necessary with the soon-to-be antiquated, bulky, inflexible catheters, ill designed for angioplasty procedures. Because of this time factor, when rumors were rampant of cardiologists' running the surgeons out of business by usurping the coronary bypass patients to perform angioplasties, cardiologist Dr. William Gaston called the idea "absolutely absurd," saying, "It took longer for you all to try to do an angioplasty than a good surgeon at Methodist to do a multiple coronary bypass."[38]

As angioplasties began to evolve from the experimental stages, Dr. Van Reet participated in the process. Creating a lasting impression on his peers as being "very good and smart," the hospital's first interventional cardiology fellow was destined to become "a super star," they all agreed. At the completion of his fellowship, he returned to the Brooke Army Medical Center in San Antonio where he continued his Army service. In early 1986, after establishing his own practice in San Antonio, he developed a very aggressive renal carcinoma and died soon after. "It was very tragic," Dr. Quiñones said. "In his honor we created the Richard Van Reet Award for Outstanding Cardiology Fellow, given to the most deserving graduating fellow at Baylor College of Medicine each year."[32]

The annual selection of only one outstanding cardiology fellow at The Methodist Hospital was to prove to be a challenging task. In the coming years, as the quality of each class of fellows continued to escalate, there were to be multiple candidates for such a singular recognition. "Within two or three years, we were attracting very good fellows," Dr. Roberts said in 1983. "I think that within six or seven years we were looking at a fellowship that was competing with anybody in the top ten programs in the country."[34]

Past fellows who previously had joined the academic staff also made significant contributions to the transformation of the cardiology section at Baylor College of Medicine and The Methodist Hospital. One in particular was Dr. James B. Young, whose fellowship training in cardiology was completed in 1979. A graduate of Baylor College of Medicine who served his residency in its affiliated hospitals, Dr. Young said he first came "under the spell of Dr. DeBakey as a medical student." As the young cardiologist's mentor, Dr. DeBakey "taught me more than anyone about being a doctor, physical examination, the 'blink' philosophy of making quick decisions and also the value of hard work. If you look at all he did in his century of existence, it is mind-boggling. He truly is the greatest physician and clinical surgeon of the last century.[39]

Throughout his training and early years on staff, Dr. Young pursued his interest in heart failure. Since heart transplants were the most viable treatment for patients with heart failure and end-stage heart disease, he mounted an internal campaign to encourage Dr. DeBakey to resume the heart transplant program. One of his convincing arguments was the fact that a new antirejection drug, cyclosporine, had been proven to suppress the immune system's rejection of foreign organs in the years since Dr. DeBakey had abandoned the program in 1970 after the death of all 12 heart-transplant recipients.

When cyclosporine received certification for unregulated use by the Food and Drug Administration in 1984, Drs. DeBakey and Noon approached the CEO of The Methodist Hospital, Larry Mathis, with their request to resume the heart transplant program. Aware there would be considerable opposition to the resumption by many of the medical staff, Mr. Mathis assembled a committee, led by Drs. John Overstreet and Lynn Bernard, two of the most influential medical staff leaders. After meeting with Drs. DeBakey and Noon, the committee was satisfied that a resumption of the program would likely prove much more successful this time around and gave their approval. Promptly thereafter came the creation of the Multiorgan Transplant Center at The Methodist Hospital and Baylor College of Medicine, with Dr. Young as its clinical coordinator and scientific director.

Referring to the original heart transplant program's demise in 1970, Dr. DeBakey explained, "Our experience at that time with 12 cases gave us results that we didn't think were sufficiently justifiable to maintain the program. However, with the advent of cyclosporine, the results of transplantation, heart transplantation, lung transplantation, as well as kidneys, have all improved significantly, and we should be able to expect a five-year survival rate of better than 50 percent, dealing with patients at the terminal stage of heart disease."[40]

The media reaction to the announcement of Dr. DeBakey's resuming heart transplants and his establishment of a large transplant center staffed by 35 doctors and clinical personnel at The Methodist Hospital and Baylor College of Medicine was unanimously favorable. Newspapers around the world reported that by these actions the legendary cardiovascular surgeon had "endorsed the general belief within the medical profession that the operation is now reliable."[40]

As the official spokesman and integral member of the transplant team, Dr. Young was to gain a modicum of recognition for his and other cardiologists' contributions, but those of others were ignored. To avoid that omission in future endeavors, Dr. Raizner recognized the need for a remedy. "At Methodist we had a very sophisticated cardiology, heart surgery program, but it was not under a single umbrella," he said. "There were great efforts, great cardiologists, great surgeons, great diagnostic, noninvasive people – just wonderfully talented people, but all the efforts were sort of independent efforts. There was a need to bring the many components that worked on heart and heart disease and heart and blood vessel disease together."[28]

Although Dr. Raizner found growing support among his colleagues in the diverse subspecialties, the opportunity to bring his unifying vision to fruition at The Methodist Hospital was to remain elusive for many years to come.

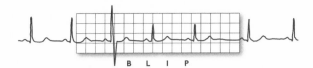

A TALE OF TWO ITALIAN CITIES

*B*y whatever means possible and with hopes of becoming one of Dr. DeBakey's patients at The Methodist Hospital, pilgrims from all over the world made their way to Houston, Texas. Many clutched in their hands a letter received from Dr. DeBakey saying that if they could make it to Houston, he would take care of them at no charge. Others arrived with funds donated to them for whatever surgical procedure was necessary. One such patient in 1969 was Valdivia Perschetti from Rome, Italy, whose benefactor was Pope Paul VI, who gave her $1,600 for a mitral valve replacement, which she successfully underwent and returned to Rome.[1]

Another patient from Italy had neither the funds nor Mrs. Perschetti's good fortune, but she did have a letter from Dr. DeBakey. Speaking no English, Carnella Giglio left her native Sicily without telling her husband she was flying to the United States to get a new heart. Arriving at John F. Kennedy Airport in New York, the four-foot, seven-inch Mrs. Giglio suffered a heart seizure and was taken to a hospital near the airport, where no one spoke Italian. Only able to keep repeating "Methodist Hospital" and "Dr. DeBakey," Mrs. Giglio soon found herself being put into a cab and sent to the Methodist Hospital in Brooklyn. With the help of New York's Italian-American League and hospital staff members, Mrs. Giglio finally was understood and she was placed on a plane to Houston, where she was to be admitted to The Methodist Hospital at no charge. Unfortunately, following a week of tests, Dr. DeBakey told Mrs. Giglio there was nothing he could do for her heart. Unable to pay for her return ticket to New York, Mrs. Giglio remained at The Methodist Hospital at no charge until staffers raised the funds for her ticket.[2]

---

1. Pope's blessing. News Dispatch. June 10, 1969.
2. Epic trip for life ends in sorrow. UPI, The Milwaukee Journal. March 9, 1973.

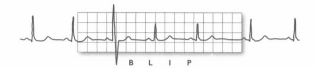

B   L   I   P

DR. DEBAKEY'S JET LAG REMEDY

*J*et lag was never a problem for Dr. DeBakey, and he often advised others of how they, too, could avoid such a nuisance. His advice was simple: When on an airplane, don't drink alcohol, don't drink anything that has caffeine, and don't eat airline food. For sustenance, bring your own bananas and granola. Although he believed that "sleep is as close to death as a living person can get and it wastes time," he was known to doze off immediately upon boarding an airplane, not waking until it landed. He believed one should go to sleep at the same time as the folks you are visiting. "That's how I avoid jet lag," he would explain, neglecting to point out he also always flew first class and, more often than not, had the luxury of two seats in which to stretch out and sleep.[1]

---

1. Wendler R. Michael Ellis DeBakey, M.D. Sept. 7, 1908 – July 11, 2008. *Texas Medical Center News.* July 15, 2008.

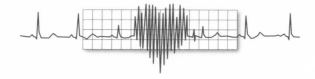

CHAPTER FOURTEEN

OPENING NEW CHANNELS
1984 - 1989

"You raze the old to raise the new."
JUSTINA CHEN

The multiple subspecialties in cardiovascular care at The Methodist Hospital and Baylor College of Medicine in 1984 mirrored an international phenomenon. With the complex, technological advances made in cardiologic diagnosis and treatment since the advent of open-heart surgery, the necessity for maintaining high levels of skills to optimize patient care had resulted in increased subspecialization.

Since many of these subspecialties had their own training requirements, professional societies, and journals, there was a tendency for each area of expertise to exist as an independent entity. Soon there were separate national conferences for electrophysiology, interventional cardiology, cardiothoracic surgery, echocardiography, and nuclear cardiology. As the multiple subspecialties of cardiology began to separate themselves professionally at The Methodist Hospital, the cardiologists began to develop their own departmental silos.

By the early 1980s, the professional fragmentation of the cardiovascular community at The Methodist Hospital and Baylor College of Medicine was palpable. There were departmental silos in invasive cardiology or interventional cardiology that included the established diagnostic studies of hemodynamics and angiography plus the newer therapeutic procedures of angioplasty, later to become known as percutaneous coronary interventions or "PCI." The other silo was noninvasive cardiology, encompassing the major imaging modalities of cardiology. There also were a growing number of subspecialists in electrophysiology, hypertension, peripheral vascular disease, lipidology, care of patients with acute coronary syndromes, heart failure, and other areas of prevention and rehabilitation.

Already established as an independent section of internal medicine at both Baylor and Methodist was "cardiovascular sciences," located in the Fondren-Brown Building. Named chief of the section of cardiovascular sciences in 1977 was Dr. Mark L. Entman, a noted scientist with many accomplishments, who had been recruited in 1970 by Dr. McIntosh to oversee the laboratories in the Cardiovascular Research Center. Dr. Entman has since been the recipient of numerous academic awards and honors including the Outstanding Research Award from the International Society of Heart Research and the NIH Merit Award.

Cardiovascular sciences was to gain its independence at Baylor and Methodist after Dr. Entman received a five-year grant of $13.4 million from the National Heart and Lung Institute in 1975 to establish the nation's first National Heart and Blood Vessel Research and Demonstration Center (NRDC). Serving as director and principal investigator of the center was Dr. DeBakey, with Dr. Gotto as scientific director and co-principal investigator. "They both decided that cardiovascular science should not be part of cardiology, but should be a separate basic research section within the department and that would be a central source for the 'Super Center,' as I called it," Dr. Entman said, recalling his initial efforts to write the grant.[1]

Dr. Entman had many conversations with Dr. DeBakey while involved in these early planning stages in 1972. "He had a better understanding of basic science paradigms and algorithms than many people who presume to call themselves basic scientists," Dr. Entman said. "And he had an almost unbelievable memory for them. He told me what he wanted. He had this vision for the future of the Fondren-Brown Building. He could envision its being a cardiovascular center, and he wanted to have his practice in the same place because he thought the influences were important."[1]

Enthusiastic about the possibility of creating a Super Center, Dr. Entman nonetheless was skeptical about receiving the grant. "I never thought we would get it," he said, noting how surprised he was when it was awarded. "It was astonishing. I was just stunned. At that time the Cardiovascular Research Center in Fondren-Brown was growing and doing well, but compared to Harvard, Yale, Stanford, Iowa, and Washington St. Louis, we were not even in the same ballpark. But what we did have was a center. We had built a center. We had research. We had a demonstration section on health and outreach. We basically had an education center. And we had research cores built to support all those things."[2]

These research cores provided the necessary resources to support scientific research. "We could also use them in the mentorial sense," Dr. Entman said. "It was patterned after the program project grant which was becoming popular, only we did it in the more expansive version. This concept was dependent on a grant because medical schools just do not have the amount of money required to support cores."[2]

When the "Super Center" in the Fondren-Brown Building opened in 1975, it was organized into three divisions: research, control and demonstration, and education. Over the following five years it implemented a unique approach to disease prevention, combining basic and clinical research with demonstration and community education. Its purpose was to translate laboratory findings into community programs for the prevention of heart disease, and more than 84 organizations participated in the center's educational and clinical projects, including junior and senior high schools, government agencies, and civic and corporate organizations. An additional three-year grant of $9.2 million was awarded in 1979 to support the NRDC through December 31, 1982.[3]

At the conclusion of the NRDC grant in 1982, Dr. Entman applied for additional funds for the specific purpose of funding the research cores for another two years, through 1985. Again successful, he was under the impression that the NHLBI was going to reinstitute the NRDC as cores in the future and not as individual grants, but instead it did something else, and somewhat abruptly.[1] "They gave us about three months notice that they weren't going to continue the program and they were going to stop our funding as of January 1, 1985," Dr. Entman said, recalling how he felt responsible for the "total chaos" that ensued in the research laboratories. "All of a sudden, these people were out without any money. Now they were very good people, and they were applying for things, but there was no way you could get funds for them in a three or four month period. So I put them on my emergency fund, figuring we'd get through Christmas and it would get taken care of."[1]

Within the following three months, there came a solution to the problem of replacing the federal funding. Announced March 1, 1985 by Dr. William Butler, president of Baylor College of Medicine, was the newly named DeBakey Heart Center. Supported by private donations and directed by Dr. DeBakey, the new center named in his honor was to continue the national heart research programs and community education as well as support core laboratories and pilot projects. An endowment campaign to raise the necessary $5 million commenced in March 1985.[4]

Serving as the scientific director of the DeBakey Heart Center at Baylor College of Medicine was Dr. Gotto, who later announced that the DeBakey Heart Center also included the multidisciplinary transplantation center under the medical direction of Dr. James B. Young. Funded in 1984 by a $500,000 matching grant from the Cullen Trust for Health Care and a gift from Claude Hamill, the multidisciplinary transplantation center was to procure, preserve, and transplant organs and tissues, including heart, lung, kidney, liver, pancreas, cornea, and bone marrow.[5] In 1985, Drs. DeBakey and Noon and their surgical team had performed this new program's first heart-lung transplant.[6]

Announced several months later by Dr. Gotto was the fact that the DeBakey Heart Center "recently" had become "a joint activity of Baylor College of Medicine and The Methodist Hospital."[7] To Dr. Entman, this affiliation was never in question, at least in his mind. Since the Super Center and the preceding Cardiovascular Research Center had always been a joint project of Baylor College of Medicine and The Methodist Hospital, it stood to reason to him that the DeBakey Heart Center would be the same. "Ever since I first came here, my laboratory has always been in the Fondren-Brown Building at The Methodist Hospital," he said, recalling his conversations with Dr. DeBakey on the subject.[2] "I felt the same way Dr. DeBakey did about the DeBakey Heart Center. He saw it as something that had no boundaries—of institutions, of departments. He thought that at the very least, it was for the entire Texas Medical Center. And that's how he preferred it—a community of scholars."[1]

As envisioned, there were to be a number of outstanding scientists and leaders produced over the years in the graduate program developed within the DeBakey Heart Center. Furthermore, these graduate students won numerous young investigator awards, including The American Heart Association (AHA) Katz Award; The AHA Marcus Award; and the American College of Cardiology Young Investigator Award.

In concert with the accolades received came the realization that the DeBakey Heart Center encompassed the field of cardiovascular sciences but did not include all of the clinical subspecialties of cardiology or many of the cardiovascular surgeons. To remedy this oversight, Dr. Raizner continued to advocate for the establishment of a separate designated heart center at The Methodist Hospital. With growing support for this concept among both private practitioners and full-time faculty, committees were formed to investigate the possibility and to submit budget recommendations to The Methodist Hospital administration. To achieve their ultimate goal was to become a lengthy process, often filled with controversy.

The difficulties in creating an umbrella entity for cardiovascular care at The Methodist Hospital resulted from the pre-existing conditions dictated by its long-term affiliation agreement with Baylor College of Medicine. The hospital's chief of cardiology, Dr. Roberts, was a full-time faculty member, and the section's highly regarded training program was identified with Baylor College of Medicine, not The Methodist Hospital. Determining the hierarchy of responsibility for an independent, all-inclusive heart center at The Methodist Hospital that offered the services of both faculty members and private practitioners proved to be problematic.

Lengthy and frustrating efforts to achieve this goal were to be expended by all interested parties during the following 15 years. After a succession of committees was formed to explore the possibilities of establishing a hospital-based heart center, the outcome of each effort was inconclusive. "We had a lot of private doctors who had nothing to do with Baylor and thought Baylor was the enemy," Dr. Raizner explained. "We also had Baylor doctors who thought private doctors were a problem. So we had a hospital that had conflicts. It was a bit of a battle to get it created."[8]

While these negotiations took place off-the-record and behind the scenes, the newly established DeBakey Heart Center at Baylor College of Medicine and The Methodist Hospital quickly gained national recognition. Beginning in 1985 and consistently thereafter, in the myriad newspaper stories about Dr. DeBakey as well as those that only mentioned his name, reference to his being the director of the DeBakey Heart Center was always included. Similarly, the ubiquitous identifying phrase for Dr. Gotto, who had served as president of the AHA in 1984, was to become a reference not only to his past presidency of that national organization but also to his current position as scientific director of the DeBakey Heart Center.

Further recognition of the DeBakey Heart Center at Baylor College of Medicine and The Methodist Hospital was to come in 1986. Having served as president of the AHA during the 1984 establishment of the AHA-Bugher Foundation Centers for Molecular Biology in the Cardiovascular System, Dr. Gotto suggested that Dr. Roberts submit a letter of intent to become one of the first participants in this innovative training program. "Tony thought that we should go for it because we already were training some people in molecular biology," Dr. Roberts said, explaining how the DeBakey Heart Center later submitted a proposal and became one of the 24 applicants accepted. "The American Heart Association was going to dwindle the 24 applicants down to five, but only award three programs. When I learned we were one of those five, I was honored to be there."[9]

Also causing Dr. Roberts to be apprehensive was his realization of the high caliber of his competition. Among the other four candidates was his former mentor at Washington University St. Louis, Dr. Sobel, and the two 1985 Nobel Prize winners in physiology at Southwestern Medical School in Dallas, Dr. Michael Brown and Dr. Joseph Goldstein. During the six weeks necessary to prepare his presentation to the AHA-Bugher Foundation selection committee, all Dr. Roberts could think about was "Brown there with this medal around his neck; how could we compete with that?"[9]

One solution was to recruit the services of a Baylor colleague who was one of the most respected leaders in the field of molecular genetics, Dr. Tom Caskey. "I went to Larry Mathis, president of The Methodist Hospital, and told him I wanted Tom Caskey to go with me to the presentation," Dr. Roberts said, recalling how he also had asked another special favor. "I asked Larry, 'Would someone from the hospital write a letter that I could read from the podium saying that every person who is willing to do a third year, in addition to the two year fellowship, that you (The Methodist Hospital) would pay the third year salary?' Larry wrote the letter, stamped it, and I took it to Dallas."[9]

The value of the supporting role played by The Methodist Hospital was to be tangible. The first three AHA–Bugher Foundation Centers for Molecular Biology in the Cardiovascular System were awarded to the DeBakey Heart Center at Baylor College of Medicine and The Methodist Hospital, Children's Hospital in Boston, Massachusetts, and University of Texas Southwestern Medical Center in Dallas, Texas. Each institution received a $1,125,000 award to provide five years of financial support from The Bugher Foundation.[10] It was an exhilarating achievement for Dr. Roberts, whose former mentor was not among the three selected. "Burt didn't talk to me for about a year," he said. "But after that he became very proud of me."[9]

When the AHA–Bugher Foundation Centers for Molecular Biology in the Cardiovascular System was instituted in 1987, it established a formal infrastructure for training in molecular cardiology at the DeBakey Heart Center. Compared to the nascent program Dr. Roberts' established in 1984, it was a considerably accelerated four-year program of two years in the laboratory and two years in clinical cardiology. It also consolidated the newly created molecular cardiology laboratory's intradisciplinary collaboration with Baylor College of Medicine's departments of cell biology, genetics, and physiology. "This would facilitate the transfer of innovative techniques developed in the basic science departments," Dr. Roberts said. "My challenge was to get investigators in basic science interested in cardiovascular disease so we could pursue a program embracing fundamental, translational, and clinical research."[11]

Over the following five years there were to be 35 trainees in the AHA-Bugher Foundation Centers for Molecular Biology in the Cardiovascular System at the DeBakey Heart Center at Baylor and Methodist. "The success of the program is shown by the more than 85 percent of our graduates remaining in academics," said Dr. Michael D. Schneider, the molecular biologist and internist recruited by Dr. Roberts to help launch the molecular cardiology laboratory in 1984. Crediting the innovative intradisciplinary aspects of the training program, Dr. Schneider said, "This integrated design has consistently proven to be effective in providing successful, independent, and competitive investigators in molecular biology of cardiovascular medicine."[12]

Within the coming decades, Dr. Schneider was to become recognized internationally for his expertise on the molecular genetics of cardiac growth and heart failure, and many of the former trainees were to establish noteworthy academic careers in molecular cardiology. "The best thing Dr. Roberts did for molecular biology here was recruiting Michael Schneider," said Dr. Entman in 2011. "He is an outstanding guy and collaborated with all of us. He was recruited to London as head of cardiovascular science for the National Heart and Lung Institute in 2007 and now is chairman of cardiology at the Imperial College of London."[2]

As the molecular cardiology program at The Methodist Hospital continued to expand, both in the laboratory and clinically, Dr. Roberts nurtured the enhancement of the academic program in cardiology at The Methodist Hospital. Throughout the 1980s there were advanced clinical and research studies by Dr. Christopher Wyndham in electrophysiology, Dr. Young in heart failure, Dr. Pratt in cardiac arrhythmias, Dr. Raizner in the catheterization laboratories, Dr. Quiñones in echocardiography, and Dr. Verani in nuclear cardiology.[13]

Each subspecialty in cardiology began to flourish during Dr. Roberts' tenure, an achievement he credited not only to the expertise of the individual cardiologists in each area but also to the hospital's generous support. "The fact that the nuclear lab became one of the top two or three in the country, the echo lab certain in the same category, could not be without The Methodist Hospital's having state-of-the-art equipment to do it," Dr. Roberts said. "It clearly very much related to what they had put in and the talent that they developed. And had they not created the right environment, people like Mike Quiñones and Mario Verani would not have put in that effort to be where they were without the support of Methodist."[9]

As the cardiology subspecialties expanded, Dr. Roberts launched an aggressive recruitment program to increase the full-time faculty in cardiology. One of the first cardiologists recruited by Dr. Roberts was Dr. William A. Zoghbi, who had just completed residency training and a fellowship in cardiology at The Methodist Hospital in 1985. "At the time I joined the faculty, color Doppler had just started," Dr. Zoghbi said, recalling the rapid onslaught of technological advances in echocardiography through the years. "Just before I started my fellowship in 1981 or 1982, I used to see Mike Quiñones in the hallway carrying strips of paper with just a few dots on them. There was no color on them, but he was just so excited about these few dots indicating that the valve was leaking. Our diagnostics were so primitive then. Nowadays you look back and say, 'Oh my God, how much we were able to interpret with so little.' It is amazing how much it has evolved. It's just amazing."[14]

Also constantly evolving was the full-time faculty in cardiology. While new recruits in the 1980s included Drs. Marian C. Limacher, Jerry Griffin, Lawrence Poliner, Janice Schwartz, Donald L. Johnston, and James Mahoney, their careers at The Methodist Hospital were to be brief. With a fluctuating number of full-time faculty, Dr. Roberts relied on the educational services provided by the voluntary faculty members in his teaching and training programs. "I probably wished in some ways that I'd had more time to role model to some of the fellows than I did," Dr. Roberts said in retrospect. "I mean I tried to do it through all the other different things I did, but there is only a certain amount of time."[9]

Prominent among those serving as role models in Dr. Roberts' voluntary faculty were members of The Chapman Group. Having established a reputation for being "exceptionally competent cardiologists," Dr. Chapman and his associates comprised the Cardiology B Teaching Medical Service.[15] With a number of teaching accolades from Baylor, Dr. Chapman cherished this responsibility during his six decades of service. His office wall was adorned with awards, and people who have known him and been schooled under his leadership recall him as a legendary teacher.

In addition to Dr. Chapman's contributions as a member of the voluntary faculty of Baylor College of Medicine, he served as a visiting professor in medical schools throughout the world. He served as president of a diverse group of medical societies in Houston and in Texas and as governor from South Texas with the American College of Physicians (ACP) and the

ACC, for which he was to receive the master award from both organizations. The Harris County Medical Society also honored him with the John
P. McGovern Award in 1996 for exemplifying the ideals of Dr. William
Osler, who pioneered the practice of modern medicine. As the recipient
of the Baylor Distinguished Faculty Award in 1978 and numerous teaching
awards, Dr. Chapman was an inspiration not only to his peers and students
but also to all of his associates in The Chapman Group, Drs. Beazley, Spencer, Cashion, Samuels, Hausknecht, Richard Heuser, and especially William L. Winters Jr.

Proving to be equally as effective in the role of teaching was Dr. Beazley,
who was always described by Dr. Winters as the "rock" of The Chapman
Group—the one sought out for the most difficult problems, whether they
be medical or other. He was very well regarded "by the housestaff for his
sensible approach to problems in cardiology and fine interpersonal skills,"
said Dr. Lynch, who served as the associate chief of medicine at Baylor College of Medicine. "He received the Outstanding Clinical Faculty Award in
1986."[15]

Another outstanding educator among the voluntary faculty was Dr. William R. Gaston, who completed his training in cardiology at Baylor College
of Medicine in the 1960s. "Don Chapman had been my mentor," he said,
recalling how the legendary teacher and cardiologist influenced his switching from child psychiatry to cardiology as a specialty. "He was an icon here
and all over the South and Southwest."[16]

After serving as chief resident and head of the teaching service at Ben
Taub Hospital, Dr. Gaston entered private practice and later became chief
of the Cardiology C Teaching Medical Service at The Methodist Hospital
for more than two decades. Similar to his mentor, Dr. Gaston loved to teach
"at the level we taught at because the motivation of these bright, young
people makes it fun," he said. "You learn more than they do. They asked you
questions. They asked you to prove what you're teaching.[16]

Because of Dr. Gaston's passionate approach to teaching, he was "an
exceptionally popular faculty member for students taking an elective in
cardiology and has been equally well regarded by residents," Dr. Lynch
said. "Among the voluntary cardiologists on Dr. Gaston's teaching service
through the years were Drs. John M. Lewis, Robert C. Fulweber, David
Gonzalez, Oscar de la Rosa, Howard Rubin, Stuart Solomon, and Milton
S. Klein, who later was to succeed Dr. Gaston as chief of the cardiology
teaching service."[17]

As with most great teachers, Dr. Gaston always was eager to learn more.

Intrigued with the technological advances made in the emerging field of interventional cardiology, he regretted not being able to join Drs. Raizner, Lewis, and Winters when they traveled to Zurich, Switzerland, in January 1980 to participate in one of Dr. Gruentzig's demonstration courses in percutaneous transluminal coronary angioplasty (PTCA). Shortly thereafter, when Dr. Gruentzig moved to Atlanta, Georgia, to become the director of international cardiovascular medicine at Emory University School of Medicine, Dr. Gaston decided to learn the procedure firsthand. "Maybe it's time for me to get involved in this," he remembered saying to himself following the 1982 development of better guiding systems, improved balloon catheters, and flexible steerable wires. "I flew over to Emory and took the course. Gosh, it was primitive then. Less than five percent of people with coronary disease would be amenable to that. But what an impressive guy Dr. Gruentzig was!"[16]

The live demonstration courses Dr. Gruentzig conducted at Emory became a continually updated outgrowth of his original courses in Zurich to advance and disseminate his PTCA technique. Unfortunately these courses came to an unexpected end when Dr. Gruentzig and his wife died tragically after a private plane he was piloting in stormy weather crashed on the way back to Atlanta in October 1985. He was 46 years of age. To honor and acknowledge Dr. Gruentzig's contributions and pioneering work in the field of cardiology, Emory established the Andreas Gruentzig Cardiovascular Center to further build upon Dr. Gruentzig's progress in the area of interventional cardiology.

Based on the strict guidelines established by Dr. Gruentzig, the number of coronary artery disease patients eligible for PTCA treatment at The Methodist Hospital was less than two to three percent in the early 1980s. "He specified that the blockage should involve one artery; it should be a very localized blockage," Dr. Raizner said, acknowledging that even though it was slow starting the program, more than 600 PTCA procedures had been performed at The Methodist Hospital by 1986. "Initially, the number of cases that met the criteria was so small, it took months to follow his criteria and we turned down more than we actually did."[8]

Another requirement for PTCA dictated by Dr. Gruentzig was the surgical standby, comprised of a skilled team of surgeons, anesthesiologists, and operating room personnel immediately available in case of complications and to prevent further damage to the heart. "Causing deaths by what we were doing was pretty uncommon, but in those early years we were saved by the surgeons, who backed us up when we caused an artery to close,"

Dr. Raizner said. "The surgeons did a bypass on that patient urgently. It was their skill and expertise that provided the safety cushion to angioplasty during those early years. And then, of course, angioplasty became safe."[8]

The safety features came into the technique in tandem with multiple technological advances in the catheterization laboratory. As the experience of the interventional cardiologists increased, the criteria for patient eligibility for PTCA expanded to include more complex blockage and multiple vessel blockage. "It was clear that we were taking on many cases that surgeons previously would have bypassed," Dr. Raizner said, recalling how the volume of cases accelerated in the late 1980s. "So we really did expand into the surgical realm. It was interesting because the ultimate success of angioplasty probably was provided by the surgeon's expertise in getting us out of trouble."[8]

The rapid increase in the number of PTCA procedures performed at The Methodist Hospital mirrored a national trend. Throughout the United States, where more than 200,000 patients underwent angioplasty in 1988, PTCA had become a major therapeutic alternative to bypass surgery.[18] Despite this unbridled growth, the volume of coronary bypass (CABG) operations had not diminished greatly, numbering more than 250,000 in 1985.[19]

Equally undiminished was the ongoing debate among medical professionals about the efficacy of CABG and the lack of scientific evidence that the surgery prolonged the life of a patient. When the results of two major studies indicated there was no significant difference among the survival rates of patients who underwent CABG and patients who were treated with drugs and other nonsurgical treatments, Dr. DeBakey publicly questioned the findings. Indicating these studies were flawed because only relatively low-risk patients were included and the most seriously ill excluded, he reiterated his longstanding advocacy of the procedure while delivering a speech in 1982. While praising coronary bypass surgery as a valuable tool in the treatment of heart disease, Dr. DeBakey stated his opinion about the controversy over the procedure's efficacy at that time: "The data clearly demonstrate that survival is increased. If there is a debate, it has to be among people who don't know the facts."[20]

Four years later, when the Knight-Ridder newspapers published a series of articles about the excessive death rates from coronary bypass surgery on Medicare patients in 200 hospitals in the United States in 1986, Dr. DeBakey again spoke his mind. Rather than criticize the articles as misleading and unnecessarily alarming to patients, as many of his peers did, he called the articles "a real service to heart surgery."[21] Pointing out there was a direct link between small caseloads and high death rates, he publicly urged the federal government to deny Medicare reimbursement for heart surgery in hospitals that perform less than a minimum of 150 operations per year.[22]

Because of the inexperience levels evident in hospitals where less than the minimum number of operations were performed, Dr. DeBakey once again advocated the creation of regional "centers of excellence." In 1989 he suggested that these centers be formed through financial incentives from the federal government and equipped with the best technology and the finest staffs. Furthermore, he proposed that organ transplants and the treatment of heart disease and cancer be performed only at these centralized high-tech medical centers.[23]

The volume of surgical caseloads at The Methodist Hospital for the treatment of heart disease far surpassed the minimum Dr. DeBakey declared as mandatory. Of the more than 36,000 surgical procedures performed there on an annual basis in the late 1980s, the most common type of major surgery had been the CABG operation.[24] During his three decades at The Methodist Hospital, Dr. DeBakey and his surgical team had admitted 13,827 patients for the treatment of arterial atherosclerotic occlusive disease, compiled the records, analyzed the data, and published the "Patterns of Atherosclerosis and their Surgical Significance" in the 1985 *Annals of Surgery.*[25]

Verification of Dr. DeBakey's steadfast opinion of coronary bypass surgery as the best treatment for most heart-disease patients came in1989. It was the published results of a 15-year observational study of 5,809 patients at Duke University that documented coronary bypass surgery was more effective than treatment with drugs and diet changes.[23] What soon became the next controversial debate in the cardiovascular medical community nationally was how to determine which patients formerly sent for bypass surgery were candidates for coronary angioplasty.[26]

At The Methodist Hospital, this therapeutic debate between cardiologists and surgeons was not as contentious as expected. To the amazement of Dr. Raizner, Dr. DeBakey became an avid supporter of balloon angioplasty. "I thought he would oppose it but it was quite the contrary," he said, recalling his astonishment at the time. "Not only did he and his team back us up, but they also referred many cases to us. I did a lot of Dr. DeBakey's patients; he was one of our best referrers for interventional cardiology. I think this was another one of his abilities to see the future, to see beyond. He was a remarkable man; he saw the future of interventions."[8]

While Dr. DeBakey and the cardiovascular surgeons at The Methodist

Hospital continued to maintain a legendary volume of CABG and other cardiovascular surgical procedures throughout the 1980s, there was to be substantial growth not only in interventional cardiology but also in each of the emerging cardiology subspecialties. With the therapeutics developed in tandem with innovative diagnostic techniques in arteriography, echocardiography, cardiac electrophysiology (EP), and nuclear cardiology, cardiologists had amassed an arsenal of tools for the diagnosis and treatment of heart disease.

In nuclear cardiology, Dr. Verani was to gain recognition throughout the decade as one of the pioneers in the field of pharmacologic stress imaging and other clinical applications of nuclear cardiology. With imaging provided by single photon emission computed tomography (SPECT), an imaging modality introduced in the 1950s that was not to come into widespread use until the 1980s, Dr. Verani and his colleagues were able to classify coronary artery disease by observing the result of the disease study and how well the heart muscle was being fed with blood. Enhanced detection of coronary artery disease allowed nuclear cardiologists to offer postcatheterization assessment of physiologic significance of intermediary coronary stenoses and evaluation of myocardial perfusion after PTCA and CABG.

With the introduction of the advanced imaging modalities of magnetic resonance imaging (MRI) and computed tomography (CT) in the late 1980s, Dr. Verani's clinical capabilities began to expand, as did the subspecialty silo of nuclear cardiology at The Methodist Hospital. Invited to join the faculty upon completion of his postgraduate training and cardiology fellowship at Baylor College of Medicine in 1987 was Dr. John J. Mahmarian, who earned his medical degree from New York Medical College in Valhalla, New York. With a clinical focus on preventing heart disease, acute coronary syndromes, and myocardial infarction, Dr. Mahmarian was to write extensively on myocardial perfusion imaging and CT angiography in the coming decades.

Since the evolving, noninvasive diagnostic techniques of nuclear medicine were complimentary to those in echocardiography, Dr. Verani collaborated with Dr. Quiñones to develop a more sophisticated approach to patient management. "Mario Verani and I became very close friends and did a lot of research together and a lot of collaboration," Dr. Quiñones said. "Mario was the third person to step into the nuclear cardiology lab, but he is the one who truly took the nuclear lab to a whole different level nationally."[27]

Propelling the recognition of the importance of cardiac electrophysiology (EP) at The Methodist Hospital was Dr. Christopher Wyndham. For the diagnosis of heart rhythm disturbances, one of the most common causes of sudden cardiac death, he employed a unique tool an electrode attached to a catheter that made it possible to record and study the origin and spread of electrical impulses inside the heart. The catheterization laboratory on the hospital's fourth floor was used for these diagnostic EP studies.. "Chris Windham was working when we had that old cath lab cradle," recalled Patty Chesnick, who had become director of the catheterization laboratories in 1983. "The facilities were archaic when judged by modern standards."[28]

To perform a particular type of intracardiac electrophysiologic study, Dr. Wyndham worked with cardiovascular surgeon Dr. Gerald M. Lawrie in the operating room to identify and map the origins of heart rhythm disturbances. Personally invited by Dr. DeBakey to become a cardiovascular fellow in 1974 after his thoracic surgical training in Sydney, Australia, Dr. Lawrie subsequently had become a member of Dr. DeBakey's surgical team in 1975. "By the time I got here, they had perfected the surgical techniques of this specialty," he said, recalling his initial impression of cardiovascular surgery at The Methodist Hospital. "There are many places today where the pure technical part is still not performed as well as it was being done here in the 1960s."[29]

One of the newest surgical techniques devised in the 1970s and finetuned in the 1980s by Dr. Lawrie was for patients with serious cardiac arrhythmias who were unresponsive to medical therapy and catheter radio frequency ablation. Between 1981 and 1985, after intracardiac electrophysiologic studies of 580 patients, Drs. Lawrie and Wyndham performed surgical intervention in 90 patients with intractable cardiac arrhythmias with favorable results. "The high success rates achieved encourage further application and refinement of these surgical techniques," they reported in 1985. "These results confirm the feasibility of relieving a variety of serious arrhythmias by surgical intervention."[30]

Further intracardiac electrophysiologic study at Baylor College of Medicine and The Methodist Hospital was to be undertaken by Dr. Antonio Pacifico, named to replace Dr. Wyndham after his departure for the University of Texas Medical School of Southwestern in Dallas in the mid-1980s. Born and educated in Italy, Dr. Pacifico received medical and cardiology training at Southwestern in Dallas followed by electrophysiology (EP) training in San Francisco. Under Dr. Pacifico, the EP program at Baylor College of Medicine and The Methodist Hospital was to continue to flourish. Joining him in 1992 was Dr. Nadim Nasir, who was Baylor-trained in cardiology and EP. For a brief time period in the early 1990s, there were four in the EP group, including newcomers Drs. Timothy Doyle and Susan Wheeler. Within a few years, Dr. Wheeler retired and Dr. Doyle left for solo practice.

In an effort to establish effective regimens to control arrhythmias and prolong the lives of people with heart disease, Dr. Pacifico founded the Texas Arrhythmia Institute in January 1994. After leaving Baylor College of Medicine to go into private practice in the mid 1990s, he had two offices, one in The Methodist Hospital in the Texas Medical Center and the other at The Methodist Willowbrook Hospital. Around the turn of the millennium, Drs. Pacifico and Nasir merged with two cardiologists, Dr. Valintine Ugolini, an advocate for preventative medicine and Dr. Pacifico's wife, and Dr. Anton Nielsen, Baylor-trained in general cardiology, and became known as the Willowbrook Cardiovascular Associates. Additional associates were to join them in the following years, including Drs. Rami Tappan and Douglas Bree, both EP specialists, and Drs. Stanley Duchman and John Isaac, general cardiologists.

Recruited from the Cleveland Clinic to replace Dr. Pacifico as head of the EP program at Baylor College of Medicine was Dr. Ron Mahoney, who also brought Dr. Dennis Zhu into the program. Together they recruited Dr. Hue The Shih, who had recently finished the EP training program at Baylor College of Medicine. After a short stay, Drs. Mahoney and Zhu moved on to other institutions and Dr. Shih entered private practice. Therefore electrophysiology at The Methodist Hospital was in the hands of private practitioners in 2005, not Baylor College of Medicine.

As a private practitioner and one of the leading clinical investigators in cardiac electrophysiology, Dr. Pacifico developed expertise in the implantation of pacemakers and the implantable cardioverter-defibrillator (ICD), a new device that was to revolutionize the treatment of patients at risk for sudden cardiac death due to ventricular tachyarrhythmias. In 2002, Dr. Pacifico published one of the first comprehensive textbooks on implantable defibrillators.[31] Another one of his passions was flying, and he frequently flew his private plane to medical meetings and on hunting and fishing excursions. He died an early, unfortunate death in November 2005 when the plane he was piloting crashed on takeoff from Hobby Airport in Houston.

Since the early 1980s, the EP specialists at The Methodist Hospital had been involved in both surgical intervention for the treatment of cardiac arrhythmias and the implantation of pacemakers and implantable cardioverter-defibrillator (ICD), procedures that took place either in the operat-

ing room or in the catheterization laboratories. "The surgeons would make
the pocket, the cardiologists would place the leads, and the surgeons would
go ahead and suture that pocket," explained catheterization laboratories director Ms. Chesnick, noting how this eventually evolved into Dr. Spencer
and other cardiologists implanting pacemakers in the catheterization laboratories without surgical assistance. "For those surgeons to 'let go' of that
procedure was a lot, I think."[28]

Radiologists at The Methodist Hospital also experienced the "letting go"
process as they began to relinquish abdominal aortogram studies and peripheral arteriogram studies to cardiologists. Unlike other hospitals where
all such cardiovascular imaging remained in radiology, there was a major
difference at Methodist. The advances made by cardiologists in imaging
procedures in echocardiography and nuclear cardiology in the early 1980s
was one of the major reasons why the imaging name at The Methodist
Hospital has done so well—because it has all been concentrated in one
department.

The concentration of specialized cardiovascular care in the coronary
care unit (CCU) at The Methodist Hospital was also to garner national
recognition in the 1980s. Named as the principal investigator of one of
the 13 participating clinical sites in a national clinical trial supported by
the National Heart, Lung, and Blood Institute, Dr. Roberts headed a team
of nine coinvestigators comprising Drs. Raizner, Pratt, Verani, and Young,
among others. During Phase 1 of the Thrombolysis in Myocardial Infarction Trial (TIMI) in 1984, the 13 clinical sites documented the outcomes
of rapid administration of intravenous clot-busting drugs streptokinase and
recombinant tissue plasminogen activator to patients with evolving acute
myocardial infarction.[32]

This exploration of the possibility of limiting or even preventing myocardial infarction by dissolving newly formed clots in the coronary artery
intravenously generated worldwide interest. Heretofore, a catheter directly inserted into the coronary artery was the only approved method of ad-
ministering streptokinase, licensed by the FDA in 1982. Because of this
limitation, it was a procedure that took place only in hospitals that had a
specialized CCU.

While intracoronary streptokinase had been administered effectively by
catheter in The Methodist Hospital CCU since 1982, both Drs. Roberts
and Pratt believed that intravenous streptokinase could be just as safe and
effective in restoring coronary flow. Documenting their recommendation of
a "large-scale, randomized placebo-controlled study" after the publication

of successful results in the preliminary studies of intravenous streptokinase conducted in Europe in the early 1980s, they stated: "These reports clearly indicate the potential for a significant impact on acute and long-term mortality since it can be administered with ease and rapidly throughout the medical community."[33]

The clot-busting effect of recombinant tissue plasminogen activator, one of the first bioengineered drugs produced for clinical use by means of recombinant-DNA techniques, had been studied only in small clinical and animal studies. Since it had not received FDA approval, the drug had limited access and was available only to the 13 participants in the TIMI trial. Quite unexpectedly, the preliminary findings of Phase 1 of the study in 1985 established that recombinant tissue plasminogen activator was the more effective and safe agent for unclogging freshly obstructed coronary vessels intravenously.[34] Since maximum benefit was achieved with rapid administration of the bioengineered drug in acute myocardial infarction patients, this thrombolytic therapy was unavailable to those patients who did not live in close proximity to one of the participants in the TIMI Study Group.

At The Methodist Hospital, this logistical problem was to inspire the creation of a unique cardiovascular service. To transport the eligible patients within a 200-mile radius of The Methodist Hospital, Dr. Spencer of The Chapman Group spearheaded the establishment of a cardiovascular aeromedical service. The referral area to be served encompassed southeastern Texas, western Louisiana, and the southwest corner of Mississippi. "I felt like if we could fly the tissue plasminogen activator in a helicopter out to hospitals where patients were having heart attacks," he said, recalling his initial motivation for the service, "if we could get it there in a decent period of time, we'd be able to administer that to the patient and then bring the patient back here and do further cardiovascular work."[35]

Further need for the aeromedical program at The Methodist Hospital became evident during Phase 2 of the TIMI Study Group (TIMI II). Beginning in July 1986, the two-year study expanded to 25 participating medical centers to determine whether the administration of tissue plasminogen activator (TPA) intravenously during the early hours of a heart attack should be followed by dilation of blocked coronary arteries with a balloon-tipped catheter. "The rapid advances in the treatment of patients with acute myocardial infarction, especially thrombolytic therapy and emergency angioplasty, have increased the desirability of having such patients moved to tertiary hospitals with 24-hours-a-day cardiac catheterization laboratories and state-of-the-art coronary care units," Drs. Spencer, Pratt, and Roberts reported in 1987.[36]

To safely transfer these patients, The Methodist Hospital Aeromedical Services became operational on March 23, 1987. It became the first such service to exclusively focus on the cardiovascular patient in Texas. With two experienced pilots and fitted with advanced cardiac life support equipment, the spacious Sikorsky 76 helicopter had a medical team comprised of a cardiovascular nurse and a cardiology fellow who was in direct communication with a cardiologist at The Methodist Hospital. The nurses on call for the helicopter service were required to be certified paramedics and advanced cardiac life support instructors and have extensive experience in the CCU, ICU, or emergency room. In addition to receiving extensive education in the use of thrombolytic drugs and their adverse effects, the nurses also had to demonstrate their ability to function properly in an airborne vehicle.

Those interested in qualifying to join the medical team underwent a unique test. "I had the honor of interviewing those staff members," Ms. Chesnick said, recalling how the program continued for seven to eight years until direct coronary angioplasty became the preferred treatment for myocardial infarction. "Jean Nelson was director of the program and part of their orientation was to go to NASA and suit up for flight simulation studies. They had to experience what was called the 'vomit comet' to make sure they could acclimate to being in the helicopter. Some of them did well, but I remember some coming back and saying 'I'm not cutting this. I can't do it.'"[28]

Another of Ms. Chesnick's responsibilities as director of the catheterization laboratories was fulfilling staffing requirements necessary for the around-the-clock catheterization laboratories dictated by the TIMI II trial. Recalling the necessity of lengthy, on-the-job training of critical care nurses recruited for the catheterization laboratory, she said, "Talk about challenges. With a helicopter dropping in patients to get TPA at all hours of the day and night we had to have newly trained call teams on standby every hour of the day and night."[28]

Since her office in the catheterization laboratory was located directly below the helipad atop the Alkek Tower, Ms. Chesnick, in more ways than one, was aware whenever a transported cardiac patient arrived at The Methodist Hospital. "It was the best of times, it really was—I'll never forget that first day when they brought the first patient in," she said, remembering how she had to establish the choreography for all challenges presented by the more than 270 transported patients in the first eight months.[36] "With the helicopter dropping in patients to get TPA at all hours of the day and night, in addition to staffing for diagnostic cardiac catheterizations and angioplasties, we had to have the operating room on standby in case something (unexpected) happened."[28]

The critical need for The Methodist Hospital Aeromedical Services and its ability to transport acute myocardial infarction patients after the initiation of thrombolytic therapy was obsolesced after the FDA approval of TPA increased its availability in outlying areas. "A lot of other drugs and techniques became commercially available and they spread out to the periphery and there was no longer the pressing need to get people here on an emergency basis to be treated," Dr. Spencer recalled, noting the service's successful two-year existence. "It worked out very well for patients who were very ill. It was unbelievable. We published several manuscripts based on the helicopter transport of patients with acute myocardial infarction."[35-37]

While there had been a low incidence of complications experienced by the transported cardiovascular patients, the possibility of those that could occur during coronary angioplasty continued to exist. "It was clear to everybody who was doing interventions that the most frightening complication was a tear in the artery where the inner lining would just not get out of the way," Dr. Raizner said. "Instead of opening the blockage, the artery would close and often we'd have to spend hours or have to send the patient to emergency surgery. And that was the traumatic part of coronary angioplasty. It was clear that something would be needed to tack these tears or dissections down."[38]

Another major problem for interventional cardiologists in all PTCA patients was the high incidence of restenosis, the reoccurrence of a blockage or narrowing of a large blood vessel or artery. In more than 25 percent of the patients treated with PTCA, the majority had to undergo another balloon angioplasty procedure for restenosis within six months. In addition to aggressive anticoagulation therapy to prevent restenosis, interventional cardiologists began to investigate newly developed technologies for better long-term results.

Laser light was tried for obstructing coronary artery plaques by the interventional cardiologists at The Methodist Hospital. Pulsed laser light was delivered through very small optical fibers bundled into flexible catheters. As the catheters were advanced through the artery, the noncalcified obstructing plaques could be ablated. But the technique was short-lived because of cost and development of more effective options.

With the encouraging results of similar devices that used percutaneous entry placement techniques, "we became interested in stents," Dr. Raizner said. "There was an interventional radiologist at M. D. Anderson Hospital named Cesare Gianturco, who had developed a stent for use in stenosis of the biliary tree. We knew him and asked if we could do some of the very basic animal work to see if this device was applicable to coronary arteries. Since we did not have the required laboratory here, we worked with him in his lab at M.D. Anderson where we developed a pig model."[38]

Through similar collaborative efforts in the early 1980s, a device for patients who were having recurrent pulmonary emboli had been conceived and developed by Dr. Gianturco and an interventional radiologist at The Methodist Hospital, Dr. Jack Roehm. "He had published a paper in 1980 about putting these wires in the inferior vena cava of dogs," Dr. Roehm recalled. "The device sort of looked like a little wire broccoli with a wire coming out of it with a button buried under the skin so it wouldn't escape. I began working with him and together we developed the first percutaneous inferior vena cava filter. And I put them in dogs and then in 1982, I put one in a human being, a patient of Dr. Jimmy Howell's, and over the next two years I put one in 29 patients."[27]

The reluctance of the two developers to claim pride of authorship by naming the device after themselves led to an unusual result. "Stanley Crawford said to me one day, 'You know, Jack, that looks like a rat's nest,'" Dr. Roehm said, pointing out that Dr. Crawford grew up on a farm and knew what a rat's nest looked like. "So I called it the 'Bird's Nest Filter,' not the 'Gianturco-Roehm Filter.' But if you look on the package that it comes in, it does say Gianturco-Roehm Filter, but it's not really called that, it's called a Bird's Nest Filter."[27,39-41]

Cook Incorporated, who manufactured the Bird's Nest Filter and the stents developed by Dr. Gianturco for the biliary track, became involved with the development of coronary artery stents. During Dr. Gianturco's initial collaboration with Dr. Raizner in the first animal studies of the new device, efforts to place a metal stent in pig arteries produced positive results when accompanied by preventive measures such as the use of Coumadin and aspirin. "It looked like it was going to work in humans," Dr. Raizner said.[42,43]

"At about the same time, Julio Palmaz, who was a radiologist, developed a stent also for the biliary tree and came up with the same idea that this stent might be applicable for the coronary arteries. He approached Richard Schatz, who was a cardiologist in San Antonio. So their efforts in San Antonio and our efforts in the animal lab here were concomitant when Dr. Gianturco and Cook Incorporated approached Dr. Gruentzig, who had moved to Atlanta, who was very interested in this approach. Unfortunately, he died in an airplane crash in 1985 and Gary Roubin, a research fellow he had brought over to do some of the testing in dogs with a stent, became the one who put the first stent in humans in Emory. We put the second stent in humans in the United States at The Methodist Hospital in 1988."[38,44,45]

Named the Gianturco-Roubin flexible coronary stent, the new device immediately underwent a multicenter study, one in which The Methodist Hospital participated from September 1988 through June 1991. The results of the deployment of one or more stents in 494 patients with acute or threatened closure after angioplasty demonstrated a high technical success rate and encouraging results with respect to the low incidence of emergency coronary artery bypass surgery and myocardial infarction. The preliminary conclusions of the study, published in the *Journal of the American College of Cardiology*, stated: "The multicenter experience suggests that this stent is a useful adjunct to coronary angioplasty to prevent or minimize complications associated with flow-limiting coronary artery dissections previously correctable only by surgery."[44]

For those patients with peripheral vascular obstructions that could not be treated by PTCA or stents, another new procedure became available in the interventional catheterization laboratory in the late 1980s. It was to become known as "Rotorooter," after the name of the company that reams out drainage pipes, because it involved the intravascular delivery of a mechanical, rotational atherectomy device consisting of a high-speed rotary burr to remove portions of impenetrable plaque and improve blood flow. "There were two people who invented that device simultaneously," Dr. Raizner said. "One of the inventors was Dr. Nadim M. Zacca, a cardiologist at The Methodist Hospital, but he never received credit for it. His collaborator filed a patent first, but unbeknownst to Dr. Zacca. He and I did the first 'Rotorooter' atherectomy in a human being anywhere in the world in a leg artery in 1988."[8,46]

Welded to a long, flexible drive shaft, the device was guided by a catheter to the obstruction in a reduced diameter configuration, expanded and rotated to remove the obstruction, and contracted to remove. "The one we used was named Rotoblator and it actually was a cutting blade where you push the opening, it looks almost like a bullet, and you push it into the plaque and the plaque goes into the window in the bullet and the knife comes and cuts it off," Dr. Raizner said, explaining how the high-speed rotary cutter was designed to preferentially scrape harder surfaces such as plaque while minimizing damage to lubricated surfaces such as endothelium, the thin layer of cells that lines the interior surface of blood vessels.[47] "We worked together on that with Dr. Noon, who did a bypass on the artery and then Nadim and I went in and did the atherectomy."[8]

Even though Dr. Raizner and his team of interventional cardiologists began to perform atherectomies with the Rotoblator and other similar devices and laser angioplasty, the advances made in coronary stents caused the technology to wane and the popularity of those procedures to be brief. The introduction of coronary stenting significantly improved the safety and early results of coronary angioplasty, but it was accompanied by its own set of disappointments. Recurrent stenosis within a stent (restenosis) remained a nagging problem. Long known was the fact that scar tissue around and in a healing wound, called "keloid," could be prevented by radiation treatment. Dr. Raizner surmised that recurring stenosis after a stent had been deployed could be prevented or inhibited by radiation. Similar thoughts occurred at the same time to researchers at Columbia University and Emory University.

The procedure to be developed was called "intravascular brachytherapy" (IVBT). Radiation was delivered through a catheter using either gamma or beta radiation. After a clinical trial provided clear evidence of its safety, several clinical trials were conducted providing evidence for efficacy in preventing restenosis.[48] This technique soon became a historical landmark as drug-eluting stents came on the scene as the primary approach to arterial stenosis and for restenosis within a previously implanted stent.

By the late 1980s, the predominant coronary intervention performed in the catheterization laboratories around the world was PTCA, numbering more than one million worldwide.[49] In the United States alone, the number of coronary angioplasties nearly equaled the number of coronary bypass operations at the end of the decade.[50-52]

After the 1989 publication of the TIMI II trial findings, in which immediate PTCA after the administration of TPA in acute myocardial infarction patients was deemed unnecessary, there was relatively minimal impact on the volume of coronary angioplasties performed. Results of that study at The Methodist Hospital and 49 other centers indicated that "prophylactic PTCA offered no advantage in terms of reductions in mortality or reinfarction over a more conservative strategy," one that was less complex and less costly.[53]

By the late 1980s, the number of PTCA procedures performed at The Methodist Hospital totaled more than 3,000 and an exponential growth in the volume of procedures seemed a certainty. In the decade since introducing Dr. Gruentzig's procedure at The Methodist Hospital in March 1980, Drs. Raizner, Lewis, and Winters had participated in its evolution, adapted to each innovative development in balloon catheters, fine-tuned each procedural modification introduced, and trained countless cardiologists and fellows in that rapidly emerging field of interventional cardiology.

One such postdoctoral fellow trained at The Methodist Hospital was Dr. Neal S. Kleiman, a 1981 graduate of Columbia University College of Physicians and Surgeons and a former resident of Baylor College of Medicine. Recruited to join the faculty after his cardiology fellowship in 1987, Dr. Kleiman became assistant director of the cardiac catheterization laboratories at The Methodist Hospital in 1989. At that time, the expanding eligibility requirements for interventional cardiology began to dictate its parameters. "We sort of settled into a pattern," Dr. Raizner said. "If it was left main or triple vessel disease, those patients went to surgery. If it was single or double vessel disease we tended to do those patients by PTCA. We later would expand into triple vessel disease and discover everything is fair game for intervention."[8]

With all the expanding parameters of the various subspecialty areas of clinical cardiology during the decade, the probability of further expansion seemed inevitable, particularly to Dr. Quiñones. Of that promising era, he said in retrospect, "In the 1980s cardiologists were beginning to have the innovation and creativity that Dr. DeBakey had in the 1940s, '50s and '60s."[54]

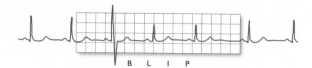

B   L   I   P

AT THE HEART OF THE MOB

*I*n *1986, Fortune magazine listed the top 50 Mafia bosses in order of importance in the United States. Two named on that list, the Tampa boss, Santo Trafficante (No. 15) and the Chicago boss, Joseph Ferriola (No. 20) would share another commonality shortly thereafter. In the late 1980s, both reportedly were treated for heart disease "by the best in Houston."[1] A patient of Dr. Denton Cooley's in 1987, Mr. Trafficante underwent triple-bypass surgery at the Texas Heart Institute but died in his sleep three hours later at the age of 72.[2] A patient of Dr. DeBakey's two years later, Mr. Ferriola became the first known member of organized crime to receive not just one heart transplant but two in as many weeks at The Methodist Hospital. Following the second unsuccessful heart transplant in March 1989, Mr. Ferriola died in the hospital at the age of 61.[1]*

Although Tony "The Ant" Spilotro was not listed as one of the top 50 Mafia bosses by Fortune, he was the Las Vegas chieftain of the Chicago mob when he underwent coronary bypass surgery at The Methodist Hospital in 1985. Known to be one of the most colorful characters in the "Outfit," he was the inspiration for Joe Pesci's character, Nicky Santoro, in Martin Scorsese's 1995 movie adaptation of Nicholas Pileggi's book, Casino. Even though he survived the heart bypass operation, "The Ant" and his brother were both dead a year later after being brutally beaten and buried alive in an Indiana cornfield by mob members on June 23, 1986.[3]

1. Hampson R, McShane L. Number of mob leaders is shrinking. AP, *Hudson Valley News.* November 29, 1991.

2. Reputed mob boss Trafficante dies. AP, *Park City Daily News.* March 19, 1987.

3. Luft K, Heard J. Joseph Ferriola, Chicago mob figure, dies at 61. *Chicago Tribune.* March 12, 1989.

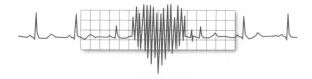

CHAPTER FIFTEEN

PREVENTION AND CONTROVERSY
1987 - 1991

"The prevention of disease today is one of the most important factors in line of human endeavor."
CHARLES MAYO

I n the 56 years since gaining his medical degree at Tulane University, the 79-year-old Dr. DeBakey was perhaps the world's best-known physician in 1988.[1] A prominent fixture in the public eye, his presence had become ubiquitous in newspapers, magazines, and television.

Heralded by President Ronald Reagan as "one of the heroes of the modern age" in a Rose Garden ceremony at the White House in 1987, Dr. DeBakey received the nation's highest award for achievement in science and technology, the National Medal of Science. Recognized as being among those who "put their genius to work and the results are phenomenal," Dr. DeBakey received praise for his "pioneering medical innovations throughout his medical career."[2]

Listed in 65 directories of Who's Who, Dr. DeBakey had authored more than 1,200 medical articles and served on 50 editorial boards. With appointments to serve on 114 advisory committees, he was a member of 100 professional organizations and the recipient of 32 honorary degrees and 150 scientific awards. As a medical statesman and surgeon, Dr. DeBakey continued to travel throughout the world, giving lectures, receiving awards, and operating on numerous heads of state as well as paupers.[1] Regardless of their stature, his patients remained his top priority.

Along with his established reputation for being a demanding perfectionist in the operating room, Dr. DeBakey also was known to be a compassionate caregiver who often developed close personal relationships with his patients. One such occasion at The Methodist Hospital in 1984 enabled the septuagenarian surgeon an opportunity to further enhance his reputation as a trailblazer. "George Noon and I performed a heart transplant on David Saucier, a National Aeronautics Space Agency (NASA) engineer," Dr. DeBakey said, recalling the serendipity of their initial interaction. In the course of his stay in The Methodist Hospital following the procedure, the engineer and the surgeons began to talk about the intricacies of mechanical heart pumps.[3]

Mr. Saucier was intrigued upon learning about Dr. DeBakey's creation and implantation of the first left ventricle assistance device (LVAD) in 1966, his abandonment of his decades-long research on a total artificial heart, and his ongoing desire to create a ventricular assist device (VAD) for long-term chronic support in end-stage heart failure patients as a bridge to transplant, bridge to recovery, or alternative to transplant. When told of the surgeons' challenge of developing a permanent axial flow pump that was small enough to be implanted in the chest but powerful enough to push blood through the thousands of miles of vessels in the body, Mr. Saucier had an epiphany. Quite unexpectedly, Dr. DeBakey said, "Saucier suggested we meet some of the NASA engineers who were experienced in developing pumps for moving fluids such as rocket fuel."[3]

Returning to his job at NASA/Johnson Space Center in Houston six months after his heart transplant, Mr. Saucier convened colleagues James Akkerman, Bernard Rosenbaum, Gregory Aber, and Richard Bozeman with Drs. DeBakey, Noon, and other Baylor College of Medicine researchers. As the NASA engineers responsible for the system used to fuel the space shuttle's main engines, they had extensive experience with axial flow motors and shared Mr. Saucier's enthusiasm about the possibility of a collaborative effort to create the first axial flow pump for intermediate-to long-term treatment of end-stage heart failure.

The memory of that initial meeting was vivid to one of those engineers. "It was interesting, the day they showed up, two great big limousines came, and there were six doctors in each of the limousines, and they had on their pinstriped suits, and there was the doctor of hematology and the doctor of hemodynamics and the doctor of hemo-this and hemo-that," Mr. Akkerman said. "And they brought a big box full of blood pumps that they had worked on, all of 'em had gears and electric motors, and I'm a mechanical engineer and it just made my heart go pitter pat to see all of this machinery."[4]

Within four years, this unique collaboration officially had begun its comprehensive research and development process to create a miniaturized, implantable axial flow blood pump. Initially called the NASA/DeBakey heart pump, this trailblazing VAD had the potential to address limitations of the existing, larger pulsatile devices in existence.

To create the first prototype, the NASA engineers worked in their spare time, at night, and during weekends. "I remember I spent most of the Christmas holidays at my computer designing the pump blades for this thing, trying to get the flow, the diameter, and the length and all in the ballpark," Mr. Akkerman said, recalling how the prototype was to be the size of a thumb and would create no pulse, just a constant flow of blood.[4] Working in tandem with researchers from Baylor College of Medicine, the NASA engineers endeavored to design and develop "a safe, effective, reliable, simple-to-operate, affordable pump that would allow recipients to move about freely with a portable controller and batteries," Dr. Noon explained. "With this type of design, the recipient could potentially recover from the effects of heart failure, be discharged from the hospital, perform the normal activities of daily living, and maintain an improved quality of life."[5]

While the ultimate results of this collaborative effort were to come later in the decade, the impact of the previous contributions of Dr. DeBakey and other pioneers in the cardiovascular field was evident in the late 1980s. Such advances enabled the accurate diagnosis of diseases of the heart, lungs, and blood to be achieved safely in virtually all patients. Although effective symptomatic treatment and prolongation of life could be provided to many, cure was possible only in a small number of cases.[6] According to the American Heart Association in 1985, more than 800,000 Americans died each year from all forms of cardiovascular disease.

Predominant among the forms of cardiovascular disease treated at The Methodist Hospital in the 1980s were complications of atherosclerosis, a disease in which plaque builds up inside the arteries in the heart, brain, abdomen, legs, pelvis, and kidneys. While Dr. DeBakey and his team of cardiovascular surgeons were performing more than 5,000 heart surgeries annually, Dr. DeBakey continued to believe the key to conquering heart disease would be prevention and not surgical intervention.[7] This also was the consensus of the cardiologists and other physicians at The Methodist Hospital who devoted a majority of their efforts to the diagnosis and treatment of the different diseases resulting from atherosclerosis. A paramount quest in the 1980s and early 1990s was to develop preventative measures for coronary heart disease, coronary microvascular disease, carotid artery disease, peripheral arterial diseases, and chronic kidney disease.

The precise cause of atherosclerosis, one of Dr. DeBakey's career-long pursuits, remained elusive. His pioneering cardiovascular research during the previous four decades had yet to produce a conclusive answer. One breakthrough came in 1983 when he and Dr. Joseph L. Melnick, a molecular virologist at Baylor College of Medicine, reported evidence of cytomegalovirus involvement in arterial walls of some patients with atherosclerosis.[8] "Since replicating virus was not detected, this finding suggested that the occurrence of cytomegalovirus early in life may initiate the lesions that later cause atherosclerosis," Dr. Gotto said. "Extending this line of investigation, Dr. DeBakey and colleagues in 1987 reported patients with atherosclerosis have higher-than-normal levels of antibodies to cytomegalovirus."[9]

As research efforts into the origin of atherosclerosis continued unabated in the early 1980s, the four major risk factors for heart disease—obesity, high blood pressure, smoking, and unhealthy eating habits—had already been established in the 1950s. The American Heart Association began recommending a "prudent diet" to lower blood-fat levels for all Americans in 1961, and a national commission of medical experts first defined the specifics of a heart-healthy diet in 1970. Since there was minimal evidence that reducing cholesterol and LDL-C with diet or drugs would reduce cardiovascular events, the medical experts called for government-sponsored studies to determine the facts. In the meantime, the experts concluded there should be "'safe and reasonable' changes in diets to lower cholesterol levels in hopes of stemming the current 'epidemic' of heart disease."[10]

The "first conclusive evidence" that lowering blood cholesterol can help prevent heart attacks was established in 1984 at the conclusion of the 10-year study conducted by the National Institutes of Health's (NIH) Coronary Primary Prevention Trial. The study took place in the NIH's 12 Lipid Research Clinics, including the one established at The Methodist Hospital and Baylor College of Medicine under the direction of Dr. Gotto. As president of the American Heart Association in 1984, Dr. Gotto announced that the key message of this study was "if all Americans would reduce their blood cholesterol levels by 25 percent, this would eventually lead to a 50 percent reduction in the incidence of coronary heart disease."[11-13]

Further recommendations from a consensus of the physicians and scientists at the American Heart Association included an urge to physicians to obtain measurement of blood fats in all their patients. This was to include total cholesterol and its components, high-density, low-density, and very-low density lipoproteins and triglycerides. National surveys indicated that 80 percent of the general public had heard of the condition of "high blood cholesterol," but only 3 percent knew their cholesterol levels—meaning that 70 to 80 million Americans were unaware of their cholesterol level and had not taken action to have it checked.[14]

Addressing this challenge as president of the American Heart Association, Dr. Gotto suggested a government-sponsored mass-screening program at offices, schools, stores, and airports similar to one initiated for high blood pressure in the 1970s. "It could achieve a dramatic reduction in the death rate from coronary heart disease, which is the No. 1 killer in our country," he said. "It might save as many as 250,000 to 300,000 lives a year."[15]

Following the published results of the NIH Primary Prevention Trial in January 1984, the National Heart, Lung, and Blood Institute announced the creation of the Consensus Conference on Lowering Blood Cholesterol to Prevent Heart Disease, which in turn enacted the National Cholesterol Education Program (NCEP). Established in 1984, the NCEP was to educate the medical profession and the general public and raise awareness and understanding about the benefits of lowering cholesterol levels by all possible means.[14]

When word of this new program first circulated in Washington, Mrs. Lasker and her "noble conspirators" at the Lasker Foundation recognized an opportunity to expand the parameters of their populist lobbying efforts. Based on their successful impact on the National High Blood Pressure Education Program in the 1970s, they knew an independent lobbying body would be able "to revitalize a broad based constituency."[16]

In 1985, the independent lobbying group known as Citizens for Public Action on Cholesterol was formed with Mrs. Lasker as honorary chairwoman, Dr. DeBakey as chairman, and Dr. Gotto as chairman of its medical advisory panel of cholesterol experts. Under the direction of Mr. Gorman, who also had served as director of Mrs. Lasker's high blood pressure lobbying body in Washington, the Citizens became a legislative action network to "encompass this new cholesterol offensive" and to procure funds and state support for its specifically tailored strategies for a mass-oriented cholesterol education program.[16]

As public awareness began to increase following such education programs and the "know your cholesterol level" campaign launched by the NCEP, an effective treatment to lower cholesterol levels remained limited. Since pharmaceutical intervention was considered to be "high risk," physicians continued to prescribe reduced intakes of saturated fat and cholesterol, increased physical activity, and weight control.[14]

Recognizing there was a need for specific information about healthy eating habits, Dr. DeBakey, Lynne Scott, chief dietician, Dr. John Foreyt, a clinical psychologist who served as director of the diet clinic at The Methodist Hospital, and Dr. Gotto published *The Living Heart Diet* in 1985.[17] Destined to become a best-selling book, it was the result of five years of research with 5,000 patients at The Methodist Hospital. "To the best of our knowledge," Dr. DeBakey said upon publication of the book's recommended, low-cholesterol lifestyle, "These are the things that we can do now to reduce the risk of heart disease."[18]

As for future treatment to lower cholesterol, answers were expected to come through research. Enabled by a $14-million, five-year grant received from the National Heart, Lung, and Blood Institute in 1987, Dr. Gotto and his colleagues expanded their research. This grant established a National Research and Demonstration Center at Baylor College of Medicine and The Methodist Hospital specifically targeting atherosclerosis. In essence, it was a revival of the defunct "Super Center" that ended in 1982 after seven years of funded research on heart and blood vessels. Through work perfected in the new center, Dr. Gotto said, "We hope we not only prolong life, we believe we are improving the quality of life."[19]

As the appointed chairman of a year-long study involving 13,000 people at the 12 national Lipid Research Centers in the United States in 1987, Dr. Gotto was able to show that screening large groups of people for high cholesterol at shopping malls, medical facilities, schools, and work sites can accurately identify those at risk for heart disease.[20] When a 1987 survey by the NIH indicated that fewer than 10 percent of all Americans knew their cholesterol levels and an estimated 55 percent of the untested had higher levels than desirable, Dr. Gotto once again proposed a mass-screening effort. "Motivating everyone to know their cholesterol number is the first step in controlling high cholesterol and preventing heart disease," he said. "Large scale screening is a means of achieving this and our study has demonstrated these programs work and are valuable."[21]

The merits of Dr. Gotto's proposal, as well as the aggressive education program mounted by the NCEP, became the fodder for an ongoing debate within the medical community. Although most physicians were in agreement that high levels of cholesterol, in general, were undesirable, many questioned whether there were clear indications of the risks involved and adequate evidence of the benefits achieved by lowering the levels with drugs. At that time, most physicians considered atherosclerosis to be an inevitable accompaniment of aging, about which nothing much could be done.[22] Therefore, many questioned the efficacy of cholestyramine, the "drug of choice" recommended by the NCEP in its 1987 treatment guide for those unable to achieve the proper cholesterol level through a medically supervised diet.[23]

To this debate Dr. DeBakey was to contribute his own research-based evidence that proved to contradict recently concluded studies of the role of cholesterol in heart disease. In an April 1987 press conference following his receipt of an award for outstanding contributions to cardiovascular medicine from Cedars-Sinai Medical Center in Los Angeles, Dr. DeBakey said that 30 years of observation of more than 15,000 patients had led him to conclude that cholesterol was not the central cause of atherosclerosis. Responding to this statement, Dr. Gotto reportedly replied that although there may be more important factors than fat and cholesterol in surgery patients, "all the evidence runs in the other direction."[24]

Although of differing opinions on the subject of cholesterol, Drs. Gotto and DeBakey agreed the definitive cause of atherosclerosis remained unknown. They also concurred that dietary cholesterol was one of the important risk factors, along with hypertension, smoking, obesity, exercise, diabetes, stress, and behavior patterns. In their coauthored book, *The Living Heart Diet*, they concurred that it "was possible to follow a prudent diet and also eat well," as demonstrated in the heart-healthy cuisine served at Chez Eddy, the restaurant created and introduced by Dr. Gotto in 1981 at The Methodist Hospital.[25] Nonetheless, based on his extensive research of former surgical patients, Dr. DeBakey had formed a decidedly different opinion about the benefits of achieving the perfect cholesterol levels, saying, "People should lower their cholesterol to protect themselves, but should not be shocked if they still have heart disease."[24]

His was an opinion that was to be oft repeated during the continuing cholesterol debate. Having taken place mainly within the medical community, the heated discussions evolved into a public controversy in 1989. Publicly voicing criticism of the NCEP, its leaders, and the necessity of its guidelines was an article authored by journalist Thomas J. Moore titled *The Cholesterol Myth* in the September 1989 issue of *Atlantic Monthly*. His conclusions about whether or not decreasing cholesterol levels would reduce coronary events were the headlines superimposed on a cartoon drawing of a frustrated diner with his mouth taped shut with Band-Aids: "Lowering your cholesterol is next to impossible with diet, and often dangerous with drugs–and it won't make you live any longer."[26]

Described as a "blistering attack" by those supporting the NCEP, the article pointed out how "the dissenters have been overwhelmed by the extravaganza put on not just by the Heart Institute but by a growing coalition that resembles a medical version of the military-industrial complex." After identifying Dr. Gotto as one of the five leaders of this coalition, the author pointed out that each of these cholesterol experts and investigators was very active in the lipid field and implied that their laboratories "were heavily involved in research funded by Merck." This veiled accusation was followed by this statement: "There is no reason to doubt the honesty, sincerity, and expertise of any of these men."[23]

When doctors, scientists, and drug companies refuted these published claims, the author retorted that all such naysayers were in cahoots as members of the "Cholesterol Mafia."[27] The public's reaction to this iconoclastic article was measurable, both immediately thereafter and decades later when the September 1989 *The Cholesterol Myth* cover was to be identified by *Atlantic Monthly* as one of its top-selling issues of all time. The negative publicity not only impacted the efforts of the NCEP but also inspired the House of Representatives Committee on Energy and Commerce, Subcommittee on Health and the Environment to convene a December 7, 1989 hearing at which both Mr. Moore and Dr. Gotto testified.

Chaired by the Hon. Henry A. Waxman, the subcommittee had convened because of its "particular interest in trying to learn the truth" about various aspects of the national cholesterol program. Testifying that the hazards of cholesterol had been greatly exaggerated, Mr. Moore reiterated his published opinion that the "national campaign to lower cholesterol is a serious and expensive mistake and will push millions of Americans into a program of medical treatment that is expensive and risky without delivering benefits." In rebuttal, Dr. Gotto stated cholesterol was a national health priority because "numerous epidemiologic and laboratory studies have confirmed the continuous, positive correlation of elevated cholesterol levels to increased heart disease and clinical studies have shown that cholesterol modification by diet or drugs can lower that risk."[28]

Even though this congressional investigation resulted in no charges, there continued to be widespread professional and public criticism of the widespread educational and treatment offensive endorsed by the NCEP. In the medical community, where Dr. Gotto was recognized as one of the experts in cholesterol and atherosclerosis, several prominent cardiologists continued to question the program he championed. Many argued that without a completely safe cholesterol-lowering drug, the safe and effective treatment of a prudent diet and exercise did not warrant the necessity of "the presently advocated dramatic cholesterol campaign of uncertain value but tremendous cost."[29]

Not everybody bowed at the altar of atherosclerosis. Most of the 20,000 board-certified cardiologists in the United States were preoccupied with the implementation of new and exciting diagnostic and interventional tools at that time. Along with the diagnostic innovations established in echocardiography, nuclear stress testing, coronary angiography, and invasive electrophysiology testing, the advanced therapeutics of pacemakers, angioplasty, and implantable defibrillators had enabled cardiologists to offer specialized care for an expanding range of cardiac problems.

With such diversified areas of interest, the professionalism of cardiology in the late 1980s and early 1990s and the delivery of high-technology care was, according to Dr. Winters, "in stark contrast to the early days of the subspecialty when my father spent two weeks training with Dr. Paul Dudley White in the early 1930s. He then purchased an electrocardiographic machine and called himself a cardiologist. There was no grand plan that shaped cardiology. Individuals and organizations exercised their options continuously in response to scientific advances, patient demand, economic incentives, and government initiatives."

To help all cardiologists remain current and competent in all factions of this continuously expanding field, educational resources were provided by The American College of Cardiology (ACC), the specialty's professional society founded in 1949. Since its inception, cardiologists at Baylor College of Medicine and The Methodist Hospital had been actively involved with the society. Dr. Don Chapman, one of the first members of ACC in 1949, served as governor of South Texas with the American College of Physicians and the American College of Cardiology and was awarded the title of Master in each society. After Dr. Chapman put Dr. Winters' name in the pot, he was to follow Dr. Chapman's footsteps in both organizations.

Already actively involved with the local chapter of the American Heart Association soon after his Houston arrival in 1968, Dr. Winters was named president of the Houston affiliate in the early 1970s. While in office, he endeavored to promote physician education through a professional education committee. Prior attempts to do so had failed miserably, and few participants came to the scheduled conference. To remedy the problem, several AHA members decided to concentrate education on just the committee members themselves. So was born the Houston Cardiology Society.

After the charter was drawn up and bylaws established, charter members of the Houston Cardiology Society included Dr. Winters and, among others, Drs. Spencer, J.K. Alexander, and Robert Hall. Monthly dinner meetings at The Doctors Club were held nine months of the year, with each meeting the responsibility of one of the major hospitals in Houston, both in the Texas Medical Center and suburbia. To their great surprise, attendance grew from a dozen or more in the beginning to as many as 80 to 100 attendees. While mostly cardiologists, those attending also were interested in cardiovascular pathology, cardiovascular surgery, cardiovascular radiology, and general medicine. Attendance stayed healthy until several years later, when the format began to change under new leaders. Instead of case presentations from the hospital medical staffs, invited speakers changed the format and attendance gradually declined. Over the years, the society gradually faded away.

After serving as governor of the Texas chapter of the American College of Cardiology (ACC) in the 1980s, Dr. Winters became chairman of the ACC's board of governors in 1981. Asked to run for vice president in 1987, he was elected, becoming president in 1990. "I think the influence the physicians on The Methodist Hospital staff have had on the American College of Cardiology has been pretty impressive," Dr. Winters said. "Initially there was Dr. Chapman in the 1960s, followed by Dr. Henry McIntosh, who served as president in the 1970s, and then my presidency in 1990 and, more recently, Bill Zoghbi in 2012. When it comes to ranking hospitals, one of the major criteria is reputation, which includes the reputation of the people on staff. I think our role at the American College of Cardiology has had a major impact in the medical community."

Dr. Winters' presidency represented the prominent role of private practitioners in the ACC. Of its diverse membership of physicians from the fields of cardiology, cardiovascular surgery, pediatrics, radiology, pathology, and anesthesiology, the greatest number of members was in private practice. At any given time during its existence, private practitioners comprised approximately one-third of the board of trustees. Says Dr. Winters, "I believe strongly that the role of the private practitioner in the College will expand even further in the years to come as the College agenda broadens in response to the issues facing the profession. These challenges demand effective leadership and because time commitments can be substantial, leadership requires personal sacrifice."[30]

To meet the time constraints of serving simultaneously as president of the ACC and governor for South Texas for the American College of Physicians in 1990, Dr. Winters turned to his colleagues in The Chapman Group to cover his office and hospital practice. "The anticipated time commitments of my duties caused my sacrificing my time in the catheterization laboratory, where I had participated in the first angioplasty performed at The Methodist Hospital in 1980," he said. "After 22 years as one of the early interventional cardiologists at the hospital, I was never to resume catheterization procedures following my time in national office."

"As president of the American College of Cardiology, I probably traveled 60-70 percent of that year. It was fun. I visited practically every state in the country. I traveled to England, Japan, Italy, and several other European countries. It was wonderful. I listened to a lot of lectures and I gave a lot of lectures. In so doing, I gained perspective on what was going on in the country in the medical field in general and in cardiovascular care specifically. At the time, varying aspects of the ongoing cholesterol debate continued and many were unaware that the conclusion of the controversy was imminent."

The solution to the lengthy debate about the priority of lowering cholesterol levels was to come partially from a steering committee of nine independent medical investigators convened in 1990. Led by Dr. Gotto, the investigators began an eight-year in-depth study of cholesterol-lowering statins, a potent inhibitor of cholesterol biosynthesis. Named the Air Force/Texas Coronary Atherosclerosis Prevention Study and scheduled to be completed in 1998, the study was made possible by a research grant from Merck & Co. Inc., the developer of Mevacor, known generically as lovastatin, the first statin drug available on the U.S. market in the late 1980s.[31-33]

The definitive results of Dr. Gotto's 1998 group effort in primary prevention followed those of the Scandinavian Survival Study that examined patients who already had established coronary heart disease.[34] Completed in 1994, it was the first truly large-scale, randomized, double-blind trial to show that aggressive treatment with simvastatin, another statin drug developed by Merck, not only reduces coronary heart disease mortality but also decreases all-cause mortality. This study's findings heralded the advent of the statin era and, since the wisdom of decreasing blood cholesterol no longer was doubted, the lengthy controversy was to come to an end.[35]

Such a scientific advance was unforeseeable in 1990 but was indicative of how cardiovascular care continuously evolved. In order for cardiologists to exercise their options in response to such breakthroughs, Dr. Winters utilized his ACC presidency to stress the importance of the ACC's mission to foster optimal cardiovascular care and disease prevention through professional education, promotion of research and leadership in the development of standards and formulation of health care policy.[36] To address one of the specific challenges facing the ACC in 1990, he often spoke about the newly instated American Board of Internal Medicine requirement for cardiology fellows to be recertified every ten years, emphasizing the priority of the college's program of continuing education to insure intellectual and procedural competency.

Already an active member of the staff of volunteer educators at the

ACC's Heart House at that time was his colleague at The Methodist Hospital, Dr. Miguel Quiñones, who had been teaching his own course in echocardiography since the early 1980s. "Those were the days when Heart House would have four to six echo courses a year because echocardiography became a very, very popular topic for courses," recalled Dr. Quiñones, who later served as chairman of the Heart House Educational Committee, which puts on all of the courses at the Heart House. "Because a lot of physicians wanted to train and retrain or re-update on echocardiography, we started with one course and subsequently had a second one. We started to use educational videotapes in the mid to late 1980s and early 1990s that were really popular."[37]

It was Dr. Quiñones who later introduced his colleague Dr. William Zoghbi to the ACC. "He had two courses in echocardiography and he invited me to be on the faculty in the mid 1980s," Dr. Zoghbi said, recalling the beginning of his meteoric rise within the society. "I later preceded Mike Quiñones on the ACC Board of Trustees, even though he was my mentor."[38]

Having two people from the same hospital and laboratory on the ACC board of trustees was unusual when Dr. Winters nominated Dr. Quiñones to serve simultaneously with Dr. Zoghbi. "They told me I was crazy to nominate him, but my reply was, 'What have we got to lose?' When they said, 'Nothing,' we nominated him and he got it. I also nominated Bill Zoghbi to be vice president and that worked out really well, too," said Dr. Winters. "It would be two other colleagues from The Methodist Hospital whom I found myself unexpectedly emulating in my role as president of the American College of Cardiology. Much like Drs. DeBakey and Gotto, whom I always praised as the two emissaries of this institution and terrific leaders, I found myself in my first, really in-depth involvement with the advocacy of physicians."

Although Congress had promised at the inception of Medicare in 1965 that it would refrain from exercising "any supervision or control over the practice of medicine or the manner in which medical services are provided, or over the selection, tenure or compensation of any officer or employee of institution, agency or person providing health services," spiraling costs had rendered this ideal untenable.[39] Since the inception of Medicare, Congress had permitted physicians to bill what they normally charged their privately insured patients. To reform that method of payment, known as the "customary, prevailing, and reasonable" (CPR) charge, Congress passed the Consolidated Omnibus Budget Reconciliation Act in 1989, a comprehensive law that reforms Medicare payments to physicians. Beginning in 1992, the

CPR method was to be replaced gradually by a fee schedule based on a re-source-based relative value scale (RBRVS).

Rather than being based on traditional charges for specific services, the relative value scale devised by a congressionally mandated study at Harvard School of Public Health was one based on actual costs. Supported by a contract with the Health Care Financing Administration and with the American Medical Association's cooperation since its 1986 inception, the Harvard study team developed a scale that would weight such factors as the value of doctors' time in performing a given treatment, the length of their training, and their outlays for office expenses such as rent, heat, and equipment as well as a geographic variable and malpractice expense. The stated intent of the resulting Physicians Fee Schedule was to raise payments for the allegedly underpaid family and general practitioners while reducing payments for surgeons and other specialists, whose services allegedly were overvalued.[40]

The results of the Harvard study group's survey of cardiovascular services were released to the ACC for review and comment in 1990. Indicative of the college's reaction to the study's findings and the proposed Physicians Fee Schedule was one prominent member's documented observation: "What was put forth as an attempt to reallocate and equalize payments to physicians has become a maneuver to reduce the federal budget without thought to the devastating effects on the future of American medical practice."[41]

To address its concern that the issue of quality and appropriateness of care was not addressed in RBRVS, Dr. Winters announced that the college had convened an ad hoc committee of members and technical consultants to address this omission as well as all of its analytical concerns. "Refinement of the RBRVS will be ongoing," he reported to the membership of the college. "It will be fine-tuned over the next several years. Several refinements are necessary to establish reliable total work values, particularly related to cardiovascular services."[42]

When some members of the House Ways and Means Subcommittee on Health in 1990 believed the new physicians fee schedule would do little to curb the rising costs of health care, Dr. Winters was asked to address one of the major sources, the increased volume of service. Acknowledging cardiovascular medicine's prominent and critical role in health care of those enrolled in Medicare, he stated that with America's aging population, the increase in the demand for cardiovascular services was inevitable. Because of the positive impact of the advances made in cardiovascular care, as documented in the 1990 Department of Health and Human Services Annual

Report, he pointed out that the age-adjusted prevalence rates for heart disease decreased by 33 percent between 1980 and 1987.

"Even with the death rate associated with cardiovascular disease decreasing over the previous 20 years, I stated that more than 67 million Americans had cardiovascular disease in 1987, of which 18 million people over the age of 65 and more than 80 percent of those died of the disease," Dr. Winters stated. In addition, he continued, "More than 50 percent of all heart attacks occur in those 65 years or older. The elderly are increasing in number, especially those over age 85, and this group utilizes health care services at a far greater rate than do younger age groups."[43]

The primary concern of the ACC in 1990 was that the medical services be provided to patients effectively, competently, and in a timely fashion. In an effort to achieve this goal and to influence medical practice in a positive and cost-effective manner, clinical practice guidelines for diverse techniques and procedures were developed by the college in conjunction with the American Heart Association. Already in place were guidelines for coronary angiography, stress testing, ambulatory electrocardiography monitoring, coronary angioplasty, pacemaker implantation, and early treatment of myocardial infarction.

The ACC's establishment of practice guidelines "leads to a supposition that eventually reimbursements will be tied to them," Dr. Winters explained at the government hearing. "To date, however, there is no information indicating how much money, if any, can be saved with the use of practice guidelines. They are not meant to provide 'cookbook' medicine; the hope is that guidelines might reduce the need for intrusive utilization review, at the same time allowing physicians to make independent judgments."[43]

After the hearing, however, Dr. Winters surmised that the impact of his testimony was to be limited: "That some legislators did not believe such guidelines would be an effective deterrent in slowing the growth of demand for medical services was clearly evident to me, an opinion that was to be validated by actions taken several months later." In an effort to slow the growth of medical costs of procedures performed on the elderly and disabled patients insured by Medicare and to help balance the federal budget, the House Ways and Means Committee announced an amendment to the law. Projecting a savings of $725 million over four years in Medicare payments to doctors, legislators proposed eliminating payments for one of the basics of cardiovascular care, routine electrocardiograms.

This unexpected legislation astonished heart specialists around the country, who collectively exclaimed in a *New York Times* article, "Such a law was harmful to the patient and unfair to the physician."[44] After Congress voted to eliminate payment for interpreting routine electrocardiograms for Medicare patients beginning in 1992, no one took responsibility for its origination. Committee members blamed the White House; the White House retorted it originated in the committee.

"Forming my own opinion about the source of the idea, I believe that Congress, in the middle of the night, decided to cease payment for the reading of the electrocardiograms," Dr. Winters speculated. "They decided that it was so easy to read, that you didn't need to be paid for it anymore. Well, as one can imagine, that caused a bit of a stir, but it was just the beginning of the government's involvement in the payment of physicians."

This last-minute decision by Congress to eliminate payment of a cardiovascular service before assessing its impact on the practice of medicine was a dangerous precedent to establish. Wary that the tremendous efforts put forth by the ACC to more appropriately reward physician work through the Medicare payment process could possibly be for naught, Dr. Winters remained suspicious about the conversion factor ultimately decided by Congress. Because of this apprehension, he reported the following opinion to the ACC: "It may render inconsequential the enormous work and the endless time of hundreds of thoughtful individuals."[42]

Whatever the outcome, Dr. Winters was to become an active participant in the process of its implementation. When the American Medical Association/Specialty Society RVS Update Committee (RUC) was formed in 1991, he was appointed by the ACC to serve as its representative. Comprised of 26 physicians, of which 22 represented medical specialties, the RUC was created to provide input from the physician community to the Centers for Medicare and Medicaid Services (CMS). Required by statute to review the RBRVS at least every five years and issue updates annually, the CMS agreed to accept recommendations from the RUC with respect to the relative values to be assigned to new or revised codes. In its first year, the majority of the submitted recommendations from the RUC were accepted, and over the following years it was to become recognized as "the committee that helped set all of the standards of payment for physicians."[45]

When Dr. Winters stepped down as president of the ACC in 1991, the "electrocardiogram issue" remained unsolved. The existing nonreimbursement policy galvanized generalists and heart specialists into forming an orchestrated campaign to express their concerns to Congress. Members of the ACC were urged to contact their legislators and explain the justification for separate reimbursement for electrocardiogram interpretation.

Other doctors, such as family physicians and general internists who also interpreted the tracings of an electrocardiogram, joined the heart specialists in a coalition that would expand to include more than 20 professional societies and health care organizations.

Framing its argument in terms of access and quality care and addressing the legislators "on behalf of the millions of Medicare patients," the coalition composed a detailed request to Congress. Signed by each participant, the letter explained how electrocardiograms "are an essential diagnostic tool for detecting heart abnormalities. In the absence of expert interpretation by a qualified physician, however, the results of an electrocardiogram test are meaningless."[46] The coalition's efforts would finally come to fruition in 1993 when President Bill Clinton signed a bill that restored separate payment for electrocardiogram interpretation.

The gradual implementation of Medicare's realignment of payments to physicians had commenced the previous year. Within the following decade there was to be a transformative impact on individual physicians as well as on particular specialties, academic physicians, graduate medical education and physician specialization, quality of care, physician incomes, physician autonomy, and on various other aspects of medical practice.[47]

In the midst of this lengthy transformation process throughout the 1990s at The Methodist Hospital, Dr. Raizner's mission to create a unifying identity for cardiovascular services began to gain the necessary momentum required for realization.

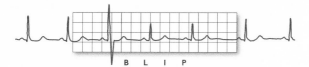

B L I P

CARDIOLOGY BY THE BOOK

When Dr. Winters served as president of the American College of Cardiology (ACC) in 1990, the college celebrated its 40th-year anniversary. To celebrate this event, the ACC board of trustees approved a motion to have a history of ACC recorded, and the college historian, Dr. Bruce Fye, agreed to do this work. To his credit, Dr. Fye recommended that the topic be broadened to encompass the history of cardiology in the United States and thus was born American Cardiology - The History of a Specialty and its College, published by John Hopkins University Press in 1996 to strong reviews.

1. Hampson R, McShane L. Number of mob leaders is shrinking. AP, *Hudson Valley News*. November 29, 1991.

2. Reputed mob boss Trafficante dies. AP, *Park City Daily News*. March 19, 1987.

3. Luft K, Heard J. Joseph Ferriola, Chicago mob figure, dies at 61. *Chicago Tribune*. March 12, 1989.

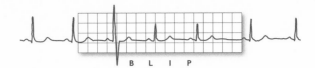

A PRECOCIOUS PROCLIVITY

*D*r. DeBakey's lifelong, insatiable intellectual curiosity and desire "to manifest
an all-inclusive interest in matters of the mind" first became evident during
his childhood. Much like his father, he became fascinated with mechanical gadgets,
taking them apart and reassembling them skillfully.[1]

With a predilection for the wonders of gadgetry, Dr. DeBakey was to develop
The DeBakey Roller Pump and a multitude of innovative surgical tools. Among
the more than 70 instruments that he either invented or improved during his 75-year
career were blood transfusion needles, suture scissors, clamps, and cardiovascular
forceps. Commonplace today in cardiovascular operating rooms around the world
are the DeBakey clamps and the DeBakey forceps, designed with atraumatic teeth to
stop the flow of blood during surgery without damaging the vessel itself.[2]

As was the case with most of Dr. DeBakey's accomplishments, his ubiquitous
surgical tools inspired more than a few urban legends—one of which concerned a
dinner in the 1980s hosted by Medical College of Virginia's chairman of surgery,
Dr. Lazar Greenfield, and honoring Dr. DeBakey. While most of the chief surgical residents and senior residents in attendance were tongue-tied while in the famous surgeon's presence at the dinner table, one suddenly spoke up and said, "Dr.
DeBakey, when I'm doing a vascular bypass and need a forcep, I ask the scrub nurse
for a 'DeBakey.' What do you ask for?" After a long pause, in which Dr. DeBakey
was said to have composed his thoughts, he allegedly replied, "Son, if I hold out my
hand for an instrument and the nurse doesn't know what I want, she's fired."[3]

---

1. DeBakey L, DeBakey S. Michael E. DeBakey, M.D.: beloved brother, master mentor,
   compatible colleague, professional paragon. *Methodist DeBakey Cardiovasc J.* 2009;5(3):
   49-56.
2. The Surgical Post: Michael DeBakey (1908-2008). Platts & Nisbett website.
   http://www.plattsnisbett.com/wordp/?p=135. Accessed October 2, 2013.
3. Carrico TJ. Random Writings: dinner with Big Mike. Tom Carrico blog/website. http://
   tomcarrico.blogspot.com/2011/08/dinner-with-big-mike.html. Accessed October 2, 2013.

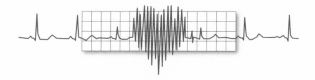

CHAPTER SIXTEEN

ADAPTING TO THE EVOLUTION OF HEALTH CARE
1990s

"Your life does not get better by chance, it gets better by change."
JIM ROHN

In tandem with Medicare's accelerated efforts to control the costs of health care in the early 1990s came other cost-containment measures implemented by a rapidly expanding number of managed care organizations.

The once fledgling managed care movement in the United States had received a major boost after the 1973 enactment of the federal Health Maintenance Organization Act. After coining the term "health maintenance organization (HMO)" as a substitute for "prepaid group practice," the act authorized start-up funding and ensured access to the employer-based health insurance market. Evolving throughout the 1970s and the 1980s, the resulting HMOs had played only a modest role in the financing and delivery of health care before the 1990s.

With a goal of reducing the spiraling costs of insuring employees against illness, a large number of HMOs identified that one critical component to savings was limited access to specialists, the "overpaid providers inclined to use too much technology and perform too many procedures."[1] To accomplish this goal, many managed care organizations contracted primary care physicians to assume the responsibility for overseeing the medical care of HMO members and to serve as the "gatekeepers" to specialized care.[2]

This abrupt change in unrestrained access to specialists marked the beginning waves of a sea change in the traditional relationship between doctors, patients, providers, and payers. Employing a managed-care lexicon, featuring such dehumanizing terms as "consumer" for "patient" and "provider" for "physician," nonpractitioners and bureaucrats were to

transform a once-revered, centuries-old profession into a common pur-
veyor of essential goods.

An outspoken critic of HMOs in the early 1990s was Dr. DeBakey,
who found such organizations to be more interested in financial rewards
than health maintenance. "Corporate America is appropriating health
care in this country with the sole purpose of making a profit, by brutally
squeezing doctors and hospitals financially, and by restricting, and even
denying, high-tech care to patients," he said.[3] "The effect has been to
move the profession of medicine toward a trade or a business and to drive
a schism between the healer and the ailing, whose partnership is essential
to a successful outcome."[4]

The cost-containment policies enforced by HMOs, such as suppressing
specialized and therapeutic measures, created circumstances that had "potentially grave consequences for the quality of health care given individual Americans and for the long-term integrity of the medical profession,"
Dr. DeBakey said, indicating his concern about the threat such policies
posed to the viability of academic health centers.[5]

With managed care organization's increasing insistence on stemming the
flow of patient referrals to specialists, the income generated by clinical faculty at academic health centers was steadily declining, jeopardizing medical
education and research. To create public awareness of the side effects of
"mismanaged health care," Dr. DeBakey, in his role as chancellor of Baylor
College of Medicine, joined forces with Dr. William G. Anlyan, chancellor
of Duke University, to coauthor an editorial to stress the imperative of preserving and sustaining the activities of academic health centers.[5]

In a concisely detailed presentation published in newspapers throughout the country, the two chancellors explained how managed care organizations' cost-containment policies had the potential to jeopardize future
medical education and research. "For several decades, the major portion
of the cost of medical education has been subsidized by income generated
from health care, either from the pool of professional fees earned by the
clinical faculty or from the income generated by affiliated teaching hospitals," they stated. "Monies generated from professional fees and healthcare operations have also substantially subsidized medical research, particularly new projects that open up promising unexplored vistas."[5]

In addition to managed care organizations' limiting the quality of
health care by serving as "gatekeepers" to specialty care, another "equally
pernicious cost-cutting strategy" identified by Drs. DeBakey and Anlyan
was the rapidly expanding utilization review process. "Before the doctor

can proceed with tests and treatment his education and training deem appropriate, he must get the approval of a nurse or clerk, or perhaps a high school dropout sitting at a computer mechanically consulting a rigid data base," they stated in the editorial. "The doctor's request may be rejected if the clerk reading the computer program decides it is 'not necessary.' Where is the logic in requiring a physician, who invests about one-third of his life in formal medical education and training, to obtain approval from a corporate clerk at an 800 number before he can administer to his patient? The logic is obviously absent, but the tragic results for patients are real."[5]

Since the government enacted a similar review process for the care of Medicare patients, the two chancellors lamented that important decisions about health care were not being made by well-trained physicians but by medically untrained people who never see or examine a patient: "The government decides whether the patient can be admitted to the hospital, can have surgery, can have an assistant surgeon during the operation and can be admitted to the intensive care unit, as well as how long the hospital stay may be."[5]

Congress began focusing on Medicare's hospital insurance program when soaring hospital costs were threatening to bankrupt Medicare in the early 1980s. To slow the growth of these costs in 1983, legislation was enacted to establish a prospective payment plan, one in which hospitals were paid a fixed fee for treating a specific illness identified in "diagnostic related groups," or DRGs. "Rather than reducing payment for hospital services by some arbitrary percentage rate, the new DRG system established incentives to change hospital behavior," said Senator John Heinz, chairman of the United States Senate Special Committee on Aging in 1984. "In order to be successful under this new system, hospitals must provide services more efficiently, at lower cost, and only when necessary."[6]

By 1986, the specific amount of the DRG payment had been established in more than 470 conditions or medical procedures. Because these flat fees were estimates of an "average" cost, should expenditures for the patient's care exceed the average, the plan specified that the hospital or the patient was responsible for the difference. Should it be less, the hospital stood to profit. According to a spokeswoman for Senator Heinz, "Congress intended for hospitals to use the money they made on the patients whose treatment cost less than the average to pay for those whose treatment was more expensive."[7]

These ever-mounting restrictions and intrusions into every decision regarding patient care had a "deleterious effect on our profession by diverting our attention from our primary concern—our patients," said Dr. DeBakey in his presidential address to the Southern Surgical Society in 1990. "Some hospitals spend as much as $2 million each year on quality assurance activities imposed on them, without observing any improvement occurring in patient health care."[8]

At The Methodist Hospital, the nation's largest private tax-exempt teaching hospital with more than 1,500 beds in 1990, Dr. DeBakey was intent on preserving the traditions of American medical research, training, and treatment endangered by the intrusion of such hostile forces. "You've got people with no experience in medicine deciding whether a patient should be operated on or how long they should stay in the hospital; all of a sudden they're empowered," Dr. DeBakey said, stating that such impositions impeded the optimal delivery of services.[9] "We would not allow an unqualified clerk to recommend repairs for our car, so why would we settle for one when it comes to our own health?"[10]

Such an intrusion into Dr. DeBakey's personal care of a patient at The Methodist Hospital was known to invoke the surgeon's legendary ire. When advised on the phone by "some clerk" at an insurance company that he should discharge a 90-year-old stroke victim, Dr. DeBakey reportedly snapped, "You come here and tell the patient's relatives you want her transferred to your care. Otherwise, butt out."[9]

Excluding itself from any extensive involvement in the managed health care market throughout the 1980s was The Methodist Hospital. As other Houston hospitals contracted with insurers and employers to provide services at reduced prices in return for an assured flow of patients, Larry Mathis, The Methodist Hospital's president, repeatedly declined to participate, stating he would rather compete on quality of care, not price.[11]

Taking the opposite approach was The Methodist Hospital's next-door neighbor in the Texas Medical Center, the Texas Heart Institute at St. Luke's Episcopal Hospital. Seizing a business opportunity to benefit from the growing cost-consciousness of the market, Dr. Cooley created the "first-ever packaged pricing plan for cardiovascular surgical procedures" in 1984. It was an innovation that was to garner him recognition as "the Sam Walton of heart surgery."[9]

The genesis of Dr. Cooley's plan to offer a package of discounted rates for heart operations and cardiovascular treatment was a request he received simultaneously in the early 1980s from a large, self-insured, Houston-based conglomerate, Tenneco, Inc., and a large national managed-care company, CIGNA.[12] With heart disease as the leading cause of American deaths and the nation's employers alone paying more than $2.5 billion in health care benefits for heart bypass surgery, not including the benefits for post-surgery disabilities, both Tenneco and CIGNA were exploring the possibility of establishing a global payment package to include a flat-fee to cover all costs, including physician and hospital charges.[13]

The response to these requests was an organ-specific, all-inclusive payment package covering 16 selected cardiovascular surgical procedures at Texas Heart Institute, an innovative approach Dr. Cooley later would describe as "a radical, new approach to health care" and "one of my major accomplishments."[14] His unique concept of bundled services, shared risk, and single payment was established as CardioVascular Care Providers, known as CVCP, in 1984.[12]

Available on a contractual basis to managed-care programs, self-insured businesses, and other health insurance entities, CVCP included a flat fee for coronary bypass surgery of $19,100, including a 10-day hospital stay. Even though this discounted fee reportedly was 52 percent less than the national average of $39,811 and 63 percent less than the rates charged in Washington, Oregon, California, and Alaska, Dr. Cooley was certain the high standards of cardiovascular care at Texas Heart Institute would be maintained.[15] His confidence was based on past experience, he said, pointing out the institute's large volume of patients in which "we'd learned to be very efficient yet provide exceptional care."[16]

When critics in the medical profession noted Dr. Cooley's packaged-pricing plan "flies in the face of the conventional medical dogma that quality and cost are inevitably correlated," many nonetheless praised his concept and the specialized focus of his "open-heart-surgery factory."[17] Several cardiovascular surgeons were more critical, particularly Dr. DeBakey, who commented to a reporter with The New York Times: "Sure, you can cut costs. But you get what you pay for."[9]

Such a response was to be expected. In Dr. DeBakey's oft stated opinion, the higher ambitions of academic health centers to pursue research, training, and the best treatment required thinking in terms of quality, not in volume, low-cost care. Therefore, he reasoned, agreeing to provide services at reduced prices in return for an assured flow of patients from health insurers and employers was not the right direction to take. "All this about trying to compete with HMOs, as far as I am concerned, from an academic standpoint, is futile," he said. "I keep saying to people concerned about HMOs: 'if you build a better mouse trap, they will beat a path to your door. Concentrate on excellence."[18]

Personifying his philosophy was Dr. DeBakey's four-decade track record as chairman of the Department of Surgery at Baylor College of Medicine. The pursuit of excellence was what motivated his building and maintaining a very stable department, particularly in cardiovascular surgery, where he had promoted and protected his productive faculty. Of the dozen cardiovascular surgeons on staff at The Methodist Hospital in 1990, more than half had been on faculty there since the early 1960s and 1970s and all had had remarkable careers.

One such surgeon was Dr. Jimmy F. Howell, who joined Dr. DeBakey's team after his fellowship training with Drs. DeBakey and Cooley in 1963. "DeBakey was a pretty shrewd fella' and he really knew how to get good talent," said Dr. Howell, recalling the expertise of those recruited during the beginning years of cardiovascular surgery at The Methodist Hospital. "Oscar Creech was the first that DeBakey hired in his department and the second was Denton Cooley and the third was Stanley Crawford, who was a Harvard man, and the fourth was Arthur Beall, who was from Emory, and the fifth was George Morris, who was from University of Pennsylvania. And then he developed Ed Garrett from his residency here and hired him. Ed and I were working partners with DeBakey for a few years."[19]

Having been trained in pediatric heart surgery by Dr. Cooley, Dr. Howell performed 50-75 congenital heart operations annually with Dr. DeBakey at The Methodist Hospital in the early 1960s. When the hospital's pediatrics department eventually was dissolved, all children seeking medical and surgical treatment were referred to Texas Children's Hospital, where Dr. Cooley had "set up shop" as chief of congenital heart disease surgery.

Also in the early 1960s, Drs. Garrett and Howell began seeking a surgical solution to coronary occlusive disease. The clinical investigations of these two pioneers in coronary artery surgery resulted in the first successful coronary artery bypass graft operation, later known as CABG. Within the coming decades, it was to be among the most common operations performed in the world.[20] By 2006, Dr. Howell alone had performed more than 14,000.[19]

Beginning in the early 1970s and continuing throughout the 1980s, the volume of CABG procedures at The Methodist Hospital continued to increase. "There was just a ton of cases; it was not unusual for me to do seven or eight a day," Dr. Howell recalled. "We started at 7:00 or 7:30 in the morning and operate until 10:00 or 11:00 at night, and do whatever we needed to do—go home and get a little sleep—and come back and go back to work."[19]

The successful clinical application of cardiopulmonary bypass in CABG and other open-heart operations at The Methodist Hospital enabled the development of new surgical therapies. "Arthur Beall was the man who really was instrumental in developing the heart-lung technician team at The Methodist Hospital," said Dr. Charles H. McCollum, who trained with Dr. DeBakey and joined his surgical team in 1966. "Arthur was a very bright fellow and knew a lot about instrumentation."[21]

Focusing his interest on expanding the utilization of cardiopulmonary bypass during cardiac surgery, Dr. Beall investigated using other solutions to prime the bypass pump to eliminate drawing blood from donors before surgery. To decrease postoperative morbidity, he designed filters to remove dangerous debris produced by the bypass pump. For postsurgical heart failure, Dr. Beall explored the concept of ventricular assist devices for circulatory support.[22]

At The Methodist Hospital, the pump, known as the heart-lung machine, was owned by Baylor College of Medicine. Since the salaries of the perfusionists also were the responsibility of the college, only faculty had access to those services in the early 1960s. After four surgeons recently trained in Dr. DeBakey's residence program exited to establish their own association to practice cardiac, thoracic, and vascular surgery, the necessary equipment that would enable them to do so was purchased by The Methodist Hospital. "In the mid-1960s, the practice of cardiac surgery outside of a medical school was a foreign concept, but to his credit, Dr. DeBakey did not try in any way to prevent this direct competition with the Baylor surgery department," recalled Dr. Walter S. Henly, who along with Drs. Robert C. Overton Jr., John B. Fitzgerald, and Don C. Quast founded Houston's first private practice cardiovascular surgical association. "While he stopped short of possibly endorsing our endeavor, Dr. DeBakey made no overt effort to hinder our progress. Perhaps he was secretly proud that a group of his trainees was taking this step, which obviously had to come some day."[23]

Remembering the day the new heart-lung machine was uncrated and assembled at The Methodist Hospital was Dr. Fitzgerald, who had first learned to operate a pump-oxygenator while serving in the Air Force assigned to the Experimental Surgery Department of the School of Aerospace Medicine. "I had plenty of time to tinker with it and learn how to set it up and operate it," Dr. Fitzgerald said. "Therefore, by default, I became the perfusionist for our team."[23]

Such an accomplishment was indicative of the pioneering mindset established by Dr. DeBakey. "I think I missed the excitement and the grinding that was going on over here," said Dr. McCollum, who had joined the surgical associates in the late 1960s but returned to Baylor College of Medicine and The Methodist Hospital in the early 1970s. "It was sort of the center of vascular surgery, and a lot of things were being done in the cardiac area as well. It was a very dynamic, busy place – just an exciting place to be and be a part of."[21]

This dynamism also lured a young surgeon from Sydney, Australia, who had just completed his residency in thoracic and cardiovascular surgery. When serving as a visiting professor in Sydney, Dr. DeBakey met Dr. Gerald M. Lawrie and invited him to spend a year with him in Houston. After accepting the invitation, Dr. Lawrie not only completed his cardiovascular fellowship in 1975, but also joined Dr. DeBakey's personal staff at his request. Working side by side, they were to be associates for more than three decades, working together on a daily basis and accumulating extensive experience in the surgical management of end-stage and complex cardiovascular disease. Continually awestruck by the vast number of patients referred to Dr. DeBakey's care over the years, Dr. Lawrie likened the vast outpouring to that of the miracle seekers to Lourdes, "He gets sent the most incredible cases."[24]

Among those cases treated by Drs. DeBakey and Lawrie were notable figures such as the Shah of Iran, the president of Turkey, and the abdicated king of Belgium. Having experienced the rewards and challenges of treating VIPs, Dr. Lawrie echoed his mentor when he stated, "The patient is always first. Everything else is secondary, including the surrounding publicity. Regardless of a patient's status, remember that underneath all the hoopla, these patients are just ordinary people trying to get restored to good health."[25]

The welfare of all patients with peripheral vascular disease was enhanced by the development of noninvasive techniques and instrumentation for the management of peripheral and cerebral vascular disease in the early 1970s. Drs. McCollum and Noon recognized the need to have a vascular laboratory at The Methodist Hospital, although only a few were in existence in 1976 and "there wasn't a lot of enthusiasm for it" among their associates, Dr. McCollum said. "Over the objections, some pretty strong objections, from some of the people in our department who thought there was no future in a vascular laboratory, we finally convinced The Methodist Hospital. And really the only reason we got it was George Noon was able to raise the initial funding for the equipment."[21]

Opened in 1977 under the codirectorship of Drs. Noon and McCollum was the Peripheral Vascular Laboratory in the Brown Building of The Methodist Hospital. The purpose of the laboratory was to determine whether a patient's symptoms were of vascular origin and to evaluate peripheral vascular occlusive disease. The noninvasive testing was not a substitute for preoperative arteriography but rather an additional clinical parameter to complement the anatomic information provided by arteriography. "In the beginning it was basically an arterial study on a treadmill," Dr. McCollum said, pointing out how rapidly technology improved in the following decade. "The technology available in the vascular laboratory was superb. Ultrasound came in and then Doppler ultrasound and it's just been having exponential growth in the lab. It's even used to follow intraluminal graphs for abdominal aortic aneurysms; Stanley Crawford was known as 'Mr. Aorta' at that time."[21]

More than 605 patients had undergone thoracoabdominal aortic aneurysm surgery performed by Dr. Crawford at The Methodist Hospital by the late 1980s. The international gold standard for surgical management was the "inclusion technique," introduced by Dr. Crawford in 1974.[26] "Stanley didn't develop thoracoabdominal aortic surgery, but he refined it so it was a very practical thing that could be done reasonably safe," Dr. Howell said, recalling his colleague's pioneering treatment of complex aortic disease. "And then he did the thoracic aortic aneurysms. Oh, he did them all. I mean that's what I'm talking about. He did the whole aorta, from top to bottom. And he published his book that is probably the milestone in aortic surgery. It made him very famous."[19]

Coauthored with his son, Dr. John L. Crawford II, *Diseases of the Aorta: An Atlas of Angiographic Pathology and Surgical Technique* was published in 1985 to critical acclaim.[27] One review, published by *Archives of Surgery*, was written by Dr. William H. Pearce, a vascular surgeon and professor of surgery at Northwestern University Medical School in Chicago, who exclaimed "the beautifully and abundantly illustrated" book was "spectacular!"[28]

Furthermore, Dr. Pearce complimented the thoroughness of the book's 12 chapters that covered a broad spectrum of aortic diseases from degenerative aneurysms to aortic dissections, Marfan's disease, coarctations, redo aortic surgeries, aoritits, trauma, and aortic tumors. "Each chapter is organized in a similar fashion, beginning with the pathophysiology of the disease, followed by clinical manifestations, diagnosis, preoperative evaluation, the history of surgical treatment, and the current surgical management," he wrote. "At the conclusion of this book, one has the feeling of having completed a surgical rotation with Dr. Crawford."[28]

In agreement with such high praise were the numerous vascular surgeons trained by him as well as those from around the world who had traveled to The Methodist Hospital to observe the pioneering surgeon known as the "godfather of major, complex aortic surgery" in action.[29] As the mentor to one former thoracic resident, Dr. Joseph S. Coselli, who joined Baylor College of Medicine in 1984 as his associate, Dr. Crawford ensured the longevity of his legacy. In the coming decades at The Methodist Hospital, Dr. Coselli, who specialized in the evaluation and surgical treatment of diseases of the aorta, was to become world-renowned in aortic surgery, performing more than 6,000 repairs of the aorta and more than 2,700 repairs of thoracoabdominal aortic aneurysms.

Another legacy of Dr. Crawford, in his position as director of the Vascular Surgical Fellowship Training Program, was the vascular conference held at 7:00 AM every Wednesday morning for many years at The Methodist Hospital. Invited to attend were those interested in peripheral vascular disease: surgeons, cardiologists, radiologists, pathologists, and internists. Conferences were crowded. The format was primarily case reporting. What made it so popular and fascinating, aside from the cases reported, was the audience participation Dr. Crawford achieved by direct questions put by him to specific individuals in the audience. Everyone could expect to be queried at some time or another. The repartee was often spirited and the learning curve very high. The conferences were never quite the same after Dr. Crawford left the scene.

In addition to being in a league of his own as a technical surgeon and teacher, Dr. Crawford also shared his knowledge and experiences with surgical societies and organizations on the local, state, national, and international levels. A proven leader, he served as president of the Houston Surgical Society, the Southern Association for Vascular Surgery, the North American Chapter of the International Society of Cardiovascular Surgery, and The Society for Vascular Surgery, of which Dr. DeBakey was a founding member.

After serving as governor of the American College of Surgeons for six years, Dr. Crawford was chosen to deliver the prestigious John Gibbon Lecture about his experience with thoracoabdominal aneurysms. Felled by a disabling stroke in January 1991, he was unable to give the lecture, which was presented by his associate, Dr. Coselli.[30] His partial disability also precluded Dr. Crawford from presenting the John Homans Lecture in

1991 to the Society for Vascular Surgery. In a poignant ceremony attended by Dr. Crawford in a wheelchair, this tribute to his surgical teachers, "Stanley Crawford's Heroes in Vascular Surgery," was presented by his son.

After Dr. Crawford's death at the age of 70 in October 1992, the Society for Vascular Surgery honored his leadership by designating the annual forum he had established to address socioeconomic and research efforts as they impact vascular surgery the E. Stanley Crawford Critical Issues Forum. "Indeed, with his passing we have lost a giant and one of our heroes of surgery," said the society's Dr. Calvin B. Ernst. "Those who knew him and were touched by his quiet and gentlemanly greatness are much the better for it. He will be sorely missed, but his legacy will live on, perpetuated by grateful patients and an indebted profession."[31]

The contributions made by Dr. Crawford revolutionized aortic surgery. In addition to the inclusion technique, he was the first to successfully replace the entire aorta with a Dacron graft. Among his other accomplishments, he introduced the repair of ascending aortic aneurysm, repair of arch aneurysm, repair of aortic dissection, treatment of Marfan's syndrome, and treatment of peripheral vascular disease. "He moved the management of difficult and vexing aortic problems to the realm of everyday treatment," said Dr. Hazim J. Safi, who joined Dr. Crawford as an associate in 1983. "He shunned publicity and was averse to giving interviews to the media. Part of this was his shy personality, and part was his constant remembrance of the humble roots from which he came. Apart from Dr. DeBakey, no one else besides Dr. Crawford has had a bigger impact on my career. I tried on many occasions to thank him, but he would always shun the compliment and say, 'All I did was crack the door open; the rest is you.'"[32]

Also leaving a lasting impression during his lifelong career at The Methodist Hospital was Dr. DeBakey's first surgical resident. "George Morris was an innovator," Dr. Howell said. "He was an intellectual and a very good surgeon. He did the first successful dissecting aneurysm of the ascending aorta in the world. His main interest was the study of mechanisms for relief of renal artery hypertension, accomplished with a bypass graft or endarterectomy of the renal arteries, but also a good deal of renal dialysis work was done. And George was very interested in the parameters of all types of renal artery innovations and procedures."[19]

As a teacher, either in lectures or by example, Dr. Morris emphasized technical excellence and the highest standards of patient care. "He was deeply committed to helping others learn and inspiring them to achieve," said Dr. Cooley, who had worked closely with Dr. Morris in the 1950s, the period in which their calculated risks resulted in great strides in cardiovascular surgery. "He was a pioneer in cardiovascular and peripheral vascular surgery and he freely shared his time, knowledge, and expertise with hundreds of medical students, residents, and fellows. Recognized internationally for his teaching ability as well as his surgical skill, he was also a visiting professor at numerous universities worldwide."[53]

At the peak of Dr. Morris's cardiovascular surgical volume at The Methodist Hospital during the 1980s, he employed Dr. P. J. Asimacopoulos, a surgeon from Greece, to help manage his service. After laboring long hours with Dr. Morris for more than a decade, Dr. Asimacopoulos returned to Greece in early 1990s to become chairman of a cardiovascular surgical program in a large private hospital in Athens.

Throughout Dr. Morris's career at The Methodist Hospital, he was known for his demeanor during surgical procedures. When he was operating, the climate could be tempestuous if his assistants were not fully engaged. Often the results were memorable, as indicated by the hilarious list of Morris-isms developed by the operating room staff over the years. "I no longer have the list, but I probably would not dare repeat them anyway," Dr. Winters confided.

Another graduate of the DeBakey training era was Dr. Raphael Espada, who, upon finishing the surgical residency in cardiothoracic training at Baylor College of Medicine in 1977, joined Dr. Jimmy F. Howell in practice. They worked together for 17 years before he and Dr. Howell ended their relationship, but Dr. Espada continued in practice at The Methodist Hospital until 2007. A native of Guatemala, Dr. Espada annually spent many hours in Guatemala treating underprivileged patients requiring cardiothoracic procedures. For this work, he received honors and rewards from Guatemala, Mexico, Brazil, and the International Rotary Society. In 2007, he was chosen to be the vice presidential running mate of Alvaro Colom in the September Guatemala presidential election, which they won. After serving a five–year term ending in 2012, Dr. Espada continues his medical career in Guatemala.

The career path chosen by Dr. Espada, as well as that of the hundreds of other surgeons who subsequently received part of their surgical training under Dr. DeBakey, perpetuated the master surgeon's passion for excellence in all aspects of surgery, clinical care, teaching, research, education, and the community. As a role model, "Dr. DeBakey didn't just talk about the importance of excellence," Dr. Lawrie said. "He truly pursued it, relentlessly, in all these areas."[34]

Another unique aspect of Dr. DeBakey's cardiovascular program was its all-encompassing approach to an emerging surgical specialty that rapidly had become sub-specialized. Although cardiac and vascular services eventually were separated in most surgical programs around the world, Dr. DeBakey steadfastly objected to conforming to that premise "for the simple reason that I consider the cardiovascular system a unified system."[18] Therefore, the surgical efforts of Dr. DeBakey and each of his associates were not confined to a one specific area of cardiovascular or thoracic expertise. "He did it and we continued to do it," Dr. Noon said, recalling his own involvement in general cardiovascular and thoracic surgery and transplant surgery in the 1960s and thereafter. "Today most that are graduating are either vascular surgeons, cardiac surgeons, thoracic surgeons, or general surgeons, but they are not doing it all as we were able to do because of the way Dr. DeBakey brought up the program."[35]

Many who trained in the program with Dr. DeBakey went on to become the "master surgeons of their communities," who, in turn, trained a whole new generation of surgeons all over the world, said one of his former trainees, Dr. Kenneth L. Mattox.[36] In appreciation of the vast scope of Dr. DeBakey's program and his unrelenting goals of excellence, a group of his former trainees got together to honor their teacher in 1977. To perpetuate his vision through scholarship, training, and recognition and to provide a forum for international scientific exchange, they founded the Michael E. DeBakey International Cardiovascular Surgical Society, subsequently renamed the Michael E. DeBakey International Surgical Society.[37]

By the early 1990s, members in this surgical society resided not only in the United States but also in myriad countries all over the world. Such demographics illustrated the fact that the number of surgeons from outside the country trained by Dr. DeBakey rivaled the number from within. With all his students and residents, beginning with Dr. Morris in 1950 and throughout the following four decades, Dr. DeBakey said he endeavored to impart "the spirit of surgical endeavor, of surgical standards of excellence, of surgical ethics, and integrity that I have tried to reflect in my everyday life. You see, my surgical contributions opened the way for others to perfect them. But when you train people, you are in a sense providing for your immortality because if you are able to instill these concepts, investigative efforts, ethics, standards, and pursuit of excellence in the new generation, then you have succeeded in continuing your spirit after you leave, because all of us are going to be here for a relatively short period of time."[18]

The ability to manage his own time effectively became a concern to Dr. DeBakey in the early 1990s. Having served as chairman of the Department of Surgery at Baylor College of Medicine for 45 years while juggling his medical duties, academic activities, and his obligations as a medical statesman simultaneously, the 84-year-old surgeon decided to devote more time to his own research projects and to pursue new challenges. In making the decision, he reassured his colleagues, "This won't change my life."[38]

When Dr. DeBakey announced his plans to step down as chairman of the Department of Surgery in January 1993, it was to be the first of many profound changes at Baylor College of Medicine and The Methodist Hospital. Since estimated U.S. health care expenditures for 1992 totaled $838.5 billion, 14 percent of gross domestic product, the newly elected President Bill Clinton was beginning to formulate a comprehensive health reform plan "to curb the monster of spiraling health care costs" and provide universal health care delivery to all Americans.[39]

While there was mounting speculation nationally about the scope of the Clinton Administration's plan, the chief executive officer of The Methodist Hospital expected the sweeping reform to be all encompassing. "When you start to change something as large and complex as the health care industry, you have to realize it affects every hospital, every doctor, drug manufacturers, the institutions that finance them; it's all in a package bigger than the economy of Italy," Mr. Mathis said. "It touches on everyone's lives."[40]

In anticipation of legislated health reform mandates, Mr. Mathis embarked on a program to streamline the hospital's operations in 1993. For The Methodist Hospital to remain competitive in the cost-conscious environment of managed care and federal cutbacks, "efficiencies are being sought in all expense areas, not only from the work force, but also from areas such as supplies and purchasing," Mr. Mathis explained. "As we consider our options, some functions will be downsized or eliminated, inevitably resulting in staff reductions."[41]

After cutting the pay of critical care nurses and other nursing staff to reduce costs, he initially planned to downsize the number of staff strictly by early retirement and attrition. However, in September 1993, he announced the first of 1,200 jobs to be cut, including nurses, nurses' aides, phlebotomists, technicians and office clerks. Another cost-saving maneuver implemented was the closing of Chez Eddy, the gourmet heart-healthy restaurant created by Dr. Gotto and Mr. Bowen in 1981.

Although the recipient of many awards, including one from the American Heart Association for its innovative approach to food and health, Chez Eddy struggled to remain open, maintaining a respectable luncheon trade daily but only drawing a minimal crowd for dinner each night. From its inception, Dr. Gotto and Mr. Bowen remained committed to keeping the restaurant open regardless of whether it was profitable. "It's helped the hospital's image of being concerned about disease prevention and good nutrition," said Dr. Gotto, who coauthored with Helen Roe and Babette Fraser a compendium of the restaurant's recipes in *The Chez Eddy Living Heart Cookbook* published in 1991.[42]

When asked to pen a foreword to Dr. Gotto's cookbook, Dr. DeBakey enthusiastically agreed to participate. "Chez Eddy is a restaurant I have patronized since its opening in 1981," he wrote. "It was conceived by my colleague and friend Tony Gotto, one of the world's leading researchers in cardiovascular disease. As he listened to dieting patients, he, too, was struck by their sense of deprivation—an attitude that often prevented the kind of compliance necessary to manage their illness. Chez Eddy cuisine is a manifestation of Tony's belief that heart-healthy dining need not be restrictive or bland. The meals may be simple to prepare, but the difference they will make in your diet will assuredly make you a convert."[43]

Although unable to inspire the masses, the pioneering healthful gourmet restaurant did generate disciples among Houston restaurateurs, many of who expanded or altered their menus to include health-conscious fare.[44] Chez Eddy was not the only sacred cow to lose its status under Mr. Mathis's aggressive program to streamline The Methodist Hospital. Also deemed expendable was The Methodist Hospital's long-standing policy of not accepting contracts with managed care organizations. Concerned about the increasingly unstable environment health care providers were encountering, Mr. Mathis indicated that The Methodist Hospital was willing to adapt, but "the question is how to change."[45]

This decision to reassess the hospital's position on managed care was predicated by the growing number of Houston employers who had turned to managed care to control the cost of providing health care for workers and families. By the early 1990s, three out of four insured Houstonians were getting their medical insurance from restricted managed-care plans.[46] To facilitate the negotiations of contracts with managed care health plans in the future, Mr. Mathis encouraged physicians from The Methodist Hospital, Texas Children's Hospital, and Baylor College of Medicine to create a hospital-physicians network in 1993. Subsequently, this network's initial contract negotiated with a preferred provider organization became the first managed care health program accepted at The Methodist Hospital and became effective in January 1994.

As the transformation of the health care environment at The Methodist Hospital evolved, the Baylor College of Medicine search committee formed to find Dr. DeBakey's replacement continued its efforts. With Dr. DeBakey's paradoxical desire to continue his surgical practice, his research, his teaching duties, his academic responsibilities as chancellor, and his role as head of the DeBakey Heart Center at Baylor College of Medicine and The Methodist Hospital, the committee's already difficult challenge became even more complicated. Having served as a member of the search committee, Dr. Winters remembers the prophetic advice given by an executive with a professional search company, who told the committee, "You realize the person who will replace Dr. DeBakey will only last two or three years. It's almost impossible to bring somebody else in and have him survive because, number one, DeBakey is still here and number two, his successor will try to set up things his way that people won't accept."[47]

To achieve its goal, the search committee expended its efforts for more than 18 months. Stepping into the role of interim chairman of the Department of Surgery in July 1993 was Dr. Bobby R. Alford, chairman of the Department of Otolaryngology, who was to remain in that capacity until the July 1994 appointment of Dr. John C. Baldwin. Having previously served as chief of cardiothoracic surgery at Yale University School of Medicine, the 45-year-old Harvard University graduate and Rhodes Scholar had received his medical degree at Stanford University and his particular expertise was in cardiac transplant surgery. Assuming Dr. DeBakey's previous responsibilities as chairman of the Department of Surgery, Dr. Baldwin also served as chief of surgical services at Ben Taub, Texas Children's, and Veterans Affairs hospitals as well as chief of surgery at The Methodist Hospital, a position never held by Dr. DeBakey.

Heretofore, serving as chief of surgery at The Methodist Hospital for more than 29 years was Dr. John W. Overstreet, a highly revered general and thoracic surgeon who had stepped down in 1993. He was the only private practitioner to serve as a chief of service at The Methodist Hospital while all others were Baylor College of Medicine department chairs, as specified in the longstanding affiliation agreement. The reason why this notable exception to the rule existed remained a mystery. "All I know is when the negotiations between The Methodist Hospital and Baylor

College of Medicine were finalized back in 1970 there was an agreement that John Overstreet would remain chief of surgery as long as he remained active," recalls Dr. Winters. "I don't know why that took place, but he was so highly respected here that nobody had the courage to ask him to step down, I guess."

The legendary esteem in which Dr. Overstreet was held at The Methodist Hospital was to continue unabated after the arrival of his successor. Upon his retirement in 1997, he was presented with the hospital's Excalibur Award acknowledging him as the physician on the medical staff who exemplified the best of the medical profession, demonstrated respect, empathy, and caring in his interactions with patients, family, and staff, and supported the mission of the hospital. To honor his contributions in perpetuity, The Methodist Hospital renamed this annual Doctor's Day tribute the John W. Overstreet, M.D., Award in 1998, and the first awardee was nephrologist Dr. Juan J. Olivero. The following year, Dr. Winters was honored with the second annual award.

As Dr. Baldwin began to acclimate to his new surroundings and responsibilities, as well as the challenges presented by having two such exemplary predecessors, efforts to pass the Clinton Administration's health reform legislation failed in Congress. Its September 1994 demise came as no surprise to many medical professionals, particularly Dr. DeBakey, who found fault with its underlying premise. "I opposed the Clinton proposal largely because of its complex bureaucratic structure and complete governmental domination, not only of decisions regarding the delivery of health care but also, to some extent, medical scientific and educational activities," he said. "One of my major concerns with the Clinton proposal, as well as with the changes taking place today, is the threat to the academic health centers."[3]

In Dr. DeBakey's oft-stated opinion, the cost-containment efforts of the rapidly changing third-party payment system of managed care financially threatened the future of medical education since graduate medical training in the United States was financed largely by revenues from patient care in teaching hospitals. Although he rarely received patients through the referral process, Dr. DeBakey decried the deleterious effect the gatekeeper policy of managed care had on patients not referred to specialists at teaching hospitals by their physicians.[18] Because of his established reputation, patients traditionally had come directly to him as opposed to being referred by a physician. Following the advent of managed care, he was told by many who wanted to see him that they were forbidden to do so by their health plan. "In more than 50 years of surgical practice, I have been dismayed at the recent escalating, tragic conflict between medical and financial priorities," he observed. "The disparate goals of physicians who were trained to put the patient's welfare first and those of the profit-driven, insurance-owned medical corporations are rapidly disillusioning physicians and patients alike."[48]

The once-legendary volume of cardiovascular patients at The Methodist Hospital eventually was to be impacted not only by the cost-containment restrictions enforced by managed-care plans and Medicare but also by competition from the increasing number of institutions and facilities devoted to cardiovascular care. In the beginning decades of open-heart surgery, The Methodist Hospital and the Texas Heart Institute at St. Luke's Episcopal Hospital were among the few institutions in the southern United States that specialized in cardiac surgery. By the early 1990s, numerous open-heart programs had become available throughout the country, and in Houston alone there were multiple others.

Also competing for heart patients with cardiovascular surgeons in Houston and across the nation were the interventional cardiologists who performed balloon angioplasty in the catheterization laboratory to achieve myocardial revascularization. The 1990 national statistics published by the Centers for Disease Control and Prevention's National Center for Health Statistics clearly demonstrated the exponential growth during the previous decade of this alternative to surgery. While the number of coronary bypass graft procedures (CABG) had increased nationwide to more than 262,000, the number of coronary angioplasty procedures had grown ten-fold from less than 2,000 following its inception in 1979 to 285,000 in 1990.[49]

This "extraordinary" growth was attributable "not only to demonstrated clinical benefit but also to continuing technical advances that have led to improved techniques and higher success rates over time," according to a 1993 task force of the American Heart Association and the American College of Cardiology. Stating that coronary angioplasties during the late 1980s and early 1990s had been performed most often in patients with single-vessel coronary disease, this committee reported "increasing numbers of patients with multivessel disease and those who have undergone surgical bypass are also being treated, but coronary bypass surgery is used most often to treat multivessel coronary disease, with a majority of patients receiving three or more bypass grafts."[50]

In line with the national statistics, the number of coronary angioplasties performed in the catheterizations laboratories at The Methodist

Hospital steadily increased as the volume of surgical bypass procedures began to lessen, as did other cardiovascular surgical procedures. By the early 1990s, having become the largest nonprofit hospital in Texas with 1,527 beds after the November 1989 completion of the John S. Dunn Tower, with 16 operating rooms and 338 beds, The Methodist Hospital, which previously had not accepted managed care contracts, continued to maintain its 71 percent occupancy rate.[51] The major effect of the growing popularity of managed care in the community was to become increasingly evident when patient referrals began to decrease incrementally.

For those cardiologists in private practice within The Chapman Group, the erosion in the number of their physician-referred patients at The Methodist Hospital had occurred gradually throughout the 1980s. This attrition was attributed to emerging competition rather than the restrictions of third-party payers. "When I came to Houston, patients came to us from all around the southwest part of the country," said Dr. Winters. "Then, little by little, as facilities grew in other cities, patients didn't think they needed to come to Houston, or they didn't think they needed to come here. So our referring practice with physicians shrank year by year. We kept accurate records and we could see we were losing more and more referring physicians. Fewer and fewer patients were coming from elsewhere."

To generate additional patient referrals, The Chapman Group recognized the need to extend its base of operations. Having predominantly practiced at The Methodist Hospital during the previous four decades, establishing its identity at other hospitals throughout the Houston area became a priority. Next door at St. Luke's Episcopal Hospital, the group began to increase its recognition by admitting managed care patients whose health care policies did not allow them to receive care at The Methodist Hospital.[45] In other area hospitals, their various approaches to enhance awareness of their group were inventive, but each proved to be less than ideal, ultimately causing dissention within the once-cohesive group.

The other private practice cardiologists were not oblivious to the changing environment. As the number of well-trained private practice cardiologists working at The Methodist Hospital increased, so did their interest in participating more fully in the revenue-sharing activities that pertained to their own patients. Heretofore the interpretation of ECGs, echocardiograms, treadmill testing, Holter monitoring, and nuclear stress testing had been the purview of the academic cardiologist, and the academic faculty was resistant to changing this plan for logistical as well as economic concerns.

Tracking the timely reading and reporting by the multitude of cardiologists was seen as a logistical nightmare. It quickly became clear that the reading of ECGs could be managed, and Holter monitors and regular exercise testing in the hospital were uncommonly ordered so as not to pose a significant barrier. While discussions dragged on for several months about the interpretation of echocardiograms and nuclear stress testing, guidelines for the training of cardiologists to interpret these tests were published, disenfranchising most cardiologists on the medical staff who did not have the requisite training. Those few cardiologists who did qualify were not denied the privilege but rarely pursued the credentialing process to do so. Thus, the issue slowly faded away.

One creative concept to extend The Chapman Group's presence in the community was championed by Dr. Spencer in 1985. It was a mobile catheterization laboratory in a 48-foot trailer. Fully equipped and leased from MedCath, a North Carolina company who provided the driver and necessary technicians, the trailer was designed with expandable sides to enable the creation of a 14- by 20-foot procedure room comparable to a small laboratory in a hospital. "To me, it seemed like an excellent idea to do catheterizations out in the little hospitals on the periphery–say one day a week–and, if necessary, bring these patients back to Methodist to have the coronary intervention, such as angioplasty or stents performed here," Dr. Spencer said, recalling his initial enthusiasm about the promising future for the laboratory-on-wheels.[52]

The MedCath mobile catheterization service also was expected to dovetail perfectly into The Chapman Group's new satellite clinics established in the periphery hospitals to improve the flow of patients to The Methodist Hospital. Even though the difficult logistics were daunting, the mobile lab was beneficial for a while. The Chapman Group would go to Jasper, Polly Ryon Hospital in Richmond, Baytown, and Houston's Rosewood Hospitals, taking turns one day a week to hold a clinic in these institutions.

Since Baylor College of Medicine cardiologists and the other private practice cardiologists were experiencing the same patient population shift, they too were expanding their footprint in surrounding towns some 50 to 75 miles away from the Texas Medical Center. Many were in the same towns as The Chapman Group, but on separate days. The satellite clinics took them out of the office and out of the hospital a whole day or more at a time and put a fairly heavy strain on those who were left behind. "But," says Dr. Winters, "it generated interest around, at least in the towns to which we went, and we came to know a lot of doctors and a lot of patients."

Also deemed ineffectual after a year of underwhelming results was the mobile catheterization laboratory made available to the periphery hospitals in and around Houston, Bay City, Angleton, and Baytown. "It was a good concept that didn't quite take off, and I was a little disappointed in that," Dr. Spencer said. "The upshot of all of that was that we did very few catheterizations in that cath lab and brought very few patients into The Methodist Hospital secondary to that, but in the process of traveling around, I did learn all about how physicians practiced cardiology in southeast Texas."[52]

While continuing its efforts to increase referrals in the early 1990s, The Chapman Group experienced difficulties that were exacerbated by both its limited amount of manpower and internal conflict among its five cardiologists. Since the late 1980s, Dr. Chapman had continued coming to the office each day, but he had semi-retired, remaining active in teaching and writing but no longer seeing patients. The group was constantly trying to reinvent itself, but the problem, says Dr. Winters, was that "our efforts stretched us too thin and the aims and goals of the group began to diverge along the way. Bill Spencer and I were pushing hard to expand, but Mark Hausknecht and David Samuels were not enthusiastic. Caught in the middle was Dick Cashion, who packed up and left Houston to work in College Station. He left in the middle of his term as president of The Methodist Hospital Medical Staff. And so we just decided we'd go different paths after awhile."

The opportunity to blaze a new trail previously had been offered, but Dr. Winters had turned it down. For several years Dr. Gotto often had queried about the possibility of his joining Baylor College of Medicine to enhance the clinical arm of the cardiology section, to which Dr. Winters replied that he was not particularly interested in becoming a full-time faculty member. It was an offer Dr. Gotto also made to Dr. Spencer several times previously, but also to no avail.

The extenuating circumstances within The Chapman Group provided Drs. Spencer and Winters with an incentive to leave private practice and return to academia, a career move neither of them could have foreseen in the 1980s. Disillusioned and at loose ends, they decided to meet with Dr. Gotto to ascertain the status of his previous offers. Having left academia some 30 years before in Pennsylvania because of the politics he encountered there, Dr. Winters remained apprehensive about returning to anything similar. Taking into account academia's traditional turnover rate among department chairs in search of career advancement, he also needed reaffirmation of Dr. Gotto's commitment to remain in his leadership role.

After receiving Dr. Gotto's assurances that he had "no intentions of going anywhere else anytime soon," both Drs. Spencer and Winters were persuaded to join Baylor College of Medicine as full-time faculty. Their decision was to have an unanticipated repercussion. When they left The Chapman Group in September 1994, Dr. Chapman came with them because he didn't want to stay behind. In essence, he was returning to the roots of his Houston career. In so doing, The Chapman Group, the practice he had created and built 40 years before, continued under its professional name, Houston Cardiovascular Associates, under the capable leadership of Dr. David Samuels.

"As for my own nostalgic return to academia, I was to have an epiphany within days of joining the Baylor College of Medicine faculty, one that genuinely surprised me," Dr. Winters states. "It soon became apparent that the politics that I'd encountered some 30 years before were still around, only in different form in a different school."

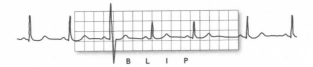

B   L   I   P

SOVIET DIPLOMACY

*I*n *appreciation of his multiple trips to the Soviet Union and to thank him for his help and collaboration over the years, a group of Soviet physicians presented Dr. Gotto with a gift for his wife, a beautiful amber necklace of obvious value. Overwhelmed by such generosity, Dr. Gotto graciously thanked them and carefully packed the necklace in his suitcase before heading to the airport. While going through Soviet customs before exiting the country, Dr. Gotto was surprised when customs officials seized the necklace, telling him that such jewelry should not be taken out of the country. "Dr. Gotto came very near to being imprisoned," Dr. DeBakey said. "He was detained for many hours and was closely questioned by the authorities."[1] Distressed by such a predicament and concerned about telling the generous Soviet physicians that their gift had been confiscated, Dr. Gotto asked the customs officials for a written document detailing the transaction, which he received. Months later, the Soviet physicians somehow retrieved the seized necklace and were able to return it to Dr. Gotto.*

---

1. SoRelle R. Dr. Gotto gets tip of hat as he leaves Baylor for Cornell post. *Houston Chronicle.* December 22, 1996.

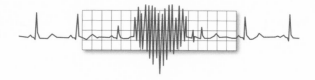

CHAPTER SEVENTEEN

CHANGING OF THE GUARD
1994 - 1996

"There are as many worlds as there are kinds of days, and as an opal changes colors
and its fire to match the nature of the day, so do I."
JOHN STEINBECK

B aylor College of Medicine was not immune to the politics endemic to
academic centers. The highly competitive environment of these centers of learning has proven to be fertile ground for the development of intense politics, often described as "backstabbing" or "cutthroat" and "more
vicious than government politics."[1]

Another universal trait of academic politics was its often-inexplicable
volatility. Recalling his years as a professor at Harvard University, former
Secretary of State Henry Kissinger once said, "I formulated the rule that the
intensity of academic politics and the bitterness of it is in inverse proportion to the importance of the subject they are discussing."[1]

Exposure to any such behind-the-scenes discussions at Baylor College of
Medicine was not common for the private practitioners at The Methodist
Hospital. As was the case in most academic centers, the public remained
generally unaware of any of the particulars of faculty politics. More apparent to Houston doctors was the town-gown conflict, one that commenced
when Baylor College of Medicine moved to Houston in the late 1940s,
escalated after the 1970 affiliation agreement, and continued to fester in
the 1990s.

A frequent source of irritation to private practitioners at The Methodist
Hospital was the stipulation in the 30-year affiliation agreement that established that, with the exception of surgery, the college's department heads
were to serve as chiefs of the correlating service at the hospital. Responsible
for generating 70 percent of the revenue at The Methodist Hospital, private

practitioners took umbrage at having a faculty member in such an authoritative position.

Another bone of contention in the affiliation agreement was the mandatory requirement for private practitioners to become members of the
voluntary faculty and teach medical students and residents. Having served
as teachers since the formative years of Baylor College of Medicine, many
Houston doctors felt such efforts had been essential to the growth of the
college but also had been underappreciated. Comprising a majority of the
teaching faculty, the private practitioners complained they received minimal recognition for their contributions. By the early 1990s, there were several Houston cardiologists who refused to teach while the disgruntled others
continued to do so. Lamented one, "Very few of us have ever received a
letter of thanks or recognition, much less a plaque after 25 years of service,
such as given by The Methodist Hospital."[2]

To address this subterranean sentiment, Dr. Bobby Alford and Dr.
William L. Winters Jr. negotiated an agreement between Baylor College
of Medicine and The Methodist Hospital to permit the secretary of The
Methodist Hospital medical staff, almost always a private practitioner, to
serve on the Baylor Executive Faculty Committee. The first designated
representative was Dr. Richard Cashion, then secretary of The Methodist
Hospital medical staff. Unfortunately, he felt he was never able to exercise
any influence on attitudes toward the volunteer faculty and the agreement
lasted only several years before succumbing to indifference by both parties.

Recalling this and other escalating town-gown conflicts in the early
1990s, Dr. Raizner said each faction openly had become distrustful of the
other. Among the private practitioners, "for some reason, there was a great
deal of concern about Baylor as the big elephant that was going to take over
everything at Methodist Hospital," he said, noting that this level of para-
noia had existed for decades. "The Baylor doctors also were paranoid and
I was sort of in the middle. I had a full-time appointment at Baylor, yet my
income was derived from private practice. I was on both sides of the fence.
And on both sides I heard the same story. Baylor assumed that Methodist
favored the private doctors so much that they felt threatened. And the private doctors thought Methodist leaned toward the Baylor doctors and they
felt threatened."[3]

While defections from one camp to another had been known to occur,
it traditionally was one from gown to town, when a fellow or resident completed his training, but rarely the opposite. The most prominent exceptions
to that norm were Drs. Spencer and Winters, who became the first two

town-to-gown conversions in cardiology in 1994. Aware that their decision to join Baylor College of Medicine would be frowned upon by their peers in private practice, both defectors nonetheless were caught off-guard by the immediate reaction of their former peers.

"I thought our personal relationships with referring doctors would be preserved and that we would keep doing what we did. I was surprised how rapidly I learned otherwise. My naivety shone brightly," recalls Dr. Winters. "Once we arrived the large practices we brought with us began to dwindle because physicians who formerly had referred patients to us when we were in private practice stopped because we had gone to Baylor. It never occurred to me it would happen. It was a town-gown thing….overnight there was a cessation of referrals from doctors right here in the hospital. It was very interesting."

Although this sudden drought of referrals was unexpected, both doctors knew the number of patients referred by private practitioners to specialists at Baylor College of Medicine traditionally had been minimal at The Methodist Hospital. A common town-gown problem at most teaching hospitals, the general perception among private doctors was that academics were too involved in teaching, research, and publishing to take care of their patients properly.

Another commonality of these town-gown conflicts was that each faction embraced its own philosophy of how to practice medicine. As Dr. Winters explains, "To simplify the whole concept I would say the town physicians took care of their own patients, they wrote their own orders, and they did their own thing. On the other hand, academic physicians shared their practices; they would teach in sections and not continuously; they would spend more time writing than taking care of patients. It's changed some over the years, but each group practiced differently, and still do to some extent."

The philosophical differences of academic cardiologists and those in private practice at The Methodist Hospital had been a constant source of debate since the advent of open-heart surgery in the 1950s. Because of the pioneering efforts of Dr. DeBakey and his team, there had been an unprecedented volume of cardiovascular surgical patients, each of whom required the diagnostic and medical management services of a cardiologist. Since the academic cardiologists at the time were few in number, the demand for their services from Dr. DeBakey's patients alone far exceeded the supply. As a result, the private practitioners, those in The Chapman Group as well as many others, rose to prominence.

While the two groups, the private practitioner cardiologists and academic cardiologists, each had its own philosophy, their collective role in the evaluation and medical care of patients with cardiovascular disease at The Methodist Hospital was clearly defined within the medical community but often indiscernible to the general public. Partially responsible for this during the advent of open-heart surgery was the media's inability to grasp the distinct responsibilities of cardiologists versus those of cardiovascular surgeons, often resulting in the misidentification of Dr. DeBakey as a "famous cardiologist."[4]

This rarely corrected misnomer was to appear sporadically in print throughout Dr. DeBakey's career. Probably the most prominent example occurred in the fall of 1996 when Dr. DeBakey agreed to go to Moscow to examine Russia's first president in the post-Soviet era, Boris N. Yeltsin. After surviving a heart attack and "rapidly deteriorating and going into early heart failure," President Yeltsin had been told by his Russian doctors he would not survive coronary bypass surgery. Refusing to accept that prognosis, he reached out to Dr. DeBakey, a frequent visitor to the Soviet Union during the cold war.

After undergoing a thorough examination, President Yeltsin insisted that Dr. DeBakey share his expert opinion at a hastily called Kremlin press conference. To the convened media, Dr. DeBakey declared the president could withstand a coronary bypass operation and expressed his complete confidence in the abilities of the Russian heart surgeon, Dr. Renat S. Akchurin, whom he previously had trained at The Methodist Hospital. Even though his former pupil referred to him as the "Leo Tolstoy of cardiovascular surgery," the 88-year-old surgeon announced he would only be serving as a consultant during the procedure. In several articles generated at that press conference and published internationally, Dr. DeBakey was described as "an American super-star cardiologist" who was to serve an "unacknowledged role as an international monitor whose presence should stifle any wild allegations of a plot if Mr. Yeltsin dies."[5]

In reporting President Yeltsin's recovery and imminent release from the hospital after the successful quintuple bypass performed by Dr. Akchurin, the *Associated Press* in Moscow stated: "Dr. Michael DeBakey, the American cardiologist who supervised his operation on 5 November, said yesterday that Mr. Yeltsin was 'out of the woods' and on his way to a complete recovery."[6]

Regardless of the recurring misidentification of Dr. DeBakey as cardiologist in the 1990s, public awareness of the discipline of cardiology and the specific role played by cardiologists in cardiovascular care had increased exponentially in the last half of the 20th century. The advances made in

medical science and technology, therapeutic methods, and procedural innovations not only increased awareness but also transformed the practice
of cardiology.

This transformation at The Methodist Hospital commenced with the
arrival of Dr. McIntosh, the first faculty Chief of Medicine, as stipulated in
the 1970 affiliation agreement, and had been ongoing under the leadership
of Dr. Roberts since 1982. Throughout its evolution, the focus of the Baylor
College of Medicine cardiology service had been on clinical cardiovascular
research, clinical trials, publishing, and teaching.

Already recognized as a center of excellence in cardiovascular care
through its association with Dr. DeBakey, the cardiology service at The
Methodist Hospital also had established itself as a pioneering clinical and
scientific research center in many of the rapidly evolving subspecialties of
cardiology. Of the 1,172 hospitals considered for inclusion in *U.S. News
& World Report*'s annual ranking of the top 40 hospitals by specialties in
1993, The Methodist Hospital had been ranked 23rd in cardiology. Before
changing its methodology in the late 1990s, the magazine based its hospital
rankings on three factors: its reputation among physicians, mortality rates,
and objective factors such as the ratio of physicians to beds.[7]

While such national recognition of the cardiology service at The Methodist Hospital was long overdue in the opinion of the hospital's cardiologists, particularly Dr. Raizner, the achievement was bittersweet. The mixed
emotions were due to their being outranked by the Texas Heart Institute at
St. Luke's Episcopal Hospital. Included in the top ten hospitals in cardiology since the inception of the magazine's annual rankings in 1990, the Texas
Heart Institute had been catapulted into national awareness by its introduction of bundled payment for coronary bypass operations in the 1980s.

In charging a flat $13,800 for the surgical procedure and the required ser-
vices of cardiologists for each patient since 1984, the Texas Heart Institute
had established a non-Medicare package price substantially lower than the
average Medicare payment of $24, 588. Since 63,000 of the nation's 250,000
coronary bypass procedures were Medicare beneficiaries in 1987, Inspector
General Richard P. Kusserow of the U.S. Department of Health and Human
Services publicly stated, "If we were to fly the beneficiary and spouse to Texas
first class, put the spouse up in a first-class hotel and give them an economy
rental car we'd come out cheaper than Medicare does now."[8]

Convinced the Health Care Financing Administration (HCFA) could
decrease its annual Medicare bill by more than $192 million by instituting
such packaged pricing, the inspector general suggested the implementation

of a study, an idea that belatedly was endorsed in 1991. Originally proposed to the HCFA by Dr. Cooley in 1985, but not acted upon until the number of Medicare beneficiaries escalated 60 percent in the late 1980s, the nationwide study was to grow from four U.S. hospitals to a total of seven in 1993, including the concept's originator, the Texas Heart Institute at St. Luke's Episcopal Hospital.[9]

As a participant in the HCFA pilot project, the Texas Heart Institute fortified its already outstanding reputation. Chartered in 1962 by Dr. Cooley, it had become known after the advent of coronary bypass surgery in the late 1970s as "one of the nation's most highly regarded bypass surgery centers."[8] While the top-ten ranking of the Texas Heart Institute in *U.S. News & World Report* came as no surprise to those familiar with Dr. Cooley's past accomplishments, it was nonetheless a source of frustration to Dr. Raizner, who questioned why The Methodist Hospital continued to be overlooked. "We were doing more research and more publications," he said, after comparing the stats of the two hospitals at the time. "Our clinical volumes were as good or higher, and yet nobody really recognized us as a heart center."[3]

The differences between the two institutions were obvious. Right from the start, Denton Cooley let everyone know what he was doing. From the beginning years of the institute's charter, he made it his mission in life and was very successful. There was no such individual at The Methodist Hospital to have that mission. While Dr. Raizner was closer to it than anybody, he did not have the same stature or backing as Denton. Instead, says Dr. Winters, "we were a diverse assortment: you had the Baylor people, you had the Methodist people, you had the private practitioners, you had the surgeons, you had the cardiologists, and nobody was in charge. They all had their own agenda. There was no one person to bring it all together."

With such disparity, the individual accomplishments of each cardiovascular group or specialist took precedence over where they had taken place, whether it was Baylor College of Medicine, The Methodist Hospital, or a cohesive entity therein. A singular example was Dr. Antonio Gotto. In both basic science and clinical cardiovascular research, Dr. Gotto was known worldwide as a leader in lipid and lipoprotein research and in the application of this research to the care of patients with cardiovascular disease.

Peers acknowledged the academic cardiologists at The Methodist Hospital as being among the recognized leaders in each of their distinct areas of expertise. Collectively spanning five categories of clinical cardiology, the faculty at The Methodist Hospital included interventional cardiologists Drs. Raizner and Kleiman; noninvasive cardiologist Dr. Pratt, who did not perform catheterizations or coronary angiography but focused on some combination of electrocardiography; Drs. Quiñones, Zoghbi, and Nagueh in echocardiography; Drs. Mahmarian and Verani, in nuclear cardiography and stress testing; electrophysiologists Drs. Dennis W. X. Zhu, Hue-The Shih, and Spencer, who performed invasive catheter-based procedures to diagnose and treat complex heart rhythm disturbances and inserted permanent pacemakers; and Drs. Gotto, Christie Ballantyne, and associates, who focused on a combination of cardiac rehabilitation, risk, and prevention.

In addition to the clinical laboratories at The Methodist Hospital for interventional cardiology, nuclear cardiology, echocardiography, and electrophysiology, faculty also could be found in the basic science laboratory for molecular cardiology and genetics, dedicated to the application of the techniques of molecular biology to cardiovascular research. Established by Dr. Roberts in 1982 and one of the first of its kind in the United States, the molecular cardiology laboratory had gained recognition for initiating a human molecular genetics program to identify familial hypertrophic cardiomyopathy (FHCM), the most common cause of sudden cardiac death in the young.

While a number of outstanding scientists had joined the cardiology service at The Methodist Hospital in the molecular cardiology and genetics laboratory, Dr. Roberts continued to recruit academic cardiologists to the clinical faculty. Succeeding Dr. Young, who left for the Cleveland Clinic, and serving as the medical director of the heart transplant center in 1984 was Dr. Guillermo Torre-Amione, a former internal medicine resident and cardiology fellow at Baylor College of Medicine who also had a Ph.D. in immunology from the University of Chicago.

Another academic cardiologist who joined the faculty at the completion of his internal medicine and cardiology training at Baylor College of Medicine was Dr. Sherif F. Nagueh, an echocardiographer who garnered praise from residents as an excellent teacher in the CCU. Also new to the faculty was former Baylor College of Medicine cardiology fellow Dr. John M. Buergler, an interventional cardiologist, and his wife, Dr. Karla Kurrelmeyer, who joined Dr. Nagueh in the echocardiography laboratory.

With the accelerated focus on cardiovascular research, both scientific and clinical, clinical trials, and teaching, this disparate group of academic cardiologists practiced a limited amount of general clinical cardiology: the diagnosis, medical management, and prevention of cardiovascular disease. To do so in 1988 they utilized the clinical facilities of the internal medicine clinic, located in the newly opened Smith Tower.

Smith Tower was owned and managed by The Methodist Hospital. The 505,000-square-foot, 25-story professional office building and outpatient facility was adjacent to the well-established Scurlock Tower, opened in 1980, and the hospital and its clinical laboratories, both easily accessible via covered, air-conditioned bridges over the street.

While most of the cardiology faculty concentrated on research, the one academic cardiologist to whom patients were a priority was Dr. Gotto, who had a huge private practice. Recalls Dr. Winters, "You couldn't meet anybody who didn't say they were his patient. Everybody in Houston thought they were one of his patients, and they probably were. He did see a lot of patients, but whenever he had a problem, he referred them to a specialist. He always had two or three general internists working with him, two of which were Drs. Peter Jones and Ellison Wittels."

While the sharing of clinical space for outpatient care previously had been adequate for the minimal needs of the other academic cardiologists, the impracticality of this arrangement was obvious to the two new general clinical cardiologists on the Baylor College of Medicine faculty in 1994. "We both brought large private practices and we reasoned that we also wanted a clinic where we could have noninvasive testing, such as treadmill, echo, nuclear testing and so forth and so on, done right there under our supervision," said Dr. Spencer.[10]

Even though Smith Tower had been fully leased since its 1988 opening, the 19th floor became available in 1994 and the opportunity to create a customized "Baylor Heart Clinic" was realized. "Baylor was kind enough to renovate the space and put in some very nice offices for us," said Dr. Spencer, who noted there also was space created for his former associate Dr. Chapman. Named the clinic's first director, Dr. Spencer later recalled its auspicious beginnings and resulting longevity: "I thought then, and I think today, the clinic's design is very comfortable and functional."[10]

As these and other efforts to prioritize patient care in the practice of academic cardiology at The Methodist Hospital were instigated by the two defectors and fully supported by Drs. Gotto and Roberts, cardiologists in private practice took notice. Some were sufficiently enticed by the ongoing transformation of the service to contemplate, albeit briefly, their own defection from town to gown, but the majority remained skeptical.

While others thought about joining Baylor, Drs. Bill Gaston and John Lewis were the first, coming on board shortly after Drs. Winters and Spencer. Each of the new faculty members had a separate and distinct motivation. Dr. Gaston loved to teach and wanted to concentrate his full-time efforts to educating students, residents, and fellows. On the other hand, Dr. Lewis likely saw it as an opportunity to have call relief, something he did not have when he practiced alone. He practiced only several more years and then retired due to failing health. He died in San Angelo January 13, 2010.

Having previously served two decades as chief of one of the voluntary teaching services in cardiology at The Methodist Hospital, Dr. Gaston believed his becoming a full-time teacher to be a seamless transition. In a conversation about his motivation, Dr. Gaston recalled his and Dr. Winters' collective contributions as members of the voluntary faculty: "Well, heck, we did the teaching anyway. If you look at the report card of the full-time faculty from the fellows and the interns and the residents and the students in the past, we always did better than they did. You know, technology makes you look better than you are and I used to tell the fellows when I gave their fellowship exam every year, 'I know you want us to teach you how to do these procedures, but I hope you realize the most important thing we're trying to teach you is when *not* to do these procedures.'"[11]

In addition to his teaching abilities, Dr. Gaston also brought with him a large private practice, as did Dr. Lewis. In spite of the town-gown conflict and the resulting cessation of patient referrals from private practice physicians, the general clinical cardiologists in academic cardiology at The Methodist Hospital were able to maintain a loyal patient base and began to thrive in their newly created surroundings on the 19th floor of Smith Tower.

Concurrent with the incremental changes taking place in the practice of academic cardiology at The Methodist Hospital was a seemingly overnight transformation of the hospital itself, spawned by the ongoing upheaval wrought by managed care. One of the largest non-profit hospitals in the country, with more than 1,000 beds and 800 affiliated physicians, it had been one of the last hospitals in Houston to join a managed care network in January 1994. After contractually agreeing to provide medical services at discounted prices with two established provider organizations in January, the hospital had yet to sign a contract with a health maintenance organization by June.

To the surprise of industry insiders, officials of The Methodist Hospital instead announced an aggressive plan to create its own insurance company, managed care organization, and physician organization. As detailed by an official spokesman in June 1994, this reorganization was to centralize and combine the delivery and financing of modern health care and transform the hospital into an integrated delivery system.[12]

When rumors rapidly began to circulate in the Texas Medical Center that The Methodist Hospital also was "reassessing" its relationship with Baylor College of Medicine, a hospital spokesman addressed these speculations in a published interview. Confirming that the hospital's board was considering a decrease in the amount of funding and resources it provided for medical research and education, the spokesman said such reassessment was required for the hospital to be competitive "with those institutions that don't have that research and teaching commitment."[12]

Another of the hospital board's strategic efforts to remain competitive involved the merging of The Methodist Hospital with St. Luke's Episcopal Hospital. The initial step of this complex process was the two institutions' September 1994 signing of a letter of intent to consolidate into a new Methodist/Episcopal hospital. Even though the merging was projected to result in the largest heart program in the country, the seamless blending of the disparate group of cardiovascular specialists at The Methodist Hospital and Dr. Cooley's organized program at the Texas Heart Institute was expected to be one of the proposed merger's major hurdles. Eventually, when the negotiations were put on hold after five months, one participant, who wished to remain anonymous, told a reporter that they had "hit some snags" and that the merger "turned out to be more troublesome than people expected."[13]

While the blending of the established hierarchies of the two heart programs was a daunting challenge to negotiators, the major obstacle reportedly was more universal in scope. Affecting the entire merger was the inescapable probability of an insoluble town-gown conflict. Chiefs of staff at St. Luke's Episcopal Hospital were private practitioners elected on a regular rotating basis, as opposed to those at The Methodist Hospital who were appointed chief upon becoming named a department chair at Baylor College of Medicine.[14] The probability that this stipulation also was an integral aspect of the merger caused one Houston physician to express his and his colleagues' doubts to the media: "Doctors on the St. Luke's side are concerned that this is supposed to be a merger but that on the medical side, Baylor will dominate the medical staff."[13]

This apprehension was to be expected. The voluntary faculty at The Methodist Hospital often had expressed fears about the possibility of academic physicians' monopolizing the hospital's services. To alleviate these apprehensions in 1994, Dr. Gotto had instituted the election of a deputy chair of each department to serve in conjunction with the appointed faculty chair for a three-year term. The entire Department of Medicine, volunteer and academic, elected Dr. Winters to serve alongside Dr. Gotto as the first deputy chair of internal medicine. Recalls Dr. Winters, "A major responsibility of the deputy chair, among others, was to address grievances; it was not a lot of fun. After one three-year term I chose not to run again."

Even with the possible inclusion of Dr. Gotto's deputy chair program at the newly merged hospitals, the uncertainties about the precise involvement of Baylor College of Medicine continued to escalate. One contributing factor was the announcement of the 86-year-old Dr. DeBakey's relinquishment of his role as chancellor to Dr. William T. Butler in December 1995.[15] As chancellor emeritus, Dr. DeBakey became responsible for heading the small faculty group charged with recommending Dr. Butler's successor as president. Approved and announced by the board of trustees in January 1996 was the appointment of Dr. Ralph D. Feigin, who also was to continue as its chairman of the Department of Pediatrics as well as physician-in-chief at Texas Children's Hospital.

The direct impact of this change in leadership at Baylor on the ongoing merger negotiations between The Methodist Hospital and St. Luke's Episcopal Hospital was never disclosed. After the two institutions failed to reach a mutually acceptable conclusion in 1996 and abandoned the concept, the specifics of its negotiations remained confidential. Rather than pursue merging with another institution, the board and administration of The Methodist Hospital began to concentrate its efforts on becoming an integrated health care finance and delivery system. In recognition of this strategy, The Texas Annual Conference of the United Methodist Church approved changing the name of its hospital operating system, which also included the operation of the Diagnostic Hospital and the San Jacinto Methodist Hospital, to the Methodist Health Care System.

As the system's chief executive officer in June 1996, Larry Mathis announced the building of a network of three community health centers with physicians' offices, day-surgery facilities, and some beds for overnight stays. "As part of our plan to be a full-service, area-wide, single-signature provider, we will build our own facilities instead of affiliating," he explained. "We have no choice if we want to be an area-wide network."[16]

In order to accomplish this mission, Mr. Mathis embarked on an aggressive plan. After previously championing The Methodist Hospital's resistance to entering the managed care market, he belatedly had signed the first contract with a health maintenance organization, Cigna HealthCare, in March 1995. In spite of this slow beginning, the pace rapidly accelerated soon thereafter. By September 1996, contracts had been signed with 39 other managed care plans, covering more than 2.5 million people. Also implemented in that time period was the hospital's own health maintenance organization to compete for contracts with employers. The measurable re-sult of this revised approach to managed care was a 24 percent increase in the hospital's patient admissions in 1996.[17]

To further increase future patient flow and "to gain an edge" in the grow-ing managed care market, Mr. Mathis and Dr. Feigin coordinated with their respective boards of trustees to establish the Baylor/Methodist Primary Care Associates. In addition, the two entities formed a joint management coun-cil to identify ways in which they could work more closely together to cut costs and become more efficient. Predicting this jointly announced alliance would result in a closer association regarding research, development, and clinical services, John Bookout, chairman of the Methodist Health Care System board, said, "We're singing from the same sheet of music now."[18]

With this initial phase of The Methodist Hospital's successful shift into managed care accomplished, Mr. Mathis announced his plans to step down as chief executive officer of The Methodist Health Care System in Sep-tember 1996. Having served in his administrative role since Mr. Bowen's retirement in 1983, the 53-year-old executive long had planned to retire by age 55. "It is a very stressful job and the industry is in significant turmoil," he said.[17]

Having advanced his retirement plans by two years, Mr. Mathis said he would remain at the hospital until the board's recruitment of his successor, a process expected to require six to nine months. The ideal candidate, ac-cording to Mr. Bookout, was an individual whose established expertise in managed care would guide the newly transformed institution into the next century.

Seemingly unaffected by the state of flux in the evolving integrated de-livery services of the hospital were its cardiovascular specialists. As was the case throughout the country in the mid-1990s, the impact of managed care on the practice of cardiology had been minimal. National surveys at the time indicated that with the exception of the West Coast, where managed care originated and flourished, Medicare fee-for-service generated more than 40 percent of cardiovascular specialists' revenues, substantially more than the 26 percent generated by the various managed care plans.[19] In ret-rospect, says Dr. Winters, "none of us really knew much about managed care at that time."

What took precedence in the thoughts of the academic cardiologists was the expanded focus of the cardiology service at The Methodist Hospital. With its vibrant clinical practice installed in Smith Tower, the once dispa-rate faculty began to evolve into a more cohesive group as the individual cardiovascular specialists began working more closely together and validating each other's studies and techniques. Furthermore, the Department of Cardiology faculty were a much more collegial group than the private practice physicians, but a seismic change was about to take place.

This transformation came when private practitioner cardiologists, in solo practice or small groups, began to converge. The sole members of Houston Cardiology Associates, formerly known as The Chapman Group, were Drs. David Samuels and Mark Hausknecht. When Dr. Gaston joined Baylor College of Medicine, his former associates, Drs. Milton Klein and David Gonzalez, were alone in practice. Very quickly, Drs. Klein, Gonzalez, Rubin, Robert Hust, Frank Rickman, and Stuart Solomon joined Drs. Samuels and Hausknecht and they continued to add new members.

Having outgrown their space in Scurlock Tower, Houston Cardiology Associates was in need of expanded facilities. When Memorial Hermann Hospital and The University of Texas Medical School in Houston constructed a new office tower a block down Fannin, the Houston Cardiology Associates moved their main office to occupy the entire top floor of that new building. As of 2012, Houston Cardiology Associates now houses 15 cardiologists embracing all the cardiology subspecialties and has become the largest private practice cardiology group in the Houston area, with hospital privileges at Memorial Hermann Hospital as well as The Methodist Hospital.

Regardless of this transformation or the two groups' philosophical differences, the "private practice guys" and the academic faculty shared an identical surprised reaction to an unexpected September 1996 announcement. After serving 20 years as chairman of the Department of Internal Medicine at Baylor College of Medicine, Dr. Gotto announced his leaving Baylor College of Medicine in January 1997 to accept a position at Cornell Medical College in New York. "Twenty years is a long time to hold a job," said Dr. Gotto, who indicated Cornell previously had approached him three times before he finally accepted. "I thought I had accomplished about all I could have here. And this was in New York and Cornell was a new challenge. I thought there were opportunities there for some resources that had not been tapped or pursued before."[20]

While contemplating such a career change, Dr. Gotto had been discreet, confiding in only a few colleagues. Foremost among them was Dr. DeBakey, whose advice vividly was recalled decades later. "I was about 60 at the time and Dr. DeBakey was in his late 80s," Dr. Gotto remembered. "I told him about the opportunity at Cornell and he said, 'Well, Tony, if you decide to go there, there will be many people here who will miss you and feel your loss and none will feel it greater than I will. But you have to look at where you can be the most productive in the years to come. You've got another 30-40 years ahead of you.'"[20]

Unburdened by any ideas of mortality, Dr. DeBakey no doubt based his optimistic view of Dr. Gotto's future not only on the longevity of his own career but also on the accomplishments they had previously shared. After all, he had been in his late 60s when he coauthored *The Living Heart* with Dr. Gotto. Together they subsequently had written three books for the general public, many of which became international bestsellers. In the Russian edition of the 1997 publication of *The New Living Heart*, an update of their original book, included an inscription from President Yeltsin that declared Dr. DeBakey as "a magician of the heart" and "a man with a gift for performing miracles."[21]

As personal witness to many of those miracles over the decades, Dr. Gotto often described their professional relationship as one of the best he had ever experienced and "probably the highlight of my career." Appreciative of Dr. DeBakey's confidence in him, Dr. Gotto recalled their working together well as physicians, collaborating on the care of such important patients as the prime minister and president of Turkey and the abdicated king of Belgium. "For some reason, he seemed to take a liking to me very early on and he was always very patient with me," he said, noting they sometimes had conflicting opinions. "I knew he had a great deal of skepticism about cholesterol, and I'm not sure whether he ever fully accepted the cholesterol-lipid hypothesis, although he did go on statins after they came out."[20]

Held in high esteem by their colleagues at The Methodist Hospital and often referred to as the hospital's ambassadors to the world, this dynamic duo had never been expected to part ways voluntarily. Among those who thought such an occurrence was inconceivable was Dr. Winters, particularly since his joining of the faculty two years earlier had been predicated by Dr. Gotto's assurances that he was not going anywhere.

"From my perspective, Dr. Gotto was a victim of not only academic politics, but also the kind I had experienced and abhorred at Temple University in Pennsylvania," Dr. Winters explains. "What happened to Tony Gotto is exactly what happened to the chairman of medicine at Temple and one of the reasons I had left that institution. His demise had occurred after he had become very prominent nationally and was internationally recognized. Like Dr. Gotto, he was away from the school a lot and when he came back to renegotiate his tenured professorship, the school felt he no longer was the man for the job. That's the precise scenario I thought of when Tony told me out of the blue he was leaving to go to New York. I had no definite knowledge of this, but it was a feeling we all had."

"Decades later when I no longer was reticent to delve into Dr. Gotto's motivation for leaving, I asked him why Baylor College of Medicine had not enticed him to remain," Dr. Winters continued. "I asked him, 'Did you have a sense that Baylor thought that you had contributed as much as you were going to contribute to their reputation at that time?' Since I was not expecting him to reply, I said, 'Before you answer, I will say I think their willingness to let you go was the first of several bad decisions that came down the line from that school.' His answer was never forthcoming."[20]

At the time of Dr. Gotto's decision to leave, no one questioned the fact that he had seized a wonderful opportunity to advance his career. Since his appointment as provost for medical affairs and the Stephen and Suzanne Weiss Dean of the Medical College at Cornell University was to be effective January 1, 1997, he remained in Houston through December. Underscoring Dr. Gotto and his wife's popularity in the community was a succession of farewell dinners in their honor.

While there was no knowledge or mention of the skullduggery of academic politics during these dinners, there often were fondly shared reminiscences of Dr. Gotto's relationship with Dr. DeBakey. One of his fondest memories was to be repeated often by those in attendance and eventually was published in a Houston newspaper. The story, in Dr. Gotto's own words, went as follows:

"During her high school years, my daughter spent a great deal of time as a patient in the hospital. When he was able, Dr. DeBakey never missed an opportunity to visit her. Often, he was the only one who could brighten her spirits. During one visit, my wife, Anita, was sewing a prom dress for a friend's daughter. Dr. DeBakey immediately asked to inspect her stitches.

'These are your basting stitches, aren't they?' he asked.

'No, Dr. DeBakey,' Anita said. 'These are my finishing stitches.'

'These are terrible,' he said. 'Let me have your scissors.'

He proceeded to rip out every stitch and then sew the dress in its entirety while my wife sat there in a state of astonishment.

Fifteen years later Dr. DeBakey was having a New Year's Eve dinner at our home in Houston. My wife cooked gumbo, which she knew he loved. And, of course, Dr. DeBakey–who never forgot anything–said to Anita, 'You may not be able to sew, but you sure cook good gumbo.'"[22]

This indelible memory of Dr. DeBakey's omnipresent quest for excellence in every aspect of his life was to serve as a humorous reminder to at least one of those determined to fulfill his mission at The Methodist Hospital. As opposed to being downtrodden by the uncertainties created by Dr. Gotto's unexpected departure or those spawned by the on-again, off-again merger with St. Luke's Episcopal Hospital, Dr. Raizner was inspired to once again voice his tireless support for the formation of a unifying entity for the cardiovascular specialists at The Methodist Hospital.

After years of having his idea fall on deaf ears, Dr. Raizner finally had listeners. Not only that, within a matter of months, he suddenly was to find himself to be considered politically correct, at least among those in hospital administration.

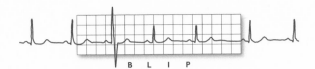

B   L   I   P

MOSCOW NIGHTS

While in Moscow in November 1996 to participate in the care of President Boris Yeltsin, Drs. Michael E. DeBakey and George P. Noon were among the guests invited to a dinner at the home of the minister of health. "During the evening, the Russian doctors would disappear at times," Dr. Noon said. "They were, unknown to us, going to smoke or play pool. While touring the home, Dr. DeBakey was shown the billiards room where the Russian doctors were playing. After watching for a while, Dr. DeBakey was pleased when the Russians, out of courtesy, invited him to play a game. He agreed. The Russians started the game. When it was Dr. DeBakey's turn, he walked up to the table and, to their amazement he promptly sunk all the balls and won the game. In Texas we would say 'he kicked their ass.' What they didn't know was Dr. DeBakey and his brother grew up playing pool in their home. He was a pool shark!"[1]

1. Winters, William L. Jr. (Methodist DeBakey Heart & Vascular Center, The Methodist Hospital, Houston, Texas). Personal correspondence with: Dr. George P. Noon (Methodist DeBakey Heart & Vascular Center, The Methodist Hospital, Houston, Texas). 2013 May.

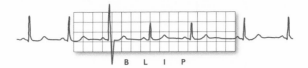

THE WINTERS CENTER FOR HEART FAILURE RESEARCH

*S*ucceeding Dr. Gotto as chairman of the Department of Medicine at Baylor College of Medicine was Dr. Andrew I. Schafer, promoted from his position as chairman of medicine at the VA Hospital in Houston. Among his several goals as the new chairman was his vision to promote research in the field of heart failure. He had the perfect person in mind to spearhead this plan: Dr. Doug Mann, who already had achieved national prominence in the field and had been under his wing at the VA Hospital. "As planning proceeded, a phone call came to me one morning from Dr. Mann," Dr. Winters said. "He described what was being planned, and out of the blue requested, and inquired, if I would accept the honor of the new research center being named, 'The Winters Center for Heart Failure Research.' The following silence emphasized my surprise and bewilderment, as I had never been involved in heart failure research. His response was that the honor had nothing to do with heart failure per se but, rather, to my 'enduring contributions to the Texas Medical Center—a sort of achievement award.'" Flattered, Dr. Winters accepted the honor and immediately began earning his keep by seeking a significant donor for the program. "That source proved to be Mary and Gordon Cain, who endowed both the program and the Mary and Gordon Cain Chair in Medicine at Baylor College of Medicine with a $5 million donation," Dr. Winters said. The chair was to be held by Dr. Mann. " After the 2005 separation of the Baylor College of Medicine and The Methodist Hospital, the chair was transferred to Dr. Biykum Bozkurt at the VA Hospital when Dr. Mann left to become chairman of the Cardiology Division of Medicine at Washington University in St. Louis," Dr. Winters said. "Dr. Bozkurt provided a summary of the center's accomplishments in 2013."[1]

---

1. Bozkurt B, Mann DL. The treatment of heart failure in the 21st century: Is the glass half empty or half full? *Methodist DeBakey Cardiovasc J*. 2013;9(1): 3-5.

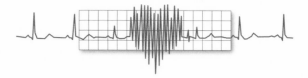

CHAPTER EIGHTEEN

A COMING TOGETHER
1994 - 2001

"Coming together is a beginning; keeping it together is progress;
working together is success."
HENRY FORD

The rapidly changing structure of healthcare delivery in the United States in the 1990s had become known as the "industrial revolution" in medicine.[1] For The Methodist Health Care System, as well as other fee-for-service-only institutions throughout the country, surviving the upheaval was dependent on its ability to transform itself into a healthcare delivery system capable of success in the world of managed care.

With its belated entrance into the managed care era in 1994, The Methodist Health Care System began its transformation by implementing the required cost-containment strategies. In the following tumultuous two years, its workforce was reduced from more than 7,000 to less than 5,000 employees.[2] After an aggressive pursuit of the managed care contracts it previously had ignored, The Methodist Health Care System had signed more than 31 provider contracts by 1996.

While rapid, it was not an easy transition. "Those years of change were extraordinarily difficult for everyone," said Mr. Mathis, recalling the administrative turmoil that ensued. "Our employees lost their sense of security. Physicians were upset, angry, and confused as their incomes dropped with the lower managed care rates and as the world of medicine they had known turned upside down. For them, and for me, the effect of change was visceral."[2]

Among the cost-containment difficulties encountered at The Methodist Hospital were those endemic to most teaching hospitals during the managed care revolution. Comprised of highly trained specialists and subspecialists equipped with the latest technologic advances, academic medical centers concentrated on the advancement of medical knowledge. With an established mission of teaching, research, and highly specialized clinical care, teaching hospitals in academic medical centers traditionally were more expensive than nonacademic hospitals and had become dependent on the revenues generated through the open-ended, fee-for-service system.[3] Before the advent of managed care, efficiency in the delivery of high-quality care was not one of its priorities.

The necessity of restructuring its priorities to include cost reductions proved stressful to academic medical centers around the country.[3] Built on layers of history and the ingrained culture of autonomy, teaching hospitals traditionally were known to be "bureaucratic, overly deliberative, and organizationally slow" and "anything but a nimble business unit," Mr. Mathis stated. "A teaching hospital is a place of competition among full-time and voluntary faculty members who vie with one another for academic prestige and for patients. Conflicts of interest and personal agendas abound. Authority is often diffuse. A confusing array of departments, institutes, divisions, centers, and programs overlap in ways that defy logic and the organizational chart. It is uniquely ill-suited to the tough, competitive managed care environment."[4]

While the primary function of managed care was the efficient delivery of high-quality care by controlling inappropriate use of resources by overseeing the process, implementing the measures required at academic medical centers was a challenge. The managed care contracts' limitation of consultants, procedures, admissions, and what Dr. DeBakey lamented as its overall "pernicious cost-cutting strategies"[5] required a paradigm shift not only in the delivery of health care at teaching hospitals but also in the attitude of those delivering it.[6]

From the onset of the implemented changes in health care delivery at The Methodist Hospital, the decrease in referrals became a major concern to the specialists and subspecialists. A predominant number of its contracted managed care plans established primary care physicians as "gatekeepers" charged with controlling access to specialists, tests, and treatments; as a result, the once-legendary volume of hospital admissions began a steady decline as the referrals diminished.

Since more than 99 percent of the physicians who previously had admitted patients were specialists and subspecialists, The Methodist Health Care System found it necessary to establish it own primary care physician network in 1996. Named the Methodist Medical Group, the group practice of 11 initial primary care physicians was projected to expand to 100 in five years. This organization of gatekeepers also had affiliation agreements with 100 additional primary care physicians who did not wish to join the private group practice. The hospital and the physicians shared ownership of a new organization created to run the business of the group practice owned by the physicians.[7]

For the steadily dwindling surgical cases at The Methodist Hospital attributed to managed care in 1997, there was another innovative strategy employed. When many contracts directed a growing number of cardiovascular surgical patients to more cost-effective hospitals in the community, five of the full-time cardiovascular surgeons on faculty expanded the availability of their services. With six other prominent Houston surgeons, Drs. Lawrie, Coselli, Howell, Noon, and Richardson formed Texas Surgical Associates, a group practice to provide cardiovascular, thoracic, transplantation and general surgical care at hospitals throughout Houston and the surrounding communities.[8]

While Texas Surgical Associates was independent of Baylor College of Medicine, Dr. Lawrie and his colleagues remained on Baylor College of Medicine faculty and continued to practice at The Methodist Hospital as well as others in the community. "The issue is continuing access to our patient base," he said. "We don't want to have to stand by and watch our patients go somewhere else because of an insurance contract."[9]

Watching patients go elsewhere was a predicament that contrasted starkly with having to place cardiovascular patients on waiting lists for surgery at The Methodist Hospital. In previous decades, admitting and performing surgical procedures on more than 100 new patients weekly had been the norm for the veteran members of Dr. DeBakey's surgical team.

Even with the great strides in cardiovascular research and technology in the intervening decades, the potential patient population for cardiovascular surgery remained formidable in the 1990s. More than 59 million citizens in the United States in 1995 had some form of cardiovascular disease, primarily heart disease and stroke. While the death rate had dropped appreciably since the 1950s, in 1995 cardiovascular disease was the cause of death in more than 961,000—as many as all other diseases combined.[10]

Before the advent of managed care, patients with cardiovascular disease freely had come to The Methodist Hospital in hopes of becoming a patient of the legendary Dr. DeBakey and his team. Many came in search of a miracle, and often found it.[11] Although still performing surgery on a limited basis in 1997, the 89-year-old surgeon did not maintain the steady schedule of surgery of his past. Having escalated his already hectic travel schedule to pursue his other interests as international medical consultant and teacher, he was away more than he was at the hospital. On the eve of his 50th anniversary of coming to Baylor College of Medicine, Dr. DeBakey remained very active on faculty but was unable to devote the time required for surgical procedures and the subsequent patient care. In his own words, "Operations tie you down."[12]

This was not to say he did not maintain his presence in the operating rooms and laboratories at The Methodist Hospital. "He's doing more traveling around and consulting than he did, but, we're still working on research," Dr. Noon said at the time, noting that the left ventricular assist device they had designed and developed with NASA was about to begin clinical trials in Europe." I would say he really hasn't given up anything because of his age. If you watch him, he's still perfectly capable of doing the things he did previously. His hands are steady. His eyesight's good. He knows what he's doing."[13]

He also was keenly aware of what he and other surgeons were unable to do. As one of the world's most recognized medical statesmen, Dr. DeBakey had become known as an outspoken critic of the limitations imposed by managed care's cost-containment policies. In an editorial printed in The Wall Street Journal in 1998, he further enunciated his opinions: "First, do no harm. That is the overriding precept of medical practice. The paramount objective of managed care—profit—is diametrically opposed to this precept. Under the pretext of containing costs, managed care has introduced strictures inimical to the physician's best judgment and the patient's best interest. This poses a grave obstacle to competent health care. Intrusive government and the interposition of corporate managed care have imposed regulations that not only are burdensome and costly (more than 20 percent of health care expenditures), but are subverting the crucial physician-patient relationship."[14]

Other concerns about the effects of managed care on cardiovascular surgery were to be addressed in other publications by Dr. DeBakey, often in a subtle way. Because of his long-established relationship with the national and international media, he often was asked to comment on breaking news stories about heart surgery. When a "minimally invasive" coronary bypass procedure (MIDCAB) captured the media's attention in 1994, Dr. DeBakey was asked by a wire service to comment on the growing popularity of the experimental procedure and its use of a small incision rather than cracking open the chest for access to the heart. His duly reported reply was a brief explanation of the history of heart surgery; how it originally had been minimally invasive due to lack of expertise; how extensive research enabled the development of techniques to treat complex heart conditions; and how dividing the sternum and parting the ribs for better access to the heart and the heart-lung machine facilitated the advent of open-heart surgery.

After explaining how opening the chest became routine with the development of extensive operations for more difficult heart problems, Dr. DeBakey concluded his observations with a thinly veiled jab at the cost-containment mandates of managed care: "Now the idea behind the so-called 'minimally invasive' is to reduce the post-operative period at the hospital and to have less discomfort after the operation. We were not doing it with that purpose in mind, originally. We were doing it in order to correct what we needed to correct."[15]

One such correction developed by Dr. DeBakey and his surgical team at The Methodist Hospital in 1964 was the first successful coronary aorta bypass graft (CABG) operation for coronary artery occlusive disease. Thirty-three years after that landmark procedure was performed, treatment of coronary artery occlusive disease had undergone extensive investigation and evolution, resulting in improved diagnosis and more effective treatment. With the newly pioneered minimally invasive MIDCAB and other off-pump innovations, the ever-evolving techniques for single-vessel, double-vessel, triple-vessel, and multiple-vessel disease established CABG as the most commonly performed major operation in the United States, with utilization growing at more than 9 percent annually, according to the National Center for Health Statistics in 1997. The following year, more than 553,000 CABG procedures were performed on 336,000 patients.[16]

At The Methodist Hospital, where untold thousands of CABG procedures had been performed since the first in 1964, the volume had decreased sizably in the decades since the introduction of coronary artery balloon angioplasty in 1980 and the subsequent development of coronary stents by interventional cardiologists. "With experience and improvements, these percutaneous devices were used more extensively than CABG surgery to establish blood flow in obstructed coronary arteries," Dr. Noon said, noting how multiple trials compared the efficacy of balloons, stents, and bypass surgery. "The success of stents in properly selected patients decreased the number of CABG procedures performed. In general, however, CABG procedures provided better long-term results."[17]

As interventional cardiologists continued to research and develop other technological advances in the less invasive treatment of coronary heart disease in the late 1990s, more and more potential surgical patients were referred instead to cardiologists for nonsurgical treatment, and many cardiovascular surgeons across the country began to question the longevity of their specialty.[18] To the contrary, when Dr. DeBakey found there was a reduced need for many of the cardiac and vascular operations he developed and introduced, "he fully supported development and refinement of these primary catheter-based procedures," Dr. Noon recalled, praising his mentor for being "yet, forever the visionary."[11]

In addition to such encouragement from Dr. DeBakey, the interventional cardiologists at The Methodist Hospital were imbued with his indomitable pioneering spirit, as epitomized by Dr. Spencer in 1996. As Dr. Roberts conducted molecular genetics research of hypertrophic obstructive cardiomyopathy (HOCM), a relatively common genetic malformation of the heart known to be the leading cause of heart failure and sudden death, a large group of his patients received pacemakers from Dr. Spencer. "It was promulgated that pacing would be a constructive therapy and we thought we were making progress, but our patients were not getting any better," said Dr. Spencer.[19]

Treatment to relieve the debilitating symptoms of ventricular septal hypertrophy included medications or open-heart surgery, a myotomy-myectomy of the septum.[20] Serendipitously, Dr. Spencer learned of an alternative treatment while attending the European Society of Cardiology meeting in Amsterdam in January 1996. In attendance was Dr. Ulrich Sigwart, a friend and former Baylor College of Medicine trainee who was at Royal Brompton Hospital in London. "He told me about three cases that he had done injecting alcohol into the first septal perforator and producing a 'controlled' myocardial infarct, which became known as Alcohol Septal Ablation (ASA), and how it relieved the obstruction of HOCM by shrinking the obstruction as the heart cell died," Dr. Spencer said, recalling his initial reaction to that innovative, yet somewhat alarming, technique. "I said to myself, 'Well that sounds like that makes imminently good sense to me and I think I ought to do that.'"[19]

Armed with a copy of Dr. Sigwart's three published cases, Dr. Spencer returned to Houston and approached the internal review board at Baylor College of Medicine with a research protocol to request permission to proceed with the experimental procedure. Given approval only if his program was funded, Dr. Spencer was hesitant, petrified about the inherent risks involved. "Shortly thereafter I told Bob Roberts I didn't want to do it," he recalled. "I said, 'I've been thinking about it and this is producing a heart attack and people are going to die and I am just scared.' He said, 'No, you have got to do it. I'm going to insist you do it.'"[19]

With no possibility of industry support, Dr. Spencer conjured up an ingenious plan. Traveling to the Temple Foundation in East Texas, Dr. Spencer
asked them for $100,000 for the first 20 patients, telling them The Meth-
odist Hospital had agreed to match their generosity. "The hospital doesn't
know this, but after they wrote that check I went back to the hospital and
told them if they gave me $100,000 I could get the Temple Foundation to
match it, so they wrote me a check, too. Well, I did that four times, raising
$800,000. I spent every cent on patient care and the first 100 patients did
not pay a cent."[19]

To get the program off and running on November 19, 1996, Drs. Spencer
and Roberts performed the first ethanol septal reduction for hypertrophic
obstructive cardiomyopathy in the United States at The Methodist Hospital using echocardiography to guide the catheter to the proper position.
Agitating saline in a syringe produced tiny innocuous bubbles when injected, thus outlining the heart muscle to be affected once the alcohol was injected. Assisting them was the technique's originator Dr. Sigwart, who had
flown in from an American Heart Association meeting in New Orleans at
Dr. Spencer's request. Advising the media gathered at the hospital that his
method of injecting pure alcohol into enlarged hearts to kill excess tissue
and reduce strain was not without pain, Dr. Sigwart said, "It hurts to get alcohol in the heart. I found the idea appealing to create a small heart attack
selectively in the area where we had too much muscle and do in essence
the same thing as is being done in surgery. It's much less invasive. You don't
have to open the chest."[21]

The apprehensions Dr. Spencer had about the procedure were to be mol-
lified by the success rate experienced in the first 33 cases. Even though there
was a "definite learning curve," the mortality rate was only one percent
and diminishing. The 30 seconds of pain experienced during the procedure was minimal, less than bad heartburn, the patients said. The results of
the procedure were immediate symptomatic and hemodynamic relief, and
the long-term results were effective.[19] Having closely followed his patients
afterward as if they were his wards, Dr. Spencer said, "Every one of them
says, 'Thank you for giving me my life back.' It's incredibly rewarding. This
procedure has been more successful than my wildest dreams."[22]

Also unexpected was the general public's enthusiastic response to the
October 1998 publication of the research results for ethanol septal reduction in Circulation, the American Heart Association journal.[20] Warned by
that journal's staff that there would be intense media interest, Dr. Spencer nonetheless was astounded when his breakthrough research appeared

on major television news network shows and in feature articles of national newspapers and magazines. "I knew I had arrived when there was a big article in the *National Enquirer* and I was quoted, except I never talked to anyone at that paper," he said. "I have that one framed at home. My wife wouldn't let me put it in a prominent place."[22]

Regardless of its popularity, because the procedure was considered experimental, managed care organizations and other insurance entities were hesitant to approve it. But since the cost was far less than open-heart surgery, approval came more often than not in the beginning. As the procedure's recognized expert in the United States, Dr. Spencer went on to perform more than 600 cases during the following three years at The Methodist Hospital and all over the world. "That is an astronomical number when you consider the number of people who have hypertrophic obstructive cardiomyopathy," he said in 2004. While the mortality rate eventually became much less than one percent, he noted, "The other risk at first was 50 percent of those patients were requiring pacemakers at first. Now it has declined to six and a half percent in the last 200 procedures I have done."[19,23]

The repercussions of Dr. Spencer's accomplishments were measurable at The Methodist Hospital and elsewhere. Even though Dr. Spencer moved to Charleston, South Carolina in 2000, he continued to perform ASA at The Methodist Hospital until 2004 and at the Medical University of South Carolina until 2010, the year he retired. With ASA, interventional cardiologists had the ability to offer yet another less expensive, catheter-based procedure as an alternative to heart surgery and continued to usurp a sizable portion of cardiovascular surgeons' patient base. Contributing to that attrition were the cost-containment measures implemented by both managed care and the government.

By the late 1990s, CABG had become one of the most expensive single treatments or procedures in the United States, consuming more of the medical care dollar than any other.[24] In addition to the costs of the surgeon in each procedure, there were those of the hospital, the laboratories, one or more assistant surgeons, an anesthesiologist, nurse anesthetists, a cardiologist, and pump perfusionists to operate the heart-lung machine during surgery. Cost-containment efforts by Medicare in the 1980s influenced the development of bundled prices for CABG and other cardiovascular surgical procedures, such as the ones developed at the Texas Heart Institute in 1984, but relatively few hospitals immediately followed suit.[25]

Within the following decade, the HCFA Heart Bypass Center Demonstration was to establish the cost effectiveness of bundled payment arrangements for CABG, proving it resulted in the more efficient provision of services, improved quality, and reduced costs.[26] At the September 1995 conclusion of the five-year project at seven participating hospitals, including the Texas Heart Institute, Medicare reported savings totaling $42.3 million, roughly 10 percent of Medicare's expected spending on CABG.[27]

Public access to CABG outcomes rapidly was becoming standard practice around the country, but it was not in evidence at The Methodist Hospital in 1997. Cardiovascular surgeons historically had not disclosed outcomes for any open-heart surgical procedures, and this nondisclosure continued unabated. "Nobody would talk about it and the surgeons did not even share the information among themselves," Dr. Winters said. " There must have been records but no one had access to them."

The protected privacy of cardiovascular surgeons' outcomes was a longstanding tradition, one that had been endorsed by Dr. DeBakey for decades. "You could not figure out anybody's mortality rates," Dr. Raizner said, echoing his colleagues' frustrations with the information void. "The surgeons only published what they wanted to publish. And there was a philosophy at the time that we were the last stop for any surgical consideration, so patients were sent in who had little or no chance of survival. But it was part of the culture here to try to save them so virtually no one was denied an operation."[28]

One of the harbingers of change for this established practice and many others at The Methodist Hospital was the newly named president and CEO of the Methodist Health Care System, Mr. Peter W. Butler, who assumed office in September 1997. Formerly chief administrative officer at the Henry Ford Health System (HFHS) in Detroit, he had overseen one of the fairly typical, large, nonprofit, integrated health systems in existence.

With commitments to a coordinated health care system that spanned the continuum of care and to proactive, longitudinal chronic disease management, HFHS comprised the Henry Ford Hospital, founded in 1915 by the eponymous automaker; six other hospitals; 1,000 staff physicians and 1,800 affiliated physicians; 30 medical centers; two nursing homes; and home hospice, home health, behavioral, and pharmacy services.[29] The Henry Ford Hospital was the sole provider of cardiac surgical services for the HFHS-sponsored health maintenance organization, one that served more than one half a million members.[30]

A prerequisite for Mr. Butler's transforming The Methodist Health Care System into the integrated health delivery system desired by its board of directors was the development of sound data about the performance of the system. To assist him in the attainment of that goal, Mr. Butler recruited a former corporate vice president of HFHS, Richard D. Wittrup, to serve as his senior advisor and to help develop systems to manage and improve accountability and to increase healthcare quality, improve outcomes, and reduce costs. While both of the former HFHS executives seemed particularly well suited for the task that lay before them, there were to be many challenges to overcome.

Clearly evident to both executives upon their arrival at The Methodist Health Care System was the resistance to change inherent in any established organizational structure. Openly expressing his preference to preserve the status quo was Ronald G. Girotto, the executive vice president, chief operating officer, and chief financial officer who had spent more than 20 years in a variety of executive and administrative positions at the hospital since 1977. Ingrained in and loyal to the hospital's traditions, he did not hesitate to openly question the prudence of implementing integrated healthcare delivery system policies.

Recalling his initial conversations with both executives shortly after their arrival, Mr. Girotto said he questioned the ability of the hospital comprised of narrowly focused specialties to transform itself into one in which primary care was to become the coordinating factor. He also expressed his misgivings about owning and operating a health plan, pointing out that inexperience in being both the provider and the payer could prove to be costly.

Prominent among Mr. Girotto's apprehensions was how to overcome the physicians' perception that the transformation to an integrated delivery system irreparably threatened their autonomy and livelihood. Having personally recruited many of the physicians, he knew them well and "knew in my heart I could not go down and look at them in the eye and try to begin to convince them this was the right thing for them to do; it was impossible." Aware that such a system had been successful in Detroit, where it had existed for decades, and elsewhere, he was wary of its ever succeeding in Houston because "The Methodist Hospital was not like other hospitals on the East Coast or the West Coast, or even here in Texas. We don't play by the same rules."[31]

Although he felt his observations to be prophetic, they went unheeded and Mr. Girotto eventually acquiesced, becoming an active, albeit skeptical, participant in the planned reorganization. One of his major contributions was to facilitate the establishment of clinical service lines. Transforming the delivery of care from one centered on specialties and procedures to one centered on medical conditions and care cycles, clinical service lines were to enable the integrated delivery of care with the goal of improving value to patients and documenting outcomes, which was becoming a necessity.

Since effective care for medical conditions usually required the combined and coordinated efforts of multiple physicians and other health professionals, the ultimate value for patients came as the result of the entire sequence of activities within the service line and not just one specialist or procedure. In addition to benefiting patients, this integration of care was known to result in an optimal organizational structure and more efficient financial management.[32]

Through Mr. Girotto's efforts to implement this proven strategy, he inadvertently was to provide the catalyst required to bring Dr. Raizner's elusive vision to fruition, a unified identity for clinical and surgical cardiovascular care. This serendipitous result followed the recruitment of 26-year-old Houston native and daughter of Baylor College of Medicine's president Dr. Feigin and Dr. Judith Feigin, Mrs. Debra Feigin Sukin.

Having earned a bachelor's degree, with honors, in health care administration from Virginia's Mary Baldwin College and a master's in health administration from Washington University School of Medicine in St. Louis, Missouri, Mrs. Sukin completed her post-graduate fellowship work at North Carolina's Duke University Hospital and Health Network. "I had just come back from Duke University, which was one of the top four cardiovascular centers in the United States," Mrs. Sukin said, recalling her initial conversation with Mr. Girotto. "I had been there to establish service lines and this was the time when clinical pathways were just evolving. The Methodist Hospital knew enough to know they needed to be there; they were not lagging too far behind others who clearly were the national leaders and Ron Girotto was interested in looking at organizing service lines within the hospital, in particular the heart service."[33]

The priority of establishing a cardiovascular service line at The Methodist Hospital in 1998 was not only to integrate its delivery of care but also to enhance its competitive edge in attracting and maintaining managed care contracts. Another impetus was the published success of the HCFA demonstration project. "In the seven hospitals that had participated in the HCFA demonstration project, the physicians and hospitals collectively worked together to achieve clinical outcomes and improve performance," Mrs. Sukin said, noting how it impacted the future. "They essentially agreed to what health care reform is today, a bundled payment. But the real emphasis was on improving outcome."[33]

The clinical information amassed on each of the more than 10,000 patients at the seven participating hospitals during the demonstration project included descriptive analyses of intra- and postoperative complications and mortality outcomes stratified by risk factor and other relevant variables.[26] These established benchmarks for length of stay, mortality, and cost for CABG were to become a mitigating factor in Mrs. Sukin's detailed planning of a cardiovascular service line.

The most prominent motivation to expedite Mrs. Sukin's efforts was to come from another source. "In the 1998 *U.S. News & World Report* listing of America's best hospitals, cardiovascular surgery and cardiology were combined for the first time," she said, stating the magazine also revised its methodology of ranking to include specialty-specific mortality rates. "The result of combining these services was Texas Heart Institute was named one of the top ten and The Methodist Hospital was nowhere to be found on the list."[33]

The exclusion from the magazine's prestigious rankings was the impetus needed to jump-start the planned proposal for implementing a cardiovascular service line. As the administrative lead in that process, Mrs. Sukin began her efforts to best understand where the strengths and weaknesses existed in cardiology and surgery by researching the data available. "You don't know what you don't know until you start measuring and looking at it, monitoring and measuring it," she said, explaining how she accessed the mortality rate data utilized by *U. S. News & World Report* for reference. "When you broke apart the surgery and cardiology outcomes, cardiology would have continued to have been recognized. When I combined the two areas, cardiovascular surgery pulled them down and all of a sudden it became apparent that everybody had to play here."[33]

Anxious to participate in the planning was Dr. Raizner, one of the few on the medical staff who instantly grasped the significant opportunity Mrs. Sukin's efforts represented. To his thinking, the goal was not just to implement a cardiovascular service line but also, ultimately, to create a heart center. His viewpoint of the researched mortality rates for cardiovascular surgery and cardiology at The Methodist Hospital was philosophical: "It was a culture and that culture was Dr. DeBakey. He was willing to experiment with lives and the things that he did had very high mortality. You had to see a goal to put up with your failures along the way. Dr. DeBakey had that vision. In cardiology, I don't think we ever had that vision. If a patient died while we were doing a procedure, we felt it for weeks afterward. The surgeons could handle that. But I think over the decades, in order to make progress, you had to have the experimental surgery of Dr. DeBakey and his surgeons."[33]

Such historical perspective and insight proved beneficial to Mrs. Sukin as she progressed in her efforts. "I worked very closely with Dr. Raizner, from the cardiology perspective, and Dr. DeBakey, obviously for overseeing the whole initiative," she said, noting how Dr. Raizner became her "partner in crime" during the lengthy planning. "We met on a monthly basis. It was really Dr. Raizner and I who were organizing this."[33]

For these two partners in crime, it was to be a daunting task, one that began with the need to convince the faculty and voluntary faculty of the merits of reorganizing the clinical and surgical cardiovascular services. "The chief of cardiovascular surgery at that time was John Baldwin and Bob Roberts was the chief of cardiology," said Dr. Raizner. "They had trouble seeing where a heart center fit into their role and there were a few among the voluntary faculty who were either opposed or passive/aggressive. They felt their autonomy was threatened."[28]

In order to present a cohesive marketing plan for the development of a cardiovascular delivery system, Mrs. Sukin and Dr. Raizner formed a steering committee comprised of cardiovascular physicians from the Baylor College of Medicine faculty and voluntary faculty and administrators from the hospital and college. Co-chairing the committee was Dr. Entman, who served as a liaison to Dr. DeBakey.

To exact a better understanding of where The Methodist Hospital stood in an operational volume perspective, locally, statewide, and nationally, the steering committee began its efforts to assess the existing capabilities of all entities involved in the proposed heart center. "We also looked at it from the NIH research component and from a full continuum to best understand where we had our strengths and where we had our weaknesses," Mrs. Sukin said, noting the need to improve coordination, cooperation, and communication among the many members of the heart team. "There also was a lack of trust and credibility between the physicians and administration."[33]

Another obstacle encountered by the committee was its inability to assess the surgeon-specific outcomes necessary for comparing not only the mortality rates used by *U.S. News & World Report* but also the benchmarks established by the CABG demonstration project. "While we all believed that Dr. DeBakey was a good heart surgeon—even the best—we had no data to support that conclusion," Mr. Wittrup was to observe in retrospect. "It was entirely possible that some heart surgeon working in obscurity somewhere had better outcomes, but there was no evidence of that, either."[34]

This seemingly insoluble conundrum constituted one of the steering committee's greatest challenges. Convinced that his fellow cardiovascular surgeons should be made aware of their own mortality data as well as their colleagues', Dr. Coselli, who was chief of cardiothoracic surgery, took it upon himself to expedite the exposure and evaluation of this data. "It probably cost him his job ultimately," Dr. Raizner said, recalling the subsequent meetings held with each surgeon to review and compare the mortality figures. "Making the heart surgeons aware of their individual data was the enzyme that catalyzed a whole change in philosophy."[28]

Mortality rates do not show that a patient may have been one who no one else would have operated on, or one who was extremely sick. To have a lower mortality rate, surgeons had to be more selective of the patients who underwent procedures. "There were surgeons whom we worked with over the years who never turned down a patient," Dr. Raizner said. "Jimmy Howell was one. Boy oh boy, did his philosophy change after our meeting. Stanley Crawford's philosophy changed; he used to do aneurysms that were ruptured. Eventually, all the surgeons changed."[35]

To generate more awareness and support for the proposed heart center, there was a combined meeting of all the cardiologists, cardiovascular surgeons, and administration executives in May 1999. Drs. Raizner and Entman stood by Mrs. Sukin's side for moral support as she presented the hard truths presented by the data. "It was a critical meeting and I will never forget it in my life," she said. "Drs. Raizner and Entman were like my bodyguards. I was 27 years old and I stood up in front of 80 physicians, including Dr. DeBakey, and showed exactly where cardiovascular services stood from an internal perspective, from a market perspective, and a national perspective. It wasn't all pretty."[33]

Perceived by many of the voluntary faculty at the meeting to be biased against them because her father was president of Baylor College of Medicine, Mrs. Sukin nonetheless remained nonplussed by the unfounded criticism. "The message we delivered was this was an incredible opportunity for everyone on the faculty and the voluntary faculty," she said, emphasizing how all the pieces of the puzzle had been built over the past five decades but had not been maximized to full benefit. "Everyone will always crowd around quality, my father used to always tell me. If you can get everyone on the same page about being the best and you can get everyone on the same page about quality, then everybody wants to play. And he was right because by the end of that meeting there was agreement that we should move forward."[33]

Over the following 12 months, the steering committee divided into different groups to work on a variety of different aspects from a clinical, research, and operational perspective. The clinical group addressed methods of delivering care in very detailed terms of developing clinical pathways and the organization of specific patients collectively in designated areas of the hospital. This process was proven to be very successful and has continued to this very day.

As the administrative group of the heart center steering committee worked in 1999 to develop an organizational plan based on the structural, marketing, and financial perspective, there was a potential glitch in the planning progress when Mr. Girotto announced his plans to retire, stepping down as chief operating officer in December 1999.

While fully supportive of the heart center concept, Mr. Girotto had maintained his skepticism about most of the major aspects of the integrated delivery system. "I had worked with Peter Butler for two years and I told the board that I can't be in that position and not advocate the system," he said. "I couldn't see how it would work because it wasn't working at that time, in my opinion. I told them it was better for Peter Butler for me not to be here as the person in charge of operations and it was better for me to move on. The board members agreed and we had a very amiable parting."[31]

Recruited by Mr. Butler to serve as executive vice president of The Methodist Health Care System in November 1999 was Dr. Lynn M. Schroth, the former chief executive officer of Memorial Southwest Hospital in Houston. In the health care arena for more than 15 years, Dr. Schroth had been an active member in an organization called University HealthService Consortium, a group of academic hospitals across the United States that had organized to develop benchmarking for quality purposes. "I convinced The Methodist Hospital to join the consortium and it was the first time they had done benchmarking on their quality," she said, noting that the outcomes were not at the levels expected. "The only ways to change that was to get the physicians focused on the patients and get the hospital resources focused on the patients."[36]

Since these changes in focus already were the established goals of the proposed heart center, Dr. Schroth wholeheartedly supported Mrs. Sukin's ongoing efforts, promoting her to vice president of operations. "She not only endorsed the heart center, but she also reorganized the entire hospital operationally to align with essentially what we had been planning for two years," Mrs. Sukin said.[28]

Over the following year, Mrs. Sukin formed a governance board for the heart center and organized the operational units. At that juncture, changes had already been implemented regarding case managements of patients, operating rooms, cardiac catheterization labs, patient care units and the ICU. The only thing lacking was approval to affix the ideal name for the heart center. "From the beginning we knew that it should be the Methodist DeBakey Heart Center," Dr. Raizner said. "But at that time, Methodist and Baylor relations were a little strained and Baylor thought it owned the DeBakey name and we could not get permission to use Dr. DeBakey's name. Eventually Mark Entman, I think, was very instrumental in getting that accomplished. But it was very interesting that something so obvious took so long to achieve."[28]

To receive approval from The Methodist Hospital board of directors for the establishment of the as yet unnamed heart center in 2000, Dr. Raizner prepared a slide show to accompany Mrs. Sukin's completed marketing plan. Included in his presentation was a slide depicting the newly released hospital rankings from U.S. News & World Report in which cardiology and cardiovascular surgery at The Methodist Hospital again failed to appear. "You may view our institution as one of the top centers in the world, but that's not how it is viewed by the public," Dr. Raizner said, challenging them to find the hospital's name on the list of the top 50 heart centers in the United States. "I think that's what sold the idea."[28]

Following his presentation, there was an honest discussion about the existing strengths and weaknesses and the opportunities outlined in the marketing plan. Together, Dr. Raizner and the board discussed whether there were any possible reasons the desired results could not be achieved. "I said there was only one great threat and it was not Baylor, not Methodist, not faculty, and not the private practitioners," he said, fully aware that competing hospitals would be the greatest challenge. "I told them the only enemy we had was our competition, and they agreed."[28]

With the heart center's local and regional competition defined through the data accumulated by Mrs. Sukin, the governance committee was able to define the opportunities presented by the establishment of a centralized service to provide a continuum of cardiovascular care. By offering primary, secondary, and tertiary services as well as prevention and rehabilitation services, all of which already were in place, The Methodist Hospital had the capability to establish and maintain a leadership position in the market place. When the board of directors endorsed the heart center, allocating the funds necessary for the establishment of its marketing plan in 2000, Dr. Raizner said, "We needed the board to recognize us as a heart center, a single entity, and now they did."[28]

Dedication ceremonies for the newly named Methodist DeBakey Heart Center took place on February 19, 2001. Presided over by Mr. Butler, Dr. Schroth, and Dr. Coselli, the ceremony paid tribute to the 92-year-old Dr. DeBakey as a "living legend," an honor he modestly deflected. "I'm living," he joked. "So the first half of that description is right."[37]

For Mrs. Sukin, Dr. Raizner, Dr. Entman, and all the members of the heart center's steering committee, the brief occasion contrasted dramatically with the many months of planning it took to bring their desired concept to fruition. When other approved aspects of the plan, including the construction of a private entrance to the Methodist DeBakey Heart Center, were postponed indefinitely, the perceived value of their original accomplishment was not diminished. The realized value was destined to increase tenfold in the coming years.

In retrospect, it can be said that the only other thing increasing noticeably at The Methodist Hospital at that time was the quiet before the storms.

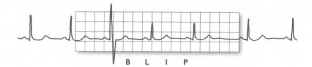

FOREIGN INTRIGUE

W orking in the DeBakey–Gotto sphere of influence was a bit like walking on bubble wrap. You never knew when something interesting would pop up because of their many worldwide connections. For example, on a Friday morning, while making his morning rounds and anticipating a quiet weekend off call, Dr. Winters received a call from Dr. Gotto, whose first statement was, "Is your passport current and readily available?" Yes, it was, Dr. Winters explained. "Good, because Dr. DeBakey and I want you to leave this afternoon on Air France for Zurich, Switzerland, to check on one of our favorite patients who had been advised by us to come to Houston for a medical consultation. However, he's hospitalized in the University Hospital in Zurich where he was taken when too ill to continue his flight from his home in San Moritz to Houston. We want you to assess the problem for us and tell us whether it is wise or even possible for him to make it here safely."

"I left for Zurich on an Air France flight that afternoon in my own first-class cubicle enclosed with a curtain and provided with a pair of Air France pajamas," Dr. Winters said. "I was to try to meet the surgeon in charge, but the surgeon was leaving for Florida that very day I was to arrive. Connections were very close, and, of course, it was too close. He left before I arrived and would be gone for the weekend. So what I thought would be a day-or-two trip turned into a weekend-long trip and, subsequently, more than a week."

When Dr. Winters finally did see the patient, it was clear he could not be transferred anywhere. "So I spent the weekend serving as a courier delivering regular updates to the family on his condition. In an extraordinary gesture of generosity, the family graciously invited my wife to come to join me in Zurich when it became apparent I was going to be there for a while. And come she did. But any decision on further medical care would await the return of his surgeon."

While waiting, Dr. DeBakey and Dr. Isadore Rosenfeld from New York City, also an old friend and family physician, both announced their intention

(continued on page 398)

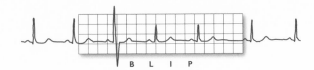

to come to Zurich. "This led to one of the most interesting nights in my life when we three had dinner at The Dolder Grand Hotel in Zurich," Dr. Winters said. "I sat entranced as those two old friends swapped hilarious stories of their careers in nonstop fashion."

"The next day, definitive decisions were made for the care of the patient, allowing the three of us to return home. He subsequently died in Zurich on Thursday, April 18, 1996, at age 86. "

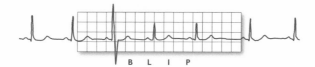

MODERATION

"*I* *weigh the same now and can wear the same uniform that I wore in the Army,*" *the five-foot, 11-inch, 160-pound, 90-year-old Dr. DeBakey told a reporter from The New York Times in 1998, noting it had been more than 50 years since World War II.*[1] *Although he and Dr. Gotto recently had coauthored a best-selling diet book, The Living Heart Diet, Dr. DeBakey believed he was living proof that good health and longevity stemmed not from a strict diet but from moderation in one's living habits. "I don't have any health secrets, but I am moderate, and I think that is the key to it," he said. "I am moderate in my eating habits, but when I eat, I try to get a variety of foods, particularly fresh vegetables and fruit, which I like very much." He attributed such food preferences to his upbringing, crediting his parents for providing him, his brother, and two sisters with a healthful diet long before it became fashionable. "They instilled in us early a taste for fresh fruits, vegetables, and other wholesome foods," he said, noting that the easy availability of seafood, including shellfish, on the nearby Gulf Coast instilled his passion for seafood gumbo, a Louisiana specialty he preferred made with fresh okra and hot peppers. "I don't eat a great deal of meat, probably once a week at the most," he said, confessing he also liked eggs, but not every day. "I usually have fish because I like it. I like rice, vegetables, and beans." Relatively trim since his youth, Dr. DeBakey maintained his weight throughout adulthood but rarely deliberately exercised, except for climbing up and down the stairs at The Methodist Hospital at a rapid pace instead of taking the elevator. Like his father, who was strongly against alcohol and tobacco, Dr. DeBakey had no desire to drink alcohol or smoke as an adult. Once, when invited to talk about his health habits, Dr. DeBakey enumerated the details of his long life of moderation. After he listed all the things he didn't do, somebody in the audience asked him, "Well, what else do you do?" To which he smiled and replied, "I pray a lot."*[2]

---

1. Altman LK. The doctor's world; Dr. DeBakey at 90: stringent standards and a steady hand. *The New York Times.* September 1, 1998.

2. Roberts WC. Michael Ellis DeBakey: a conversation with the editor, Interview with William C. Roberts. *Am J Cardiol.* 1997;79(7): 929-950

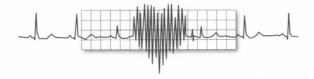

CHAPTER NINETEEN

A PARTING OF THE WAY
2001 - 2004

"Parting is such sweet sorrow
that I shall say goodnight 'til it be morrow."
WILLIAM SHAKESPEARE

When The Methodist DeBakey Heart Center was dedicated in February 2001, there were no premonitions of black clouds on the horizon for The Methodist Hospital. Only in retrospect was it clear that some of these impending storms, comprised of both the literal and metaphoric varieties, should have been foreseeable. Regardless, the havoc wreaked by each was to remain just as unfathomable after the fact as it had been at the time of occurrence.

The first deluge was to be both unpredictable and exceptional in every respect. The only "storm" with a formal name, Tropical Storm Allison devastated the entire Houston metropolitan area and beyond. Although hurricanes and lesser storms are inevitable in south Texas, experts claimed that no one could have predicted that the atmospheric disturbance that suddenly formed 80 miles off the coast of Galveston on June 5 would develop into one of the most devastating rain events in the history of the United States.[1]

Affecting more than two million people in Houston and Harris County, Tropical Storm Allison dumped more than 80 percent of the area's average annual rainfall, including a record-breaking 13 inches in one 3-hour period.[2] The resultant flooding surpassed the 100-year benchmark for the area, leaving in its wake 22 fatalities, 95,000 damaged automobiles and trucks, 73,000 damaged residences, 30,000 residents in shelters, and more than $5 billion in property damage.[1]

Prominent among the damages were those sustained by the Texas Medical Center, located on the lowest elevation in Houston. While losses were expected to total more than $2 billion, the precise amount was incalculable. At Baylor College of Medicine, where basement facilities experienced water levels of 18 to 24 feet, 30,000 lab animals drowned and countless research projects were delayed or derailed. "In the days and weeks following the flood, it was impossible to calculate the impact on research programs at Baylor, but it was clear the damage was enormous," Dr. Feigin reported several months later, predicting the losses would exceed $300 million. "Researchers in the area of cancer, heart disease, AIDS, virology, and many others lost equipment, laboratory animals, tissue samples and years of hard work."[2]

The floodwaters also inundated nearly 300,000 square feet of space on two basement levels at The Methodist Hospital, destroying four magnetic resonance imaging systems, two linear accelerators, and five nuclear medicine cameras. In addition, there was irreparable damage sustained by the hospital's pharmacy and food preparation areas, and millions of dollars worth of supplies were lost.[3] Hospital executives estimated that storm damage, including loss of business revenue, would surpass $350 million.[4]

At The Methodist Hospital, where emergency generators were located on risers outside the hospital instead of the basement, the availability of auxiliary power negated the need for a mandatory evacuation of its 690 patients.[5] Among the 183 patients willing and able to be discharged immediately was the wife of Dr. Winters, Barbara, who had undergone minor surgery the day before the flood.

"The elevators were out of service because of the limited power provided by the generators, so Barbara and I had to walk down 12 flights of stairs in the dark with all the other volunteer evacuees," recalls Dr. Winters. "At the bottom of the stairs we ran into Peter Butler, who was there in the dark to direct all of us to the safest way out of the building. All of it was unbelievable."[6]

The inconveniences wrought by the power failure, which continued intermittently for weeks,[7] including the cancellation of elective surgeries and outpatient services at The Methodist Hospital, paled in comparison to its cumulative damages in The Methodist DeBakey Heart Center. Located on the upper floors of the hospital's Fondren-Brown Building, the center was not impacted directly by the flooding but suffered significant losses in its aftermath.

The absence of full electrical power and running water resulted in unavoidable damage to the refrigerated blood samples, cell lines, and tissue cultures and the complete loss of the catheterization laboratory inventory.[6] Upon assessing the situation, Dr. Roberts surmised, "The cardiology service has certainly been delayed now for several weeks and will not be back to normal at

The Methodist Hospital for another couple of months."[6]

Although the flood waters did minimal damage to the Fondren-Brown Building, the subsequent loss of power and water service presented a problem into itself for Dr. Mark Entman and the scientists in the cardiovascular sciences laboratory. "When they turned the water back on, there were some leaks on the 8th floor and we had a deluge come down over our laboratories," he said, indicating the losses were minimal compared to those experienced in the laboratories located in the Baylor College of Medicine. "I lost some mice over at Baylor from the flooding, some of my transgenic mice in the restricted facility."[8]

Intermittent power outages during the five weeks after Tropical Storm Allison necessitated the shutting down of the eight catheterization laboratories in the Methodist DeBakey Heart Center. Providing service to 8,500 patients a year, including more than 2,000 angioplasties and more than 6,000 diagnostic catheterizations, the laboratories had just undergone a multimillion-dollar rebuild made possible by a contract negotiated with Siemens Medical Solutions. With the state-of-the-art digital imaging network systems installed, physicians in key locations throughout the hospital had immediate access to the images acquired during procedures in the diagnostic and interventional laboratories as well as afterward.[9] "The capital expenditure had been more than $14 million," said Dr. Raizner, who had overseen the installation in early 2001. "We had the greatest equipment built at the time."[10]

Despite the inability to offer its full complement of services in the five weeks following Tropical Storm Allison, The Methodist DeBakey Heart Center managed its business reasonably well. Because of the collegial relations with many cardiologists outside of the Texas Medical Center, many of whom trained at The Methodist Hospital and Baylor College of Medicine, The Methodist Hospital physicians were able to have any urgently needed interventional procedures on their patients done elsewhere. As medical director of the 75 physicians, including 45 cardiologists and 14 cardiovascular surgeons, and the 500 supporting staff in the center, Dr. Raizner remained focused on its mission "to become the benchmark heart center of the world."[11]

Emboldened by the fact that cardiovascular services traditionally contributed more than 50 percent of the hospital's net revenue, Dr. Raizner confidently projected this would not change in 2001, regardless of Tropical Storm Allison. While presenting the center's aggressive business plan to the hospital's board of directors in August, he proposed the further development of the center's clinical areas of vascular surgery, coronary artery disease/minimally invasive surgery, endovascular, genetics, heart failure, thrombosis, prevention, rhythm disorders, cardiovascular imaging, and nuclear cardiology.[11]

For the projected increased volume of these expanded programs, the space allocated to The Methodist DeBakey Heart Center was inadequate, Dr. Raizner reported to the board. Since capacity limitations already existed in all the departments, intensive care units, and research areas, he advised that the allocation of new space was crucial for future development. Aware of the significant investment required, Dr. Raizner directed the board's attention to the state-of-the-art facilities in Texas Heart Institute's new $42 million building and the Cleveland Clinic's investing $90 million in a stand-alone heart hospital.[11]

The Cleveland Clinic's new facility was indicative of the boom at that time of hospitals devoted exclusively to cardiovascular care throughout the country. "If Dr. Raizner and his fellow cardiologists and cardiovascular surgeons at The Methodist Hospital had their way, they would have had a stand-alone heart hospital," Dr. Schroth said, recalling their desire for administrative autonomy. "That would have been possible only if they were to own their hospital and they did not have that luxury."[12]

What they had instead was a hospital within a hospital—one that The Methodist Hospital's CEO had promised would have its own identity, including a designated entrance. "We don't have to have separate hospitals," Mr. Butler explained to Dr. Schroth as he approved her construction plans for the reconfigured access to The Methodist DeBakey Heart Center. "We can have centers of excellence and each can have its own entrance with a sign on the door. It doesn't matter that behind the scenes it is all part of a bigger hospital."[12]

The establishment of a separate identity for The Methodist DeBakey Heart Center was postponed as Mr. Butler and the board of The Methodist Health Care System focused on operational requirements.[13, 14, 15] However, in late September 2001 The Methodist Health Care System initiated some changes. On September 28, 2001, the board of directors announced Mr. Butler was stepping down as president and chief executive officer the following Monday, October 1. The board named Mr. Girotto as the interim acting president and chief executive officer.[16] "It was a mutually agreed upon decision by the board and the CEO," spokeswoman Nicole Rubin said in a statement released to the media. "It wasn't related to any damage by Tropical Storm Allison. Overall, Methodist is in a strong position, financially and strategically."[16]

As executive vice president of the Methodist Health Care System during the transition, Dr. Schroth was to form an opinion about the transition that would remain unchanged for more than a decade. "You can argue all day long that Peter, who had been charged with bringing Methodist into the world of managed care, didn't go about it the right way, but he definitely was a change agent that came in, shook the place up, and got them moving on the right path," she said in 2012. "I give Peter a lot of credit because he wanted to establish a system of hospitals and to me that was the one big thing of an integrated system that he did successfully. He did exactly what was needed and the whole scene had changed so that Ron could pick it up, maintain it, heal some of the wounds, get rid of some of things that were not working, and continue to move it along."[12]

As they began this new period, Mr. Girotto and Mr. Bookout turned their concentrated attention to establishing a new, 25-year affiliation agreement with Baylor College of Medicine. Their proposed agreement was intended to supersede the one-year extensions that had been enacted annually following the expiration of the original 1970 agreement in December 2000.

Throughout this transition period at The Methodist Hospital,[1] Dr. Raizner concentrated his efforts on implementing the marketing plan developed for the Methodist DeBakey Heart Center. Based on the overall marketing needs of the center, the plan included a local/national television campaign, meeting symposia support, research journal publication, heart month promotions, American Heart Association Heart Walk sponsorship, web site enhancement, and patient education materials development. Other marketing opportunities included direct mailings to physicians, support of program specific medical meetings, and other physician referral related materials.[11]

To increase national recognition of the Methodist DeBakey Heart Center in peer reviewed publications, Dr. Raizner encouraged the authors to include the center's name and its affiliation with the hospital and the Baylor College of Medicine in all submitted research papers generated by the full-time and voluntary faculty.[11] Although somewhat successful in achieving this goal immediately, Dr. Raizner found that a majority of the published research did not include the Methodist DeBakey Heart Center by name. Undaunted, Dr. Raizner remained optimistic about eventual progress, saying, "With the creation of the heart center, it looked like we had moved a little bit closer to becoming a single entity, but there's always going to be somebody on the fringe. Since everybody bought into it, we were pretty close."[10]

Major exposure in the medical profession came from the center's sponsor-

---

1. Owing to a name conflict with the Methodist Healthcare System in San Antonio, Texas, The Methodist Health Care System in Houston reverted to its incorporated name, The Methodist Hospital.

ship of programs presented at meetings of the American College of Cardiology, American Heart Association, and Thoracic Surgery Society, as recommended in the marketing plan. Through aggressive public relations tactics, the public had become increasingly aware of the center's existence several months before it was formally dedicated in February 2001. In the national news coverage of a rare cardiovascular operation performed by Dr. Mike Reardon in November 2000, a syndicated article stated "the doctors at the hospital's DeBakey Heart Center" successfully "removed a patient's heart, cut out three life-threatening tumors from the left atrium inside the heart and then successfully reinsert[ed] her repaired organ."[18]

Communicating the successes experienced in the Methodist DeBakey Heart Center, as well as its cutting-edge research and clinical efforts, became an integral part of the marketing plan to create awareness and increase recognition. Over the next few years the Methodist DeBakey Heart Center generated an escalating number of mentions in peer-reviewed publications and numerous newspapers.

Among the litany of accomplishments recognized were Dr. Raizner's participation in the collaborative research of coronary stents; Dr. Spencer's trailblazing efforts in alcohol ablation for Dr. Roberts' new concepts in hypertrophic cardiomyopathies; Dr. Zogbi's pioneering research in three-dimensional echocardiography; Dr. Quiñones' research with tissue Doppler echocardiography; Dr. Verani's breakthrough advances made in nuclear cardiology; Dr. Kleiman's improvement of common cardiac procedures through a magnet-guided catheter system; Dr. Coselli's performing his 2000th thoracoabdominal aortic aneurysm repair, more than any other surgeon in the world; and Dr. DeBakey's receiving the commercial invention of the year award from the National Aeronautics Space Agency for his contributions to the development of a miniature heart pump based on the machinery that propels the space shuttle into orbit.[19]

The ultimate recognition of the Methodist DeBakey Heart Center's collective efforts came in July 2003 with the publication of the annual list of America's best hospitals in *U.S. News & World Report*. With its outstanding nursing program featured on that magazine's cover, The Methodist Hospital was ranked among the country's top centers in ten of the 17 specialties featured. Among these was the combined service of heart and heart surgery, including clinical research, heart disease prevention, diagnosis, medical treatment, surgery and transplant services, in which The Methodist Hospital was ranked 15th in the nation.[20]

Believing this recognition was long overdue, Dr. Raizner nonetheless was ecstatic, crediting its delayed timing to recent developments. "There were really two things that were accomplished that helped us tremendously," he said, noting that the magazine's rankings were based on a cumulative score that equally weighed reputation, mortality, and a group of care-related factors such as nursing and the use of high-quality medical technology. "One was our newly installed state-of-the-art equipment in the catheterization laboratories and the other was a tremendous drop in our mortality, an indication that the era of the 'cowboy surgeon' here had ended."[10]

Dr. Winters and his colleagues were hopeful that the 2003 publication of the magazine's rankings was introducing a new era in which the focus would become much greater on the Methodist DeBakey Heart Center. "Even though the neighboring Texas Heart Institute at St. Luke's Episcopal Hospital maintained its traditional ranking among the magazine's top ten in heart and heart surgery in 2003," Dr. Winters said, "I was confident that as an entity unto itself our center would become just as well known as the one across the street."

Such optimism soon was eclipsed by a growing sense of uncertainty about the hospital's affiliation with Baylor College of Medicine. Although rumors of the impending demise of this long-time relationship began to escalate, the probability of a separation was minimal was the widely held opinion. This presumption began to change in July 2003.

By October 2003, due to the uncertainty of Baylor College of Medicine's intentions, The Methodist Hospital board had commenced site inspection tours of similar healthcare facilities throughout the United States to assess an alternative path. Explained Mr. Girotto, "We had to find out what we wanted to be if our affiliation with Baylor College of Medicine didn't play out like it had for 50 years."[21]

While the future affiliation of the school and hospital remained in limbo, it was a predicament that did not deter the disclosure of the hospital's multi-million-dollar strategic initiatives and expansion plans. Publicly announced by Mr. Girotto in February 2004 was the board's decision to construct three new facilities: The Methodist Hospital Research Institute, the Methodist Outpatient Center, and a new, 400-bed patient tower to be known as the "North Campus."[22]

The Methodist Hospital Research Institute, conceived as a necessary building block to secure being an academic medical center, would specialize in "translational" or bench-to-bedside research, that in which discoveries are translated rapidly into tangible treatment protocols for patients. Constructed adjacent to the hospital, the institute was to allow better accessibility to patients in an effort to expedite the transformation of scientific discovery into improved patient care. Focused on the medical disciplines that build on The Methodist Hospital's historic strengths in the field of cardiovascular disease, as well as cancer, diabetes, orthopedic conditions, and infectious and neurological diseases, the physician-scientists with diverse specialties and backgrounds will collaborate and share ideas to enhance the bench-to-bedside equation.[23]

The potential impact of such cardiovascular research at the Methodist Research Institute was limitless, Dr. Winters said. "Just as Dr. DeBakey's innovations in cardiovascular surgery translated into the revolutionized care of cardiovascular patients in the past, in the future the mission of the Methodist DeBakey Heart Center cardiovascular physicians and scientists at The Methodist Hospital Research Institute was to generate innovative ideas to transform cardiovascular care and to advance the fields of cardiovascular medicine, cardiothoracic surgery, cardiovascular anesthesiology, and vascular surgery."[10]

The inclusion of the Methodist DeBakey Heart Center in the 400-bed patient tower, known as the "North Campus," represented the realization of Dr. Raizner's quest to create a unifying identity for the center. "We had some tremendous architectural plans drawn up for that," Dr. Raizner said.[10] In the expansive space allocated for the Methodist DeBakey Heart Center in the North Campus were all the services required to deliver the full continuum of cardiovascular care, ranging from prevention to diagnostic through treatment and rehabilitative care. Located in close proximity to the operating rooms and the emergency room were all the center's services, including cardiology, cardiothoracic surgery, vascular surgery, cardiac anesthesia, and cardiac radiology.

In addition to the heart center in the architectural plans for the new tower, located adjacent to The Methodist Hospital in the previously occupied site of Texas Woman's University school of nursing and the Institute of Religion, were renderings of the space allocated to the new emergency department, operating rooms, endovascular radiology, a host of other services, and the newly announced Methodist Neurological Institute, the first of its kind in the region.

As to whether these announced expansion signified a resolution of the hospital's relationship status with the Baylor College of Medicine, Mr. Girotto implied to the media there were expectations of continuing the affiliation in some form, but no agreement had been made at that time. "There will always be a presence of Baylor at The Methodist Hospital," he said. "Is it equal to, greater than, or less than the current relationship? That's what we'll have to determine."[22]

Such optimism had been fortified by the behind-the-scenes resumption of the affiliation negotiations, which continued for several months. When the Baylor College of Medicine board of trustees called a special meeting on the evening of April 21, 2004, to select the hospital with the best affiliation proposal for Baylor College of Medicine, The Methodist Hospital board of directors were confident and hopeful its revised agreement was the frontrunner.

Later that evening, when informed that Baylor College of Medicine had selected St. Luke's Episcopal Hospital as its primary adult teaching hospital, where it would build its own outpatient clinic, Mr. Girotto and the hospital board members were stunned. Recalling their mutual bewilderment, Mr. Girotto said, "It wasn't easy news to take."[21]

Sharing their disbelief of the sudden dissolution of the five-decade partnership was the man who had wielded and nurtured it. Although Dr. DeBakey reportedly had espoused the necessity of Baylor College of Medicine's controlling its own destiny,[24] the 96-year-old surgeon was described as "heartbroken" by the news of the separation, his colleagues said. "It certainly saddens me," he told one newspaper reporter. "I don't understand it. I don't think it's in the best interests of either institution."[25]

Adding his thoughts was President-elect of The Methodist Hospital medical staff and a cardiovascular surgeon in the Methodist DeBakey Heart Center, Dr. Michael Reardon, who exclaimed to the media, "This ends a 50-year productive relationship for an unknown deviation in course that will have unknown consequences."[26]

These uncertainties were of paramount concern to Dr. Quiñones, who had been named medical director of the Methodist DeBakey Heart Center in 2003, succeeding Dr. Raizner. We had people with incredible seniority and titles. What would happen to them?"[27]

Also awaiting clarification was the future of the joint programs previously shared by The Methodist Hospital and Baylor College of Medicine, particularly those in cardiovascular medicine and multiorgan transplantation, among others.[28] As for the future, Mr. Girotto said, "The Methodist Hospital was unwavering in its desire to be among the top tier of the nation's academic medical centers."[26]

The board's determination to move forward with the development of The Methodist Hospital into an academic medical center became apparent within hours of its learning of Baylor College of Medicine's decision to affiliate with St. Luke's Episcopal Hospital. Having already initiated a long-range plan with the creation of the Methodist Research Institute and the Methodist Neuro-

logical Institute, the board believed circumstances necessitated that plan's ac-
celeration. With the Cleveland Clinic and Massachusetts General Hospital
as models, the board decided to launch an aggressive campaign to institute
the elements required for the transformation of the hospital into an academic medical center. "This strategic decision was enormous," Mr. Girotto said.
"Initially I did not fully appreciate the magnitude of the commitment and
how important execution became in effecting the strategy."[21]

The board knew that the establishment of an academic affiliation with a
highly nationally ranked medical school was its first priority. To ascertain what
affiliation opportunities existed nationally, Mr. Bookout flew to New York in
the third week of May to meet with Dr. Tony Gotto at Weill Cornell Medical
College to discuss what possibilities might be available. Events moved rapidly
and during their meeting agreements were reached on the structure, relationship, and conditions for an affiliation agreement. After further discussions in
Houston, Mr. Girotto and a group from The Methodist Hospital returned to
New York the first week of June for a meeting with Weill Cornell and New York-
Presbyterian Hospital to draft an affiliation agreement in compliance with
terms previously reached.[21]

Less than six weeks later, on June 23, 2004, Weill Cornell Medical College,
New York-Presbyterian Hospital, and The Methodist Hospital announced
they had entered into an historic medical affiliation.[29] Under the terms of the
new 30-year agreement, Weill Cornell Medical College and New York-Presbyterian Hospital were to become the primary affiliation of The Methodist
Hospital. This collaboration of three internationally renowned institutions
in two different states was the first of its kind. Praising this new approach
in health care delivery and medical research collaboration, Mr. Girotto said,
"Technology today makes anything possible—the sharing of information,
quality data, and collaboration on research and patient care."[29]

In blazing this new path for academic medical centers, Dr. Gotto said,
"Advances in medical education, research, and clinical care depend on our
willingness to discover new ways of doing things that broaden our vision,
making us better able to fulfill the vital missions of an academic medical center. This partnership offers many exciting opportunities for collaboration that
will benefit patients, students, physicians, and researchers of The Methodist
Hospital, NewYork-Presbyterian Hospital, and Weill Cornell Medical College as well as our broader national and international communities."[30]

While the transnational affiliation agreement gave physicians at The
Methodist Hospital the opportunity to receive faculty appointments at Weill
Cornell Medical College, its current full-time faculty would remain in New

York, as would the participants in its residency program. Although The Methodist Hospital remained committed to Baylor College of Medicine residents for the following four years, Mr. Girotto expressed an interest in establishing the hospital's own residency program in the near future.[21]

Other future plans for The Methodist Hospital were held in abeyance until the issues inherent with the dissolution of a 50-year partnership with Baylor College of Medicine were addressed. One of the major questions that remained unanswered two months after the breakup was whether members of the full-time faculty with established practices at the hospital would relocate to St. Luke's Episcopal Hospital.

After Baylor College of Medicine decided to relocate its full-time faculty to St. Luke's Episcopal Hospital, the prerequisite for any member of the full-time faculty's remaining at The Methodist Hospital was a resignation from Baylor College of Medicine, hospital executives created an alternate career path for those whose decisions remained in flux. With the Cleveland Clinic and Massachusetts General as its models, the hospital formed a nonprofit professional corporation to enable the physicians within it to maintain their autonomy while increasing their clinical practice within an academic environment. Named TMH Physician Organization and certified by the Texas Medical Board, the physician-governed organization was scheduled to become operational July 1, 2004, the day the extended 50-year affiliation agreement officially ended.[31]

Within nine days of its establishment, TMH Physician Organization welcomed its first member, Dr. Michael W. Lieberman, who resigned July 9 as chairman of the Department of Pathology at Baylor College of Medicine to become director of The Methodist Hospital Research Institute and continue as chief of pathology at The Methodist Hospital.[32]

In addition to the Baylor College of Medicine faculty who served as chiefs of service, others remained in a quandary as to which of the erstwhile partners they would pledge allegiance. Among them were those on the full-time cardiology faculty at the Methodist DeBakey Heart Center. Much like the tropical storm that preceded the separation, even though there were ample black clouds to serve as a forewarning, the cardiologists' decision was to come unexpectedly.

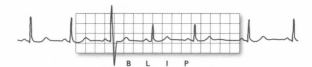

FLOOD OF '76

*T*he flood from Tropical Storm Allison in 2001 was reminiscent of the 10.47 inches of rain that fell within a few short hours on June 15, 1976. The sudden downpour flooded everything in the basement of The Methodist Hospital, including the hospital emergency generators to be used for just such an emergency if electrical power were to be lost, which, of course, it was. When we lost power, Dr. Noon was in the midst of performing a coronary artery bypass. He finished successfully while the heart-lung machine operators ran the machine by hand. The echo lab in the basement was flooded, soaking seven years of echo records. All records were successfully dried out with the helping hands of engineers at the NASA Space Center. The hospital was out of full power for only four days, and the flooding subsequently was blamed on a combination of land subsidence over the years plus an extraordinary, "once-in-a-hundred-years" deluge. That myth was shattered three years later when another tropical storm engulfed the Texas Medical Center. This time, they were better prepared as emergency generators had been moved to an upper level. On that occasion, in 1979, hospital CEO Larry Mathis recalled that his attempt to return to the hospital to take charge was slowed by local street flooding. He happened upon a canoe rental shop on the way, where he swapped his car for a canoe and paddled his way to work.

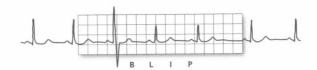

B   L   I   P

ALARMINGLY PROMPT

"*Too much to do and not enough time to do it in,*" *Dr. DeBakey once replied when asked about his legendary nonstop pace.[1] For decades he was known to accomplish the equivalent of a week's work in a day, every day. Requiring only a few hours of sleep each night, he usually was in bed by midnight, awaking at 4 or 5 AM in order to concentrate on paper work at home. Before sunrise he drove to The Methodist Hospital, spending the next eight or nine hours in the operating room. After his surgical procedures, he met with the 14 members of his surgical team to assess all of their completed procedures and discuss those scheduled for the next day. At the conclusion of the meeting, he and his team visited with the 100 to 150 hospitalized patients awaiting surgery. Upon returning to his office after these rounds, Dr. DeBakey attended to the administrative duties required of the president of Baylor College of Medicine as well as those of the chairman of the Department of Surgery. Arriving home after sunset for a late dinner, he returned to his paper work before retiring at midnight.*

An active participant in this established ritual for more than 34 years was Dr. Gerald M. Lawrie. A member of Dr. DeBakey's cardiovascular surgical team since 1974 and named the Michael E. DeBakey Professor of Surgery at The Methodist Hospital in 2008, he never ceased to be amazed at his mentor's efficient management of time. "He was always punctual, always waiting for us when we arrived at meetings," Dr. Lawrie explained. "The meetings ended punctually when his large 'Cricket' wristwatch, with a loud alarm, sounded the 'time's up' signal. He was very proud of this watch which he had seen being used by a number of U.S. Presidents including Truman, Eisenhower, Nixon, and especially his friend, President Johnson."[2]

---

1. Cromie WJ. Dr. DeBakey: he saves lives at a frantic pace. *St. Petersburg Times.* April 23, 1966.

2. Lawrie GM. Michael E. DeBakey, MD. *CTSNet.* October 21, 2008.

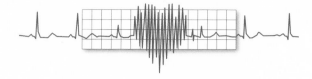

CHAPTER TWENTY

THE FORK IN THE ROAD
2004 - 2008

"If you come to a fork in the road, take it."
YOGI BERRA

The April 21, 2004, announcement of the new affiliation agreement between Baylor College of Medicine and St. Luke's Episcopal Hospital came as no surprise to the full-time faculty at The Methodist Hospital, where rumors of the impending demise of the college's 50-year partnership had been rampant for months.

Apprehensive that the repercussions from severing ties with The Methodist Hospital and affiliating with St. Luke's Episcopal Hospital would result in "a crisis of major proportions," most members of the volunteer and college faculty penned two strongly worded letters to the board of trustees at Baylor College of Medicine and the board of directors of The Methodist Hospital.[1] In essence, the missive's message was, "Don't do it; fix it."[2]

Nonetheless, the die was cast. Within four days of receipt of those letters, the Baylor College of Medicine's trustees approved the new affiliation agreement with St. Luke's Episcopal Hospital. When questioned by the media afterward about the documented opposition to severing the agreement with The Methodist Hospital, Dr. Traber replied, "When such a complex and consequential decision is considered by an institution of higher education, there will always be different views among faculty. The decision made by the Baylor board of trustees was a difficult one, but a decision made with thoughtful consideration and careful analysis of all the information before them."[1]

For many in its full-time faculty at The Methodist Hospital, the Baylor College of Medicine board's April 21, 2004, decision to affiliate with St.

Luke's Episcopal Hospital marked the ending date of an academic career. As predicted, leaving Baylor College of Medicine rather than the hospital was considered to be the only viable option to a number of those academic physicians who had developed their practices at The Methodist Hospital over the previous decades.

Preferring an alternative solution were the 11 cardiologists on the faculty who collectively had spent more than 190 years at The Methodist Hospital. Having recently developed the Methodist DeBakey Heart Center (MDHC), Dr. Quiñones, the center's director, recalled the collective determination of the cardiologists to stay there as its originating group: "We tried to see how we could stay and be part of both organizations."[3]

During the aftermath of the separation announcement, and possibly as an outcome of the mediation sponsored by the Texas Attorney General, The Methodist Hospital and Baylor College of Medicine agreed to continue some joint programs. Those programs were cell-therapy, urology, ophthalmology, ENT, and the Center for Cardiovascular Prevention.

Concentrated efforts to preserve what had taken years to establish in the Methodist DeBakey Heart Center were expended by Drs. Raizner, Quiñones and Zoghbi, who had been named interim chief of cardiology at Baylor College of Medicine after Dr. Roberts' stepping down to become chief executive officer of the University of Ottawa Heart Institute in early Spring 2004. Throughout the year following the separation announcement and amidst the ensuing custody battles between the two erstwhile partners,[4] the three cardiologists pursued all means possible to achieve their colleagues' collective goal of remaining at The Methodist Hospital as part of Baylor College of Medicine.

While waiting for the elusive approval of their preferred plan of action from both the college and the hospital, the full-time Baylor College of Medicine cardiology faculty at the Methodist DeBakey Heart Center continued to debate the merits of the alternative options available to them. When Drs. Quiñones and Zoghbi met with Dr. Traber to discuss possible joint programs for the Methodist DeBakey Heart Center and Baylor College of Medicine, Dr. Traber gave positive indications, but subsequently nothing came about and the existing options remained unacceptable. "Our choice," remembers Dr. Winters, "was to stay in private practice at Methodist or move with Baylor to St. Luke's. There was no way we were going to St. Luke's. They didn't want us. We didn't have any place over there. We wouldn't have had anything except Baylor's name."

With the separation from Baylor College of Medicine now clearly in hindsight, the hospital administration was faced with the challenge of establishing a structure for the cardiovascular surgery and medicine departments. Historically, both had been sections within the Departments of Surgery and Medicine, respectively. With strong encouragement from members of both departments, Mr. Girotto introduced an enticing organizational concept early in the spring of 2005 for the Methodist DeBakey Heart Center. It was the formation of an independent Department of Cardiovascular Surgery and Department of Cardiology, each with its own chairman, fiscal line, and administration.

Also announced in 2005 by Mr. Girotto was the reconfiguration of the hospital's construction plans for the "north campus" facilities to include sufficient space for the new departments and all the other activities of the Methodist DeBakey Heart Center (MDHC). "This concentration of resources from many disparate sources is designed to improve the delivery of care and outcomes for our cardiovascular patients, and to enhance our already well-established leadership role in cardiovascular medicine," Dr. Winters stated in an editorial published in the third issue of the *Journal of the Methodist DeBakey Heart Center.* "I congratulate those with the foresight, courage and 'attitude' to move this concept forward. To the Methodist DeBakey Heart Center, I offer my support and echo the expressive philosophy of the Home Depot advertisement which states, 'You can do it. We can help.'"[5]

For such an endorsement to appear in the *Journal of the Methodist DeBakey Heart Center* was symbolic. Having served as its editor since the publication debuted in August 2004, three months following the dissolution of the partnership between Baylor College of Medicine and The Methodist Hospital, Dr. Winters had tried to reflect his and his colleagues' desire to remain at the hospital as a faculty group. Confident this request would be granted by Baylor College of Medicine, the heart center physicians had launched the journal as a quarterly publication, but initially it had a sporadic publication schedule. Its second issue was not published until January 2005 and its third several months later in late Spring.

The publication had been in the planning stages since the formation of the Methodist DeBakey Heart Center in 2001. The medical director of the heart transplant program, Dr. Guillermo Torre-Amione, stopped Dr. Winters one day in the hall and said, "I think we ought to have a journal and you ought to consider being the editor." Shortly thereafter, Dr. Winters discussed the proposed publication with Dr. DeBakey, who was very supportive of the idea. "He gave us his blessing, but he didn't give me any ideas about articles or substance," says Dr. Winters. "He reminded me there once had been a

Cardiovascular Research Center Bulletin published years ago, but that it had died, so he emphasized the importance of having the new publication adequately funded to ensure longevity."

Inspired by Dr. DeBakey's words of encouragement, Dr. Winters next approached Mr. Girotto to request the hospital's funding of the quarterly journal and quickly received his enthusiastic support of the publication as a form of public relations. They both agreed that it should be circulated to the 35,000-plus medical professionals who were members of the American College of Cardiology, American Heart Association, Society of Thoracic Surgeons, and other prominent medical professionals throughout the country. Another decision was to forgo advertising, which the hospital supported. "As a form of PR, it's hard to beat because it represents the work of people here in the hospital as well as those elsewhere," explained Dr. Winters, adding that it also helped to maintain credibility by avoiding any potential conflicts of interest.

The first issue was dedicated to Dr. DeBakey, an honor he acknowledged in the inaugural issue: "The inauguration of the *Journal of the Methodist DeBakey Heart Center* deserves high praise, and Dr. William Winters deserves our commendation for initiating this effort," he wrote. "I am deeply appreciative of his kindness in dedicating this inaugural issue to me and in inviting me to submit a statement."[6]

While most of the articles in the premier issue were credited to faculty members of Baylor College of Medicine at The Methodist Hospital, there was no mention of the demise of those two entities' former affiliation. Also omitted was any reference to the current status of the college's faculty in the Methodist DeBakey Heart Center. Instead, and featured on page 10 of the 20-page publication, there were several paragraphs concerning the hospital's recent formation of a primary academic affiliation agreement with Weill Cornell Medical College and NewYork-Presbyterian Hospital.

In addition to describing that new 30-year affiliation agreement as one that "will draw on the strengths of all three internationally renowned institutions to enhance patient care, clinical and biomedical research, and medical education," the article spotlighted the 2004 *U.S. News & World Report* Best Hospitals Issue's ranking the Methodist DeBakey Heart Center as 17th among the top hospitals for heart and heart surgery.[6]

"Albeit subliminal, the message conveyed reflected the determination of my colleagues to preserve the status quo of the full-time faculty at the Methodist DeBakey Heart Center," says Dr. Winters. "While never stated per se, our steadfast loyalty to Baylor College of Medicine was clearly implied not only in the inaugural issue of the journal but also the subsequent one published four months later. Conversely, there was not the faintest hint given about the possibility that any of these physicians were leaving the hospital altogether."

When the third issue was published in late Spring 2005, Dr. Winters' enthusiastic support of the hospital's future plans reflected the turning point reached in the negotiations between the center's faculty with the college. Shortly before that issue was published, they had met with Dr. Jay Stein, senior vice president and dean of clinical affairs at Baylor College of Medicine. He told them their only option was to move to St. Luke's Episcopal Hospital. To stay at The Methodist Hospital required their resigning from Baylor College of Medicine. "We said we would think about it and give him our decision at a later date," recalls Dr. Winters.

Aware that their staying at The Methodist Hospital as private practitioners was welcomed by the hospital, the cardiologists were told by Mr. Girotto that their becoming full-time members of the new Department of Cardiology was dependent on their joining the hospital physician organization staff. "When we learned the hospital was launching a national search for that department's chairman, I approached Mr. Girotto to question the necessity for looking elsewhere since Drs. Quiñones and Zoghbi certainly qualified as the most likely candidates," Dr. Winters remembers.

While the 11 cardiologists continued to talk among themselves about whether they should leave Baylor College of Medicine, they eventually concurred that they could not see anything good happening if they remained, but nonetheless were apprehensive about the future. "There was a lot of concern about what the chances were of succeeding at The Methodist Hospital and my words to the group were that the opportunity to be on the ground floor of a new department, with the resources and the attitudes that were behind it, was extraordinary," Dr. Winters said. "In conversations with my colleagues, I pointed out that most people don't experience that in their lifetime. So the opportunity to be on the ground floor developing a new department with a really good solid corps to work with was extraordinary. I told them I wished I could be a fly on the wall about 30 years from now to see what's happening because I think it will be terrific"

As this drama was unfolding, a pivotal meeting took place in Mr. Girotto's office with Drs. Quiñones and Zoghbi, who presented a document outlining the Methodist DeBakey Heart Center's physicians' requirements for their joining the TMH Physician Organization. Requirement number one was that Dr. Quiñones be named chairman of the new Department of Cardiology.

Other stipulations had to do with academic support. The response from Mr. Girotto was immediate and decisive. He said, "If all of you join us as a new department, you will see more support over the next five years than you can imagine."

Motivated by Mr. Girotto's unbridled encouragement, Dr. Winters and his colleagues tentatively decided in July 2005 to become part of the new Department of Cardiology at The Methodist Hospital. After their resignation papers from Baylor College of Medicine were prepared, along with those documents required for joining the TMH Physicians Organization, each of the 11 cardiologists was given time to confer with his or her legal counsel. Since negotiations to establish alternative arrangements with Baylor College of Medicine were ongoing, the intentions of the cardiologists were not public knowledge.

Although the group's exodus was imminent, the cardiologists assumed Baylor College of Medicine was unaware of their plans. This was proven to be a false assumption in August 2005 when Dr. Quiñones was summoned to the dean's office. It was an unexpected event that that ultimately impacted not just the future of Dr. Quiñones but also that of the ten other cardiologists.

While the details of what took place in that closed-door meeting remained confidential, Dr. Quiñones confided he was "dumbfounded" when the end result was his being told he had been relieved of his duties.[7] When he returned to his office afterward he found representatives from the college already had been there to vacate his belongings. At which point he immediately went to Mr. Girotto's office to officially join the new Department of Cardiology at The Methodist Hospital.

Shortly thereafter, determined to remain together as a group and to expedite the transition as soon as possible, the remaining 10 full-time cardiologists tendered their formal notices of resignation to Baylor College of Medicine and advised Mr. Girotto of their intention to join the Department of Cardiology at The Methodist Hospital. The group included William L. Winters, Jr., John Buergler, Neal Kleiman, Karla Kurrelmeyer, John Mahmarian, Sherif Nagueh, Craig Pratt, Vinay Thohan, Guillermo Torre-Amione, and William Zoghbi. Their official start date at The Methodist Hospital was to be September 1, 2005.

Since this transition was to involve only behind-the-scene changes and not outwardly visible ones, the group was confident its implementation would be not only seamless but also indiscernible to the patients in their care. Convincing patients otherwise was an event that occurred at literally the last minute. Even though Baylor College of Medicine previously had agreed to extend all its previous resident and fellowship programs at The Methodist Hospital until June 30, 2007, an alteration to this agreement was enacted on August 31, 2005.[8]

With no advance notice, all Baylor College of Medicine cardiology residents and fellows were removed from The Methodist Hospital the day before the cardiologists officially joined the hospital faculty. The message implied by Baylor College of Medicine's abrupt actions was clear to Dr. Quiñones. When they "were pulled out and sent to St. Luke's Episcopal Hospital the night before our official start date, they were saying 'you're no longer with us, so then the fellows don't have to be with you anymore,'" he believed. "Overnight we went from having more than 20 fellows to having zero. We suddenly found ourselves very busy with a lot of the clinical activities without the prior assistance of the fellows."[9]

The experience of not having a resident or fellow between them and a patient was an eye-opening experience for those cardiologists whose entire clinical careers had been in an academic environment in which teaching and research were second nature. This sudden void of intermediaries created a valuable learning opportunity for my colleagues," Dr. Winters said. "A lot of our physicians had to practice in a way they never practiced before. To the credit of this 'team of ten,' a seamless transition of patient care did indeed follow. The realization that we suddenly were all alone began the transformation of the old Baylor College of Medicine cardiology section *at* The Methodist Hospital into the new Department of Cardiology *of* The Methodist Hospital."

After this propitious beginning, the growth and development of the new department became the responsibility of Dr. Quiñones, named by Mr. Girotto and the hospital's board as its first chairman in September 2005. His selection was embraced enthusiastically by his colleagues, who were certain he possessed the prerequisite courage, thick skin, and sated ego required to raise the fledgling department to prominence. Exemplifying these qualities when he assumed his new role, Dr. Quiñones publicly expressed how he envisioned the potential success of his efforts: "I want the department to be recognized for the individual members— not its chairman."[10]

His ability to tackle unexpected challenges quickly became evident within weeks of his first becoming chairman. To effectively address the sudden need for a new house staff and fellowships, he began to explore both the usual and unusual possibilities. "We were able to make excellent contact with the folks at University of Texas Medical Branch (UTMB) in Galveston and they were very excited about the idea of our participating in their fellowships," he said, attributing this accomplishment to extreme luck. "So together, we sent an application to the National Residency Review Committee to expand their fellowship from four-per-year to six-per-year, so that two of their fellows would always rotate through us. The first group started in July 2006 when the next cycle for the new fellows began."[3]

The medical residents' return came courtesy of the newly formed Department of Medicine at The Methodist Hospital. Under the leadership of Dr. Richard J. Robbins, who had been named chairman in October 2005, the department initiated a residency program in medicine that included a rotation through cardiology. "It was wonderful," Dr. Quiñones said, recalling the first reappearance of residents in his department in 2007. "It made us feel like we were in academic business again."[9]

It was the strictly enforced regulations in academics that governed Dr. Quiñones' pursuit to establish a fellowship program. The Accreditation Council for Graduate Medical Education (ACGME) only recognized cardiovascular disease fellowships that functioned as an integral part of an ACGME-accredited residency in internal medicine.[11] Since the new program at The Methodist Hospital had just entered the accreditation process in 2007, its provisional status prevented Dr. Quiñones' immediate submission of an application for the development of a fellowship program in cardiovascular disease.

Based on the likelihood that the residency program would not become fully accredited by the ACGME until 2009, Dr. Quiñones and his colleagues took advantage of the intervening years to design and fine-tune a comprehensive cardiovascular disease fellowship program. With a projected implementation date of 2011, the new program was designed to complete the general cardiovascular training requirements for individuals interested in pursuing a career in clinical, academic, or investigative cardiology.

The advance plans called for the phasing in of the new, three-year fellowship program to dovetail with the phasing out of the UTMB program. "When we started the UTMB program in 2006, we were very honest about our intentions to create our own program, one that would necessitate theirs being phased out," Dr. Quiñones said, recalling his motivation for that commitment. "If someone came from UTMB as a fellow and expected to complete his fellowship here, he would. We were adamant about that. We were not going to do to UTMB fellows what Baylor College of Medicine had done to theirs at The Methodist Hospital."[3]

When those Baylor College of Medicine fellows unexpectedly were pulled from The Methodist DeBakey Heart Center in 2005, each was in varying stages of a three-year program explicitly designed to focus on the expertise of the physicians therein. This interruption of their path to education was inexcusable, Drs. Quiñones and Lumsden believed. Consequently, rebuilding the structure and reputation of the cardiology and cardiovascular surgical training programs was to become their focus for the next several years. At the same time, they were simultaneously maintaining undivided attention to protecting the high reputation of the hospital for patient care. In the midst of facing these challenges in 2006 came an abrupt event of earth shaking proportion for everyone at The Methodist Hospital.

Admitted to The Methodist Hospital in early January 2006, the 97-year-old patient was unique in every respect. Self-diagnosed with an acute DeBakey type 1 dissecting aneurysm, he underwent the seven-hour surgery for a graft replacement of the ascending aorta in February. Among the 10,000 patients who had undergone this procedure before him, he became the oldest known to survive. Even more remarkable was the fact that he had been the pioneering surgeon who invented the procedure more than four decades earlier. The patient was Dr. Michael E. DeBakey.

The irony of the situation was apparent to the legendary surgeon as he spent the following eight months in the hospital for rehabilitation. Since specific details of his illness were not released to the public at his and his family's request, he became the first to speak about his ordeal. After arriving in a motorized wheelchair at the October 18, 2006, groundbreaking ceremonies for the DeBakey Library and Museum at Baylor College of Medicine, the 98-year-old made a brief speech to the astonished crowd who had welcomed his surprise appearance with a standing ovation. "I'm not sure I should be here today, I just got out of the hospital," he said before directly addressing his dissecting aortic aneurysm. "I used to be fascinated by this disease – I've written 130 articles on it – but I can tell you after personally experiencing it, I don't appreciate it anymore."[12]

Also made evident at that event was Dr. DeBakey's determination to rid himself of the "mechanical assistance" provided by his wheelchair, an accomplishment he believed would enable the resumption of his previous schedule. His achieving that goal was encouraged at the Methodist DeBakey Heart Center. In fact, when *The New York Times* asked Dr. Winters for his opinion, he responded, "I am impressed with what the body and mind can do when they work together. He absolutely has the desire to get back to where he was before. I think he'll come close."[13]

While celebrating the resiliency of Dr. DeBakey, the cardiologists in the Methodist DeBakey Heart Center mourned the loss of another nationally recognized pioneer in the care of cardiovascular diseases, Dr. Don W. Chapman, who died at the age of 90 on May 3, 2007. In the eyes of many, the legendary cardiologist and founder of The Chapman Group was the "compleat physician" long before he was recognized as such by the Harris County Medical Society's highest award in 1996—the John P. McGovern Compleat Physician Award.[14] "Early in our association, Dr. Chapman told me, 'We work hard and we play hard. It's what you do that matters, not what you know,'" remembers Dr. Winters. "Dr. Chapman will be remembered for both."

Among his countless accomplishments, Dr. Chapman is best remembered for his extraordinary teaching skills by literally hundreds of physicians who came under his influence as medical students during the formative years of Baylor College of Medicine. His role as a husband and father, mentor, role model, clinician, friend, and colleague through his 60 years of influence in this community and this country firmly established his credentials as the Compleat Physician.

As one of the first cardiologists at The Methodist Hospital, Dr. Chapman had demonstrated skills complimentary to those of Dr. DeBakey and his team of surgeons. Having deemed the consultation of a cardiologist crucial to the quality care of his cardiovascular patients in the late 1950s, Dr. DeBakey recalled, "We had several others on staff then, but Don Chapman did the most work with us, particularly in the 1960s when cardiac catheterization was fairly primitive. Well, Don got early into angiograms and some of the others had picked it up, so by the '70's we were pretty well fixed."[15]

These recollections came to Dr. DeBakey as he was in the midst of re-establishing his work schedule after his illness. Instead of resuming his normal pace within the hospital, he had begun to spend more time at his desk there. Since his offices were located in close proximity to the Methodist DeBakey Heart Center, Dr. DeBakey had the opportunity to observe firsthand the ongoing development of the center named in his honor as well as its growing number of accomplishments.

Of particular interest to Dr. DeBakey were the advances made by the former members of his surgical team in the Methodist DeBakey Heart Center. Even though he was a world-famous surgeon and considered by many to be the father of modern cardiovascular surgery, he regarded his individual contributions, such as the pioneering procedures of aneurysmectomy, endarterectomy, and coronary bypass, to be relatively insignificant "in the total scope of things" and was known to take greater pride in the accolades garnered by those he had trained.[16]

Believing his surgical contributions simply opened the way for others to refine and perfect them, Dr. DeBakey preferred that his legacy result from any newfound knowledge he shared with those surgeons under his tutelage in Houston and all over the world. "It is what you are able to transmit, it seems to me, that matters," he once said when explaining this philosophy to a colleague. "Plato is remembered for his ideas and the fact that he was able to transmit them to Aristotle. He is remembered because Aristotle was his student and was able to continue with rational ideas that Plato described and taught. If you transmit to another generation interesting new concepts, whether they are conceptually new ideas, innovations, research, or ethical concepts, then I think you have improved society, especially if the next generation can enhance them."[16]

He had become living proof of the merits inherent in the transmission of medical knowledge. The surgeon who performed his aortic dissection procedure, the exact one he had pioneered in the 1950s, was his former trainee, resident, and longtime partner, Dr. George P. Noon. The surgical director of the heart transplant program at The Methodist Hospital and professor of surgery at Baylor College of Medicine, Dr. Noon had worked with Dr. DeBakey for more than 40 years.

The decision to operate on Dr. DeBakey was made after his condition had deteriorated and he was unable to communicate. It was Dr. Noon who expressed his confidence that, despite the dangers, nothing made Dr. DeBakey a hopeless candidate for the operation except for his being 97. Convinced that "if we didn't operate on him that day that was it, he was gone for sure," Dr. Noon and his team of surgeons proceeded. "We were doing what we thought was right."[13]

The successful results of the operation were attributable to the patient who invented it, said Dr. Noon, who never doubted Dr. DeBakey's ability to survive the seven-hour procedure and recover. "From the development of procedures to diagnosing and to training the personnel, he's been able to affect medical care around the world," he explained. "He's a perfectionist and expects everyone around him to do the same. When Dr. DeBakey spoke, everybody listened. I listened, too."[17]

Like Dr. Noon, many of those who had listened to Dr. DeBakey also had emulated his pursuit of excellence. "He provided a model for my whole career, really," said Dr. Lawrie, the cardiothoracic surgeon Dr. DeBakey recruited from Australia. "This is a man who single mindedly devoted all of his adult life to helping sick people and raising the standard of teaching and research. I can only hope to do what he managed."[18]

After working with Dr. DeBakey on a daily basis for more than 20 years, Dr.

Lawrie had accumulated extensive experience in the surgical management of end-stage and complex cardiovascular disease. Subsequently and throughout his three decades as a cardiothoracic surgeon at The Methodist Hospital, he had developed special expertise in cardiac valve repair, minimally invasive cardiac surgery, blood conserving surgery, and redo operations. As Dr. DeBakey was recuperating in August 2007, his influence on Dr. Lawrie was to become exemplified. Incorporating a technique he had created 15 years earlier named the "American Correction," Dr. Lawrie pioneered the use of the da Vinci robot to successfully repair a mitral valve. "The precise movements and tiny instruments of the robot allow the surgery to be minimally invasive, allowing for a faster, less painful recovery," Dr. Lawrie said, pointing out how the four small incisions along the right side of the chest allowed the robot to slip its instruments into the chest cavity. "We have performed the American Correction for over 15 years in 1,000 patients with a great deal of success, and now we adapted the robot to our technique. It took seven months of intense training and a major team effort to be able to perform this advanced, well documented surgery with the robot."[19]

Since one of the robot's instruments was a tiny camera, the entire surgery was performed inside the closed chest, negating the need for the open-heart surgery required in traditional mitral valve repair. Therefore, the patient had less scarring, fewer wound complications, and was able to return to normal activity within a week of surgery. Certain the technique was the wave of the future, Dr. Lawrie successfully performed more than 35 robotically assisted mitral valve repairs in the following months.[20] He also predicted, "This technique is going to take over the majority of the patients as more surgeons get trained in it."[21]

Recognized for his accomplishments in 2008, Dr. Lawrie was named to the Michael E. DeBakey Endowed Chair in Cardiac Surgery at The Methodist Hospital. No doubt Dr. DeBakey was aware of his protégé's achievements. His mental recovery was far ahead of his physical response in the months after his release from the hospital. According to his colleagues, as his recovery progressed, he slowly began to resemble his former self—with the same impatience, sense of humor, detailed memory, and insistence on precision.[22] No longer performing surgery or maintaining his grueling travel schedule, he still consulted with patients and physicians, devoting any free time to concentrate on regaining his health.

Month after month he lifted free weights, pitted his muscles against resistant machines, climbed onto the treadmill, and rode a stationary bike five days a week. "I've made tremendous progress since I was so weak I couldn't get out of bed," he explained to a journalist in early 2008, exactly two years after his surgery. "I know I'm not going to be normal at 99, but I'd like to get back to a reasonably normal life. There are things I'd still like to do."[21]

His pursuit to achieve normalcy was shared with a small group of physicians at The Methodist Hospital who were monitoring his recovery for more than two years. To each of them the weekly Tuesday afternoon sessions with Dr. DeBakey were particularly memorable. Each session began with a review of his clinical status and a physical examination, and what followed on a weekly basis was extraordinary. There was a round table discussion of everything from medical subjects, embroidered by his real life experiences, to economic, political, and current events. The clarity of his mind and memory was truly remarkable.

As he had demonstrated throughout his career, Dr. DeBakey maintained his pursuit of perfection. At the age of 99, he and Dr. Noon continued their efforts to perfect the MicroMed DeBakey continuous flow ventricular assist device (VAD), designed with NASA and first introduced in 1998. As pioneers in this new frontier in mechanical circulatory support, the two surgeons had devoted more than a decade to its ongoing development. Unlike other devices available in 2008, the DeBakey VAD was much smaller, almost one-tenth the size of most of them, and had only one moving part. It required only about 8 watts of power and its application surgically was technically easier and required less intervention.[23]

Initially used as a bridge to transplant in 2001, the DeBakey VAD underwent a pivotal trial for the destination therapy indication in 2003. In 2004 Drs. DeBakey and Noon modified the device for pediatric applications. By 2005, more than 445 patients, children, and adults had been implanted with the DeBakey VAD.[24]

The proven success of the DeBakey VAD inspired an unexpected resurrection of the possibility of achieving one of its inventor's dashed dreams. "I went to Dr. DeBakey to discuss using two continuous flow VADS to create a total artificial heart," recalled Dr. O. H. "Bud" Frazier, a former trainee who was chief of cardiopulmonary transplantation, chief of the Center for Cardiac Support, and director of surgical research at the Texas Heart Institute. "Dr. DeBakey said he was surprised he hadn't thought of the idea himself.[25] At the age of 99 years, as sharp and dedicated as ever, he was excited about the potential of this new device."[26]

After gaining Dr. DeBakey's enthusiastic support, Dr. Frazier submitted a proposed grant to the NIH Bioengineering Research Partnership, a special program to encourage collaboration among medical, academic, and engineering experts. The Total Artificial Heart project was to be a joint effort by the Texas Heart Institute, the University of Houston, Rice University, and MicroMed Cardiovascular.[24]

While awaiting the grant's approval, Dr. DeBakey continued his rehabilitation in preparation for an April trip to Washington, D.C., to receive the Congressional Gold Medal, considered the nation's highest and most distinguished civilian award. When his colleagues presented him with a framed copy of the legislation passed to honor him in 2007, the clearly overwhelmed recipient said, "After learning that I was going to receive this fine honor, the Congressional Gold Medal, my pride as a citizen of the United States of America is overflowing. It is a wonderful honor and I'm deeply grateful."[27]

Although he had become known for driving his motorized scooter in the same fashion as one of his beloved sports cars, Dr. DeBakey had hoped to be free of the device before his trip. Because of the muscle loss during the months in bed after surgery, he was unable to regain the strength needed to walk into the Capitol rotunda for the ceremony. Instead, because space limitations of the Capitol elevator precluded his use of the motorized scooter, he was in his wheelchair, accompanied by family, close friends, and colleagues to receive the Congressional Gold Medal from President George W. Bush on April 23, 2008.

Upon presenting the Olympic-style gold medal inscribed with DeBakey's words, "The pursuit of excellence has been my objective in life," President Bush praised the legendary surgeon for his lifetime achievements, his surgical history of 60,000 patients, and his training thousands of doctors who went on to broaden the reach of his surgical techniques. "His legacy is holding the fragile and sacred gift of human life in his hands and returning it unbroken," President Bush said.[28]

As the sixth Texan to be honored with the Congressional Gold Medal, Dr. DeBakey joined Norman Borlaug, the Texas A&M agriculturalist and father of the Green Revolution, and the late golfer Byron Nelson, industrialist Howard Hughes, former House speaker Sam Rayburn, and former first lady, Lady Bird Johnson. In all, the congressional medal has been awarded 136 times and other recipients include George Washington, Winston Churchill, and Thomas Edison.[28]

Upon receiving the medal, Dr. DeBakey expressed his "deep-seated and humblest sense of gratitude for this high honor you have afforded me" to the president, the members of Congress, and the members of the administration and the trustees and faculty members of Baylor College of Medicine who were gathered in his honor. Speaking extemporaneously, he spoke of his childhood, his family, and the important life lessons he had learned from his parents.

Exemplifying his stature as a medical statesman, Dr. DeBakey seized the opportunity to present an idea to the gathered legislators. "Now I want to make a suggestion to the Congress about health care," he told them. "I know that you have been working on this for many, many years. In fact I was one of President Kennedy's strongest supporters when he came out with Medicare when the medical profession was strongly against. I thought it was a great idea. I still think it's a great idea. Unfortunately, its practical effect has not been that great. So I know you have sought a better health care plan for the needy. And unfortunately it has been elusive. But there is a model you should look at that I'm thoroughly familiar with because when I was in the military, I was assigned by the surgeon general to the committee that (Gen. Omar) Bradley and (Rear Admiral Jean Hodgkin) Hawley worked on in fixing up the Veterans Administration. We made many suggestions that resulted in a superb medical service. I've been familiar with the medical services of the Veterans Administration since then. In fact, I developed their research program. I assure you that you can't find a better model. For one thing, its quality of care is superior. And for another, it provides that care at half the cost of other agencies both in and out of government. So you see how efficient it is. So there must be something about what they are doing that we could use to expand our program in health care for the needy."[29]

In his concluding remarks, he extended his warm commendation for the understanding and support Congress had given medical research since the 1950s and throughout the subsequent decades. "You have no idea what you've done with medical research in improving the medical care of this country. It is the envy of the world. I hope you will continue to give it the consideration you've given it so far. Again, let me come back to my sense of gratitude and because of my sense of high treasure I have for my citizenship. Since receiving this award, my cup runneth over. Thank you very much."[29]

Among those who had traveled to the Capitol for the ceremony was Dr. Cooley, who had presented Dr. DeBakey with a lifetime achievement award during a meeting of Denton A. Cooley Cardiovascular Surgical Society on October 27, 2007.[30] When Dr. Cooley presented the award and said, "I hope this is not just a temporary truce or cease-fire (but) ... a permanent treaty between us," the media viewed the gesture as a long-awaited mending of the rift between the former colleagues. It was an observation with which Dr. DeBakey strongly disagreed. Allegedly instigated by Dr. Cooley's performing the world's first artificial heart implant without permission, using a mechanical device developed in DeBakey's lab in 1969, the supposed "feud" was "the concoction of a journalist," Dr. DeBakey said, pointing out that he had the highest respect for Cooley and what he has done.[30]

To emphasize his respect for Dr. Cooley, one week after returning from the Congressional Gold Medal ceremony, Dr. DeBakey inducted his former colleague into the Michael E. DeBakey International Surgical Society on May 2, 2008.[31] Lauding his contribution to modern medicine, Dr. DeBakey said, "Denton, it's a great pleasure for me to acknowledge the pioneering contributions you have made and have you a part of the society. I don't think I could have done it without you. In fact, I know I couldn't."[31]

Reminiscing about the 1950s, when the two pioneered treatment of aortic aneurysms together, Dr. DeBakey said Dr. Cooley had the "instincts of a great surgeon" and said they "complemented each other and worked together very effectively." In response to Dr. DeBakey's tribute, Dr. Cooley said he thought the two surgeons' "rivalry will go down in history as one of the greatest rivalries in modern medicine. I'm relieved we are again together and can be colleagues and friends again."[31]

The opportunity for the two surgeons to collaborate again was presented in June 2008 with the awarding of the NIH Bioengineering Research Partnership grant for the Total Artificial Heart project. Together with Dr. Frazier at The Texas Heart Institute, Dr. DeBakey finalized the arrangements to implant their newest experimental version of this pulseless total artificial heart. "We had planned to scrub together in September to implant the device," Dr. Frazier said, recalling Dr. DeBakey's avid desire to participate in the procedure.[26]

Once again, Dr. DeBakey was unable to fulfill his lifelong mission to implant a total artificial heart. On July 11, 2008, Drs. DeBakey and Gotto spent the afternoon reviewing the draft of their newest edition of *The Living Heart in the 21st Century*. Later in the day Dr. Noon came by for a visit. "We had a snack together; I had gumbo with peppers from his garden and he had ice cream," Dr. Noon said. "When I was leaving, I told him I was going to my grandson's baseball game and would be vacationing for a week in Aspen. He said, 'Best of luck to your grandson, and I will see you when you return from Aspen.'"[32]

Within two hours of Dr. Noon's departure, Dr. DeBakey unexpectedly collapsed and could not be resuscitated. The 99-year-old surgeon was rushed to The Methodist Hospital, where he was pronounced dead at 9:38 PM of natural causes. He died 58 days before his 100th birthday on September 7, 2008.[33]

As the news of Dr. DeBakey's death became known, tributes to his legendary career, surgical contributions, and medical statesmanship proliferated around the world. He became the first private citizen to lay in repose in the City Hall of Houston, an honor deserved by "a short list of people," said former Mayor Bob Lanier.[34] After a public memorial service at Houston's Co-Cathedral of the Sacred Heart, Dr. DeBakey was buried with military honors at Arlington Cemetery.

As lasting monuments to Dr. DeBakey, the entities that bear his name attest to the breadth and depth of his interests and his contributions: the Lasker-DeBakey Clinical Medical Research Award, the Michael E. DeBakey Center for Biomedical Education and Research, the Michael E. DeBakey Excellence in Research Award, the Methodist DeBakey Heart Center, the Michael E. DeBakey High School for Health Professions, the Michael E. DeBakey International Military Surgeon's Award, the Michael E. DeBakey Heart Institutes of Kenosha, Wisconsin, and Hays, Kansas, the Michael E. DeBakey Veterans Affairs Medical Center in Houston, the Michael E. DeBakey International Surgical Society, the Michael E. DeBakey Aviation Complex, and DeBakey Drive in Lake Charles, Louisiana (the latter a tribute to him and his parents), to name a few.[35]

In the days, months, and years following his death, countless tributes to Dr. DeBakey from his friends and colleagues appeared in national and international publications, many of which were reprinted in the *Methodist DeBakey Cardiovascular Journal*. Also appearing in that journal was one penned by Dr. Kenneth L. Mattox, who prefaced his remarks with this quote from John Quincy Adams: "If your actions inspire others to dream more, learn more, do more and become more, you are a leader." Crediting Dr. DeBakey's unique management talents for significantly contributing to his ability to so greatly impact medical education, research, patient care, policy, and community leadership, Dr. Mattox believed "his management style was a reflection of his character, unique abilities, and innovative visions" and would never be duplicated. "If, however, each of us who knew and appreciated his management techniques can adopt just a few of them, then our students, residents, medicine, and indeed the world will be all the better for it."[36]

Standing out among all the countless other tributes to Dr. DeBakey was one authored by his sisters, Selma DeBakey and Lois DeBakey. Their multipage remembrance, published in the *Methodist DeBakey Cardiovascular Journal* in 2009, concluded: "There will never be another Michael Ellis DeBakey. But this man of consummate genius and of sterling character lives on, not simply in the physical monuments to his boundless philanthropy and his ingenious life-giving contributions to humanity, but in the halls of history of the noble men who have graced this earth and have left it infinitely better than when they came, and in the hearts of all who admired and loved him. In the inimitable words of Edmund Spencer, 'The genius survives; all else is claimed by death.'"[37]

The influence of the genius of Dr. DeBakey was evident at the Methodist DeBakey Heart Center at The Methodist Hospital. Having inspired its inception and subsequent growth, the legendary surgeon was destined to remain its inspiration in perpetuity.

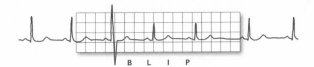

B L I P

FACT OR FABRICATION?

When Dr. Cooley resigned from Baylor College of Medicine in June 1969, journalists reported that the impetus was "Dr. Cooley's feud with Dr. DeBakey" over the implantation of the artificial heart the previous April.[1] Although both surgeons publicly denied the existence of such a rift, their denials fell on deaf ears. This was evidenced a year later when Life magazine published Thomas Thompson's article "The Texas Tornado vs. Dr. Wonderful" in its April 10, 1970, issue. On that magazine's cover, emblazoned over a close-up photo of both surgeons' faces, was this headline: "A Bitter Feud: Two great surgeons at war over the human heart."[2] Further exacerbating this erroneous public perception of the surgeons' professional relationship was Mr. Thompson's book, Hearts; of surgeons and transplants, miracles and disasters along the cardiac frontier.[3] Published in 1971, the book reportedly exposed "the famous feud between Dr. Michael DeBakey and Dr. Denton Cooley in Houston."[4]

Over the subsequent four decades, questions persisted about the status of Dr. DeBakey's relationship with Dr. Cooley. To correct this long-standing misconception about them, a medical writer from The New York Times suggested a joint meeting of the two surgeons in 2006. Although Dr. Cooley was in favor of the idea, Dr. DeBakey declined the opportunity. Believing the "very idea of a feud is a journalistic fabrication," he said that a staged meeting would only "perpetuate the fabrication."[5]

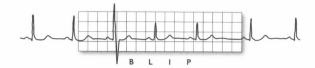

B   L   I   P

After such a meeting indeed took place the following year when Dr. Cooley pre-sented Dr. DeBakey a lifetime achievement award from the Denton A. Cooley Cardiovascular Surgical Society, the writer from The New York Times *interviewed Dr. DeBakey again, curious as to what had changed his mind. "It just seemed to be a very kind thing that they did, and I should also be kind and accept it graciously," Dr. DeBakey explained, pointing out "there was no reason to consider him an enemy. We have never had any bad words," but also "we haven't had very much in the way of communication."[5]*

1. Dr. Cooley resigns from post. *UPI*. September 11, 1969.

2. Thompson T. The Texas Tornado vs. Dr. Wonderful. *Life*. April 10, 1970.

3. Thompson T. *Hearts; of surgeons and transplants, miracles, and disasters along the cardiac frontier*. New York, NY: McCall Publishing Company; 1971.

4. Lebherz R. In touch with the human heart. *The News*, Frederick, Maryland. October 27, 1971.

5. Altman LK. The doctor's world: the feud. *The New York Times*. November 27, 2007.

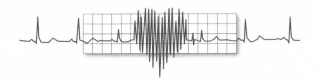

EPILOGUE

William L. Winters Jr., MD, MACC

In the minds of many, the tumultuous rupture in 2005 of a 50-year relationship between The Methodist Hospital and Baylor College of Medicine, admittedly not always harmonious, but vastly beneficial according to
nearly every consultant who had ever been engaged to analyze its positives
and negatives, led to a major overhaul in the cardiovascular service structure of the hospital.

True to Mr. Girotto's prophesy to Dr. Quiñones, hospital support for the
newly created departments of cardiology and cardiovascular surgery grew
exponentially.

Since 2005, the Department of Cardiology has grown to 22 cardiologists, and its academic and clinical programs are highly respected nationally.
Early priorities for both departments were the restoration of the education
and training programs of residents and fellows. The newly established Weill
Cornell Medical College agreement was crucial in the early recruitment of
Drs. Richard Robbins (Sloan Kettering Hospital) and Barbara Bass (University of Maryland) as department chairmen of medicine and surgery, respectively. Upon their shoulders, the subspecialty training programs would
be established once the medicine and surgery programs received ACGME
accreditation.

Dr. Judy Paukert, a Ph.D. educator with an exemplary record in graduate
medical education circles, was persuaded by Dr. Marc Boom, then COO of
The Methodist Hospital, to leave the University of Texas Medical School
in San Antonio to accept the daunting task of resurrecting the training

programs at The Methodist Hospital. To her great credit, she was imminently successful. With the help of talented program directors, 32 ACGME programs with 200 residents are in place at The Methodist Hospital at the time of this writing.

Established by Mr. Girotto was The Methodist Hospital Education Institute, an entity to guide the organization of a multitude of new non-ACGME education programs for physicians and other allied health organizations. Dr. Winters was named chairman of the education institute and chief education officer of The Methodist Hospital.

Long the overseer of the cardiology fellowship training program, conceived in 1982 and directed by Dr. Roberts during his affiliation with Baylor College of Medicine, Dr. Craig Pratt was instrumental in procuring a three-year cardiovascular fellowship accredited for a full five years (granted without even a review) commencing July 1, 2011. The first four fellows in the match process began on July 1, 2013, and the additional programs will include a two-year cardiovascular surgery program (after five years of general surgery); a five-year cardiothoracic surgery program integrated with MD Anderson Cancer Center, where The Methodist Hospital provides cardiac surgery training; a two-year fellowship in vascular surgery; a five-year vascular surgery integrated residency; and one- and two-year programs (non-ACGME) in cardiovascular imaging. ACGME accreditation for training in interventional cardiology, heart failure, transplant cardiology, and an independent electrophysiology program are expected in the near future.

Realizing it would take several years for these programs to get up and running, Dr. Quiñones approached the chairman of the Department of Medicine and chairman of the Section of Cardiology at the University of Texas Medical Branch at Galveston (UTMB) with an offer to provide additional venues for training of their cardiology fellows. His offer was accepted, and two fellows from UTMB began rotation at The Methodist Hospital in July 2006, with two more openings each year. The agreement stipulated that this arrangement would fade as The Methodist Hospital received accreditation for its own programs. The last two UTMB cardiology fellows finished in June 2013.

As arrangements were put in place for the training programs, a new organizational structure was established for cardiology and cardiovascular surgery. Dr. Quiñones became chairman of cardiology, Dr. Albert Raizner was elected as deputy chairman of the Department of Cardiology, and section chairmen were established in the following cardiology subspecialties: interventional cardiology (Dr. Neal Kleiman); heart failure (Dr. Guillermo

Torre); cardiac imaging (Dr. William Zoghbi); cardiac electrophysiology (Dr. Miguel Valderrábano); and atherosclerosis/vascular (Dr. Christie Ballantyne). A multimodality imaging center, under the overall direction of Dr. Zoghbi, was established embracing echocardiography, nuclear cardiology, cardiac and coronary CT, and cardiac MRI. Dr. Dipan Shah accepted an invitation to come to The Methodist Hospital to direct the newly created cardiac MRI section. Trained in all these modalities, Drs. Faisal Nabi, and Su Min Chang joined Dr. John Mahmarian (nuclear cardiology and CT scans) and the existing echocardiography staff. At the time of this writing, there are 24 members of the academic department: 10 original members transferring from Baylor College of Medicine (Drs. Winters, Quiñones, Pratt, Zoghbi, Kleiman, Mahmarian, Nagueh, Kurrelmeyer, Buergler, and Torre) and 14 new colleagues (Drs. Su Min Chang, Faisal Nabi, Miguel Valderrábano, Jerry Estep, Dipan Shah, George Schroth, Amish Dave, Stephen Little, Arvind Bhimaraj, Colin Barker, C. Huie Lin, Barry Trachtenberg, Sanjay Kunapuli, and Anton Nielsen). The latter two began working at a satellite clinic at the Methodist Willowbrook Hospital in North Houston. In addition, the Pearland clinic was established in 2009.

National honors began coming to members of the cardiology department. Dr. Zoghbi was elected president of American Society of Echocardiography (ASE) in 2010, after which he became president of the American College of Cardiology (ACC) in March 2012. He was also selected to participate in the 8,000-mile Olympic Torch Relay as one of the torchbearers to carry the flame across the United Kingdom in the 70-day lead-up to the opening ceremonies of the Olympic Games on July 27, 2012. The opportunity came courtesy of Coca-Cola, a philanthropic supporter of the ACC programs and also a sponsor of the Olympics games. Permitted to name several people to carry the torch along the route through England to the Olympic stadium, Coca-Cola chose Dr. Zoghbi as the ACC representative.

Elected president of the American Nuclear Cardiology Society starting in January 2011 was Dr. Mahmarian, following in the steps of the late Dr. Mario Verani who was president in 1996. Dr. Miguel Quiñones was elected vice president of the InterAmerica Society of Cardiology in 2011. He received a lifetime achievement award from the ASE in June 2012 and the Masters Award from the ACC in March 2012. Presenting this award to him was his associate and newly elected president of the ACC, Dr. Zoghbi. Dr. Sherif Nagueh became chairman of the Annual Scientific Program of ASE in 2011. Dr. Christie Ballantyne received the ACC Distinguished Scientist Award in 2013. Dr. Winters received the Texas Laureate Award from the

American College of Physicians in October 2011.

To accommodate the ever-enlarging patient population and the growing number of cardiologists in the academic cardiology department, the outpatient clinic facilities in Smith Tower's 19th floor, now under the direction of Dr. Karla Kurrelmeyer, were enlarged. Former directors of the clinic included Drs. William H. Spencer and William A. Zoghbi. Additional academic offices were established, and badly needed renovation of the entire floor was undertaken. The clinic name was changed from Baylor Heart Clinic to Methodist DeBakey Cardiology Associates in 2005.

As the training programs proliferated, so did adjunct supporting activities. The cardiology conference schedule grew to 12 weekly, including the long-standing Thursday 8:00 AM Cardiology Grand Rounds, which now included the cardiovascular surgical department on a regular basis. Established by Dr. Stephen Little in 2009 was a weekly heart valve clinic. Journal clubs involving cardiac imaging, valvular heart disease, and interventional cardiology became a regular event.

With the addition to the academic faculty of Dr. C. Huie Lin, trained in interventional adult congenital heart disease, plans are underway to establish a training program in the rapidly growing field of adult congenital heart disease.

Established in 2005 at The Methodist Hospital was the anesthesiology department under the chairmanship of Dr. Joseph J. Naples. A member of the Baylor College of Medicine anesthesiology department from 1980 to September 1990, Dr. Naples had left to become professor of anesthesiology at University of Texas Health Science Center in San Antonio. While serving there as chairman of the anesthesiology department in 2005, he was persuaded to return to The Methodist Hospital to become chairman of its newly established anesthesiology department. In addition, Dr. Alfred Groen was elected deputy chairman; Dr. Zbigniew Wojciechowski was appointed vice chairman for research and education; and Dr. Faisal Masud was appointed vice chairman for quality and patient safety.

The anesthesiology department now constitutes the third leg of the Methodist DeBakey Heart & Vascular Center and oversees the cardiovascular surgical postoperative ICU in the Fondren Building. There are 13 cardiovascular anesthesiologists and 8 cardiovascular intensivists, 3 of them with anesthesia specialty status. The department participates in several external residency programs.

Equally impressive changes also took place on the surgical side of the Methodist DeBakey Heart & Vascular Center, newly renamed in 2008 to encompass a growing activity in peripheral vascular disease under the leadership of Drs. Alan Lumsden as chairman, Mark Davies as vice chairman, and Mahesh Ramchandani, current elected deputy chairman. The first steps were taken to extend the Methodist DeBakey Heart & Vascular Center programs to the entire Methodist Hospital System.

Named president of the Society for Clinical Vascular Surgery in 2008, Dr. Lumsden also undertook the responsibility of expanding the cardiovascular surgery department at The Methodist Hospital, which eventually grew to 28 in number, including the nine in the TMH Physician Organization. While Drs. George Noon, Jimmy Howell, Hartwell Whisennand, and Charles McCollum were included in the cardiovascular surgery department at The Methodist Hospital, they retained their appointment at Baylor College of Medicine. Serving as interim chairman of cardiac surgery while a search committee seeks a permanent chairman is Dr. Jimmy F. Howell.

Collaboration between cardiology and cardiovascular surgery, long espoused by Dr. DeBakey, developed rapidly as new clinical and research projects emerged. A weekly heart valve clinic and bimonthly conference attended by members of both departments emerged. Drs. Michael Reardon and Neal Kleiman became principal investigators of the national Transcatheter Aortic Valve Replacement (TAVR) Trial using the Medtronic Corevalve. In 2013, Dr. Reardon was named the national principal investigator for the SurTAVI Trial for Transcatheter Aortic Valve Implantation in patients with severe and symptomatic aortic valve stenosis who are at intermediate risk for open-heart surgery.

The heart failure team of Drs. Matthias Loebe (surgical director of Thoracic Transplant Services), Guillermo Torre, and Jerry Estep, (both medical directors) offered multidisciplinary options for end-stage heart and lung disease, including patients with amyloid heart disease. Multidisciplinary conferences on ischemic heart disease became weekly events. Videoconferences were established with cardiovascular specialists in Berlin to compare complex cases involving left ventricular assist devices. A monthly videoconference to discuss vascular cases across Texas came into being. A videoconference discussing complex valve cases with Fortis hospitals in India was established and led by Dr. Mahesh Ramchandani.

The postoperative cardiovascular surgery ICU became fully integrated with teams that included an intensivist, cardiac anesthesiologist, cardiac surgeon, pulmonary therapist, nurse practitioner, nurse dietician, and chaplain, all board certified or trained in critical care medicine, and all under the watchful eye of Dr. Faisal Masud, the medical director of critical care.

This was a far different level of care compared to the early days when a surgical resident was primarily responsible for the ICU patients 24 hours a day for two consecutive months. Two hybrid operating suites were developed to provide facilities for complex vascular and cardiac procedures requiring catheterization facilities in operating rooms, such as endovascular repairs and transcatheter correction of valvular heart disease.

The heart failure patient remains among the sickest in the field of cardiovascular medicine. The family of an early heart transplant recipient, Mr. J.C. Walter Jr., made a substantial gift to The Methodist Hospital for which the transplant center is now named. Over the past several years, there has been substantial growth in this area: heart transplants have grown by 25%, averaging 25-30 annually; employment of left-ventricular assist devices has grown by 42% to 40-50 annually; and lung transplants have grown by 46% to around 150 annually. Dr. Matthias Loebe is the surgical director of thoracic transplantation with the able advice from Dr. DeBakey's longtime associate, Dr. George P. Noon, now retired from active surgery.

In 2010, Dr. Alan Lumsden and his vascular surgery colleagues launched the Methodist Aortic Network throughout the five Methodist Hospital System hospitals to provide multidisciplinary teams to address the variety of aortic diseases that may occur across Houston.

Minimally invasive cardiovascular surgery has been advanced under Dr. Mahesh Ramchandani. In October 2012, Dr. Lumsden introduced the Magellan™ Robotic System to treat patients with peripheral arterial disease by providing "less invasive endovascular options to a broader group of patients."

When Dr. Barbara Bass became director of The Methodist Hospital surgical department in 2005, one of her visions was to establish a simulation program to train and re-train surgeons and procedural physicians using simulated clinical environments. Her perseverance delivered the "Methodist Institute for Technology and Innovation and Education" (MITIE), occupying 40,000 square feet in the new Research Institute building. It contains multifunctional operating rooms, state-of-the-art simulators, technical training, robotics, and image-guided services. It serves surgeons young and old, echocardiographers for TEE procedures, cardiologists, and cardiovascular surgical trainees among others.

Health care and the oil and gas business are the two largest industries in Houston. Although at first glance, one might not necessarily recognize the similarities shared by these professions, Dr. Lumsden, who has a very creative imagination, speculated that the cardiovascular sciences and the oil and gas industries might indeed have much in common, as they both rely heavily on pumps and pipes. Thus was born the "Pumps & Pipes" conference in 2008 with original hosts and sponsors being the Methodist DeBakey Heart & Vascular Center, ExxonMobil and the University of Houston. The original conference, drawing 100 participants assembled at the University of Houston, has grown to more than 240 attendees in 2012. It now meets the first Monday of December in the auditorium of the new Methodist Hospital Research Institute building. Still hosted by the Methodist DeBakey Heart & Vascular Center and ExxonMobil, it now includes participants from other energy companies such as NASA, Texas Heart Institute, and Rice University.

Common ground has been found in many areas, including the remote monitoring of pipes and pumps, repair of pipes and blood vessel erosion, and pump construction (pulsatile and continuous flow), among others. A "heartbeat simulator" has been constructed under the guidance of Dr. Stephen Little with the assistance of collaborators from ExxonMobil and scientists from the University of Houston, enabling him to simulate heart valve function and, by using imaging tools, to evaluate new devices and prosthetic heart valves. The conference has gone international with a Pumps and Pipes meeting held in Doha, Qatar, in the spring of 2012 in the Qatar Science and Technology Park. Conference proceedings are now published emphasizing common challenges in the two industries and highlighting collaborations and opportunities for future interdisciplinary work.

Another first of its kind is the DeBakey Institute for Cardiovascular Education and Training (DICET) established in 2010 with a grant from the DeBakey Medical Foundation. It offers education opportunities and skill training in concert with MITIE at every stage of a medical career and training in the use of medical devices developed by industry partners. One of the first education programs developed is the "Boot Camp" for new cardiovascular trainees open to anyone interested around the country and offered in August of each year.

An E-Learning Library named for William L. Winters Jr. has been established. There are plans to provide DICET symposia and skill-training programs globally through a range of electronic resources. An Apple application will make its appearance at the 2013 Cardiovascular Boot Camp allowing interaction with the lecturers during the course and access to content and lecturers throughout the year.

The *Methodist DeBakey Cardiovascular Journal*, indexed on MedLine and PubMed, is in its ninth year of publication. In its format, as a review journal published quarterly, manuscripts are solicited from experts around the world and focus on some particular topic. A guest editor oversees each issue.

Selma and Lois DeBakey were mentors to the editors of the *Methodist DeBakey Cardiovascular Journal* from its inception. A lectureship was established at The Methodist Hospital in honor of Selma and Lois DeBakey in 2010. The inaugural speaker was Dr. Anthony DeMaria, editor of the *Journal of the American College of Cardiology*, followed by editors of *JAMA*, *New England Journal of Medicine*, and *American Journal of Cardiology*, among others—a total of nine to date.

Following the severance of its 50-year affiliation with Baylor College of Medicine, The Methodist Hospital has made impressive strides in its goal to become an academic medical center. Strong dedication to these goals by the medical staff, nursing staff, administration, and hospital employees has been the key. The "I CARE" creed championed by Mr. Ron Girotto now is nationally recognized and contributes in part to the national reputation the hospital has received. *U.S. News & World Report* in 2012 listed the hospital as number 1 in Texas, number 12 in cardiovascular specialties, and best hospital in 13 specialties. The Methodist Hospital also has been listed among the 100 best companies to work for seven years in a row by *Fortune* magazine; has received an "A" rating from the Leap Frog Group, DNV Healthcare accreditation for Quality and Patient Safety, and a Press Ganey Patient Voice Award; and has been recognized by the American Nursing Credentialing Center as a Magnet Hospital.

Vestiges of the Baylor College of Medicine/The Methodist Hospital teams still occupy space in The Methodist Hospital buildings, and collaborators still collaborate. Prominent among them is Dr. Christie Ballantyne, now chairman of the cardiology section at Baylor College of Medicine as well as director of the section of atherosclerosis and vascular medicine at The Methodist Hospital, along with his associates, Drs. Peter Jones and Vijay Nambi.

Dr. Mark Entman remains as scientific director of the DeBakey Heart Center, successor to the original "super center" funded by NIH located in The Methodist Hospital. When the super center funding was discontinued by NIH, the DeBakey Heart Center was established with philanthropic funds (1985) as a research center dedicated to research in cardiovascular basic sciences. Today, its operations are supplemented by NIH funds acquired by the DeBakey Heart Center faculty. There has always been some confusion as to whether the DeBakey Heart Center was a Baylor College of Medicine or Methodist Hospital entity. It was both. It was funded through Baylor

College of Medicine by philanthropy raised by Dr. DeBakey but housed in research space at The Methodist Hospital. At that time, Baylor College of Medicine and The Methodist Hospital, although governed by independent boards, was viewed by most as a single-functioning organization.

With the announced separation in 2004, that view was abruptly ended. However, the DeBakey Heart Center, as one vestige of a former strong affiliation, is still housed at The Methodist Hospital and continues to fulfill its mission in cardiovascular basic science research, albeit with a much smaller faculty. Over the years it has spawned many successful scientists. A grand total of 19 have moved on to other research posts and many to departmental chairs. Curiously, in a newsletter published by The Partnership for Baylor College of Medicine in 2009, the DeBakey Heart Center was described as consisting of three sections: cardiology, cardiothoracic surgery, and vascular and endovascular surgery. No mention is made of cardiovascular research efforts directed by Dr. Entman.

In contrast and as a completely separate entity, the Methodist DeBakey Heart Center officially came into being in 2001 as a way to consolidate and credit the disparate clinical and clinical research efforts of the Baylor College of Medicine faculty in cardiology and cardiovascular surgery working at The Methodist Hospital under a single rubric hoping to better publicize their work—much like the Texas Heart Institute.

Dr. Raizner and Debbie Feigin Sukin led the way. When the divorce occurred in 2004, efforts to move this concept forward accelerated, and in 2008, the Methodist DeBakey Heart Center name was changed to the Methodist DeBakey Heart & Vascular Center to acknowledge the rapid advances made in medical and surgical therapy for vascular disease.

The departments of urology, ENT, and plastic surgery along with the Center for Cell and Gene Therapy at Baylor College of Medicine retain a portion of their facilities, clinical practice, and education programs at The Methodist Hospital.

The future is bright for basic science and transitional cardiovascular research at The Methodist Hospital with the establishment of cardiovascular sciences in The Methodist Hospital Research Institute under the leadership of Dr. John P. Cooke, who transferred from Stanford University in May 2013. His research interest is in cardiovascular regenerative medicine, which in tandem with Dr. Mauro Ferrari, a world expert in nanotechnology, bodes well for advances in two of the foremost fields for cardiovascular research.

To celebrate the past and the pioneering surgical career of Dr. DeBakey, a library and museum dedicated to his life and work was opened to the public by Baylor College of Medicine on May 4, 2010. Outside in the courtyard stands a larger-than-life-sized statue of him, created by Edd Hayes. Standing tall with his arms crossed, mask around his neck, and glasses on, the statue strikes a pose familiar to all who worked with him.

As for the future of cardiovascular medicine at The Methodist Hospital, the foundation for excellence laid by Dr. Michael E. DeBakey and Dr. Don W. Chapman and their many colleagues exists to build upon – and the building blocks are in place. While scientists unravel the secrets of disease, physicians will assimilate and disseminate their discoveries to their patients always with the admonition that caring for a patient may be more rewarding than the cure. I am reminded of Voltaire: "The art of medicine consists in amusing the patient while nature cures the disease." Oh, to be a fly upon the wall 50 years hence.

As a final footnote, The Methodist Hospital officially changed its name on July16, 2013, to "Houston Methodist" to differentiate itself from the many other Methodist hospitals across the nation. At the same time it was announced that Houston Methodist once again was named by *U.S. News & World Report* as one of America's "Best Hospitals," ranked No. 14 in cardiology and heart surgery. Recognized as one of the best hospitals in 12 specialties, more than any other hospital in Texas, Houston Methodist ranked No. 1 in Texas and No. 1 in the Houston Metro area.

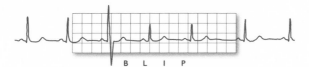

AND THE BEAT GOES ON

*T*aking center stage at The Methodist Hospital's inaugural Leading Hearts Gala to benefit The Methodist DeBakey Heart & Vascular Center in October 2009 were former Texas Congressman Charlie Wilson, the recipient of a heart transplant in September 2007, and Nobel laureate and former president of Poland Lech Walesa, successfully implanted with a biventricular pacemaker-defibrillator in February 2008.

Each had a story to tell. Earning the nickname "Good Time Charlie" for his penchant for drinking, parties, women, and mischief in the nation's capitol and all over the world, the larger-than-life Texas congressman known as the "liberal from Lufkin" was first diagnosed with cardiomyopathy —a disease that causes an enlarged and weakened heart —in 1985 by Dr. Dick Cashion at The Methodist Hospital. During the following two decades, while championing his infamous plan to fund Afghanistan's resistance to the Soviet Union, he underwent treatment for his illness. When the deterioration of his heart in the summer of 2007 necessitated his becoming a heart transplant candidate, the congressman expressed his desire to live long enough to attend the December premiere of "Charlie Wilson's War," the movie about his successful efforts abroad.

Announcing that he was feeling "tremendous" after his September 2007 transplant, he lauded the medical team, the hospital staff, and heart transplant pioneer Dr. Michael E. DeBakey. "The treatment has been absolutely superb from the person who empties the wastebaskets to the masters of the universe who master the scalpel," said the grateful recipient. "It could not have been a single more positive experience."[1] To demonstrate his appreciation to his cardiologist, Dr. Guillermo Torre, chief of the division of cardiac transplantation at The Methodist Hospital, the grateful congressman invited him to attend the highly anticipated official premiere of his movie in Los Angeles on December 10, 2007, with its stars, Julia Roberts and Tom Hanks.[2] Continued on next page

---

Note: In February 2010 Charlie Wilson died of heart failure at the age of 76.

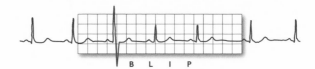

Two months later at The Methodist Hospital, Dr. Torre supervised the treatment of another patient famous for fighting communism. After being invited "to be taken care of by our team of physicians" by Dr. Zbigniew Wojciechowski, vice chair of the department of anesthesiology at The Methodist Hospital and an honorary consul to the Republic of Poland, Lech Walesa explained, "Communism wore out my heart," he said, "but I believe the doctors in Houston can fix it."[3]

To treat his symptoms of cardiomyopathy and resynchronize the contractions of his heart to improve function, Dr. Miguel Valderrábano, an electrophysiologist at the Methodist DeBakey Heart & Vascular Center, implanted a biventricular pacemaker-defibrillator in February 2008. While undergoing treatment at The Methodist Hospital, the Nobel laureate, with Dr. Wojciechowski as his interpreter, visited with former United States President George H. W. Bush, former Secretary of State James Baker, and Dr. DeBakey. "I want to regain my health so I can work a few more years and solve some more problems in the world," he told Dr. DeBakey. "Like my heart, the world needs a little fixing to make it work better than ever." Addressing the audience at the Leading Hearts Gala more than a year later, the peacekeeper with the pacemaker said, "It has been a long time since I felt this good. Dictators and oppressors should continue to fear me because I will be here for a long time."[3]

Praise for the hospital also came from the gala's honorary chairs President George H. W. Bush and Barbara Bush, who underwent heart valve replacement in March 2009. "I am very impressed with and grateful to the wonderful team of doctors and nurses at The Methodist Hospital who have helped Barbara," the former president said. "Having undergone bowel surgery there the previous November, the former first lady thanked both of her surgeons, Drs. Michael Reardon and Patrick Reardon. "I had two brothers attack two parts of my body, and they saved my life," she said.[4]

At the conclusion of the gala, the first Leading Hearts Award, established to honor a physician, individual, or organization that, through leadership, service,

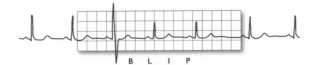

B L I P

and lifelong commitment, has made significant and continuous contributions to the advancement of care in the field of cardiovascular diseases, was presented to Dr. George P. Noon. Accepting the honor, the former student, resident, and surgical colleague of Dr. Michael E. DeBakey reiterated his praise of the genius of his mentor, who "singlehandedly raised the standard of medical care, teaching, and research around the world. He was the greatest surgeon of the 20th century, and physicians everywhere are indebted to him for his contributions to medicine."[5]

1. Hoepfner D. Saying he feels 'tremendous,' Wilson released from hospital. *The Lufkin Daily News*. October 4, 2007.
2. Carlson P. Sticking to his guns: Charlie Wilson: the wild card image was the real deal. *Washington Post*. December 22, 2007.
3. Angelle D. Peacemaker gets a pacemaker at Methodist. *Texas Medical Center News*. March 10, 2008.
4. Sewing J. Former Patients Laud DeBakey Center. *Houston Chronicle*. November 1, 2009.
5. Wendler R. Michael Ellis DeBakey, M.D. Sept. 7, 1908 – July 11, 2008. *Texas Medical Center News*. July 15, 2008.

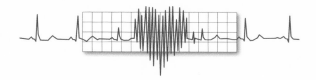

REFLECTIONS OF TWO PRINCIPALS

Antonio M. Gotto Jr., MD, D.Phil. and George P. Noon, MD

*Having played an integral role in development of cardiovascular
medicine at The Methodist Hospital, Dr. Gotto has fond memories*

For someone who spent the largest portion of his career at The Methodist Hospital and Baylor College of Medicine, this book makes fascinating reading. I congratulate Bill Winters and Betsy Parish on an outstanding job. The events are meticulously researched, and Dr. Winters has carried out extensive interviews with many of the individuals who were involved at the time. Dr. Michael DeBakey, Dr. Denton Cooley, and others not only overturned the field of cardiovascular surgery at The Methodist Hospital and in Houston in the 1950s and 1960s, but they literally overturned it for the entire world.

Dr. Cooley has recently written an autobiography that describes many of the same events from a different, but individual, perspective. One of the strengths of *Houston Hearts* is that through interviews the authors obtained so many different perspectives on the same events. The book reminds me somewhat of Lawrence Durrell's four-volume work, *The Alexandria Quartet*, in which he describes the same sequence of events from the eyes of four different individuals. What Dr. Winters has done is to forge together individual perspectives with newspaper accounts, medical publications, and his own valuable, precise, and inside view of the events that took place where he has worked for the last four decades.

I was at Baylor and The Methodist Hospital for 25 years, including 20 as chair of medicine, then resumed my relationship with The Methodist Hospital nine years ago when it became affiliated with the Weill Cornell Medical College in New York. The descriptions by the various interviewees are personalized and revealing, and they give an excellent sense of the evolution of the institution over the last 60-plus years.

It really is an extraordinary story. The two people who did the most to put The Methodist Hospital as well as Baylor College of Medicine on the map as world-renowned institutions were undoubtedly Dr. Michael DeBakey and Mr. Ted Bowen. They worked closely together and had a great deal of mutual respect, and together they made the achievements of The Methodist Hospital possible.

Of course, the ascendancy of The Methodist Hospital and Baylor College of Medicine could not have happened without the wonderful efforts of Michael DeBakey. In my opinion, he was the physician of the century. I know of no one else who had the broad impact on medicine that he had — from being a pioneer in surgery and a leader in political and social changes affecting medicine to a medical diplomat on behalf of the world. I had the extraordinary privilege of working closely with him for 25 years, traveling with him, seeing patients together, codirecting the country's only National Heart and Blood Vessel Research and Demonstration Center, and coauthoring several books, including most recently *The Living Heart in the 21st Century*, which he and I agreed to prepare on the day he died and which was completed and published after his death. Dr. George Noon kindly provided the foreword for that book, in which he describes the surgical treatment of Dr. DeBakey's dissecting aneurysm.

My wife Anita and I first met Michael DeBakey when I was a senior medical student at Vanderbilt in Nashville. He was a speaker at our Alpha Omega Alpha banquet, and I was fascinated at hearing him speak for the first time on "patterns of atherosclerosis." This was already a theme of his and remained so for the rest of his life. He described different patterns based on his surgical experience. Some patients had primarily coronary disease, others largely carotid, others aortic, and others peripheral. And some had combinations of all. He would give his lectures illustrated with slides from the many patients he treated. He was very skeptical about any significant involvement of cholesterol in atherosclerosis, and when I first moved to Houston, he thought that a level of blood cholesterol up to 300 mg/dL was normal. He gradually softened his views over the years and actually agreed to take statins after they became available. He was always exceedingly prudent about his diet, never overate, and barely consumed any alcohol.

Dr. Joe Merrill, one of the unsung heroes who helped forge an academic medical center at Baylor College of Medicine after it gained its independence from Baylor University, initially invited me to Houston in the fall of 1968, as Dr. Winters noted in this book. I decided to stay at the National Institutes of Health for a further period of time and subsequently was recruited when I was in the process of considering an offer from Cornell. I met Dr. DeBakey in Washington during one of his visits during this period and recall his advice on the subject of academic tenure. In effect, he said the only security you have in a medical school or at a hospital is that you continue to be productive. As long as you're productive, they're going to want you to stay there. This is but one of many pieces of sage advice that I received from Dr. DeBakey over the years.

Dr. DeBakey was always most generous and kind to our daughters, and one episode involving our middle daughter Jill is mentioned in the book. On one of my recruitment visits, he met with my wife Anita, my oldest daughter Jennifer, and me. When he was introduced to Jennifer, he reached out his hand to her, and she immediately grabbed his hand and arm and began swinging around. This completely horrified her mother and me, who feared she would inflict some damage to his operating hand and arm. Fortunately, this did not occur.

In the years before Dr. DeBakey passed away, I attended several of his lectures and speeches, one of them to the New York Surgical Society about various people he had operated on. This was always of great interest to the audience, and he relished relating various anecdotes. I had been involved in consultations with some of Dr. DeBakey's patients. It has been said many times, but it bears repeating, that the patient was always the center of his focus. And he literally had patients all around the world who would come seeking his help. He always did his best, poor or rich, famous or unfamous.

I saw patients with Dr. DeBakey on Sunday mornings whenever he called to request my presence. One of these was President Lyndon B. Johnson, on whom we performed what I believe was his last checkup a few months before he died. Lady Bird had called to request examinations as Mr. Johnson was coming to Houston to see the Rice-Texas football game and stay with George Brown. We saw him early on the following Sunday morning and spent most of the day with him. The former president was in a very good mood and regaled us with stories and jokes. He told us about the day he sold a television station in Austin and how he had taken more nitroglycerine pills for angina that day than any day since his last heart attack. And then he paused a minute and said, "well, with the exception of the day George McGovern visited the LBJ Ranch." Dr. DeBakey conveyed to Dr. Willis Hurst, Mr. Johnson's primary cardiologist and physician in Georgia, that he advised continuing medical treatment, not surgery, at that time.

Dr. DeBakey attracted patients from all over the world and was especially well known in the Middle East. We developed a very robust referral group of patients from Turkey, beginning with a prominent businessman who then referred another businessman friend who came to the hospital in 1978. Dr. DeBakey and I strongly advised him to have bypass surgery, but he insisted on returning to Istanbul to talk with his family. He developed unstable angina, and the family requested that I go over and try to get him stabilized to bring him back to Houston. I did this, but while on Air France three hours out of New York, he suffered a heart attack. I gave him Demerol, and we administered oxygen on the plane. The staff and passengers insisted on continuing to smoke, and we were afraid they were going to blow up the plane. Fortunately we survived, and Dr. DeBakey operated on him in November 1978. The patient lived until just a few months ago when he passed away well into his 90s. The patient felt great affection and admiration for Dr. DeBakey and subsequently referred a political friend of his.

Two years later, this individual, Turgut Özal, was elected president of Turkey, and we began receiving politicians as referrals as well as businessmen and other people. The Methodist Hospital signed an affiliation agreement with the Admiral Bristol Hospital, which has now become the Koç Hospital, and helped establish a number of laboratories. Dr. Mario Verani helped establish a nuclear cardiology laboratory. At the height of the interaction with Turkey, The Methodist Hospital was receiving approximately 200 patient referrals a year. Dr. Jimmy F. Howell operated on many of these patients and became a surgical hero in Turkey. When I sent a patient who we found out was a leading member of the Turkish mafia to Dr. Howell, he sent back word, "Tell Tony, I don't have to operate on every Turkish patient who comes to Methodist Hospital."

I was privileged to spend some time with Dr. DeBakey on the last day of his life. As mentioned above, we discussed another edition of the *Living Heart* book series, which was subsequently published after he died and in which he had wanted to emphasize prevention.

Dr. DeBakey was an icon, and his statue appropriately adorns the entrance to the Dunn Tower of The Methodist Hospital. While there is no biography at this time as far as I am aware, it is fortunate that this book on the cardiovascular history of The Methodist Hospital so admirably and ably describes and documents many of Dr. DeBakey's activities and contributions. They will be long remembered, and *Houston Hearts* will be an extremely valuable contribution after our memories fade.

Antonio M. Gotto Jr., MD, D.Phil.

*Proud of the past and enthusiastic about the future of cardiovascular surgery
at The Methodist Hospital, Dr. Noon shares his observations*

This book records the history of cardiovascular medicine and cardiovascular surgery at The Methodist Hospital, Houston, Texas, from its inception. For those of us who were part of the history and for those who were not, it is a remarkable story from the inception of The Methodist Hospital (TMH), Baylor University College of Medicine (BUCM), and The Texas Medical Center (TMC).

In the late 1940s and early 1950s, two struggling institutions moved to the Texas Medical Center. In 1947, BUCM moved from its temporary home in the Sears and Roebuck Building into the New Cullen Building. The Methodist Hospital moved to its new 289-bed hospital in 1951. When Dr. Michael DeBakey arrived in 1948 to assume the Chairmanship of the Department of Surgery at BUCM, the College did not have a primary teaching hospital, as was promised to Dr. DeBakey when he accepted the position. Arrangements with Jefferson Davis Hospital and Hermann Hospital were not satisfactory. Dr. DeBakey was planning to leave, but was finally persuaded to stay when he was successful in converting the U.S. Naval Hospital to a Veterans Administration Hospital, which was affiliated with BUCM. He moved his private practice to TMH.

With the aid of philanthropy, hard work, and Dr. DeBakey's vision, BUCM and TMH moved forward together. Under the leadership of Ted Bowen, President, TMH provided the facilities, organization, commitment, and foresight for growth and development. It takes more than bricks and mortar, however, to succeed as they.

Dr. DeBakey, BUCM, TMH, and TMC became superstars in patient care, research, and medical academia. Patients and trainees came from throughout the United States and the world. In the 1950s and 1960s, many life-saving "firsts" in cardiovascular surgery occurred, including carotid artery endarterectomy, resection of aneurysms of the aorta, and coronary artery bypass. Homograft arteries were replaced by Dacron grafts as a result of Dr. DeBakey's pioneering research. Research laboratories were booming. BUCM and Rice were working together in artificial heart research. Residency and fellowship programs were established. Research funding from the NIH, other federal sources, industry, and philanthropy provided the necessary start-up and sustaining funds. The rapid growth and resultant achievements were phenomenal. We are now in the 21st Century, entering a new era in medicine. We are witnessing the development and application of minimally invasive surgical procedures, robotics, catheter-based diagnosis and treatment, tissue engineering, genomes, nanotechnology, personalized and global medicine. This is the future on which we must now concentrate.

Before Dr. DeBakey died, on numerous occasions he expressed his disappointment in the BCM/TMH separation. Shortly before the BCM board announced its decision to separate in 2004, he addressed the TMH Quarterly Medical Staff Meeting. At the end of the meeting, a hand vote was taken, and nearly every hand was raised in support of a continued affiliation between TMH and BCM. Despite his disappointment after the announced separation, Dr. DeBakey considered TMH and BCM his professional homes for sixty years. He was proud of both. Well, what is done is done and what is past is past. It is time to focus on the future.

The growth and success of TMH were and will be a mutually beneficial relationship between the Hospital and the academic institutions in our community. The revival of such a relationship will ensure that TMH will not only be leading medicine but leading medical research. It would complement mutual achievements, reward our community leadership in medicine, politics, and philanthropy, and lead to further breakthrough advances.

George P. Noon, MD

---

1. LBJ turned to DeBakey for cardiac consultation. *Boston Globe.* Jan 31, 1973.
2. Turkish Prime Minister Turgut Ozal underwent successful triple bypass surgery at Methodist Hospital in Houston. *The Atlanta Journal-Constitution.* February 11, 1987.

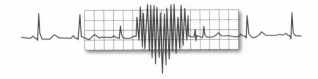

FOR RHYME AND REASON

Courtesy of William L. Winters Jr., MD, MACC

There once was a cardiologist quite witty
Known for his occasional limerick or ditty.
Treating special events with rhyme
Often memorable and sublime
He was the most well versed Doc in the city.

Since I have been penning impromptu limerick poetry since 1960, a friend was inspired to write the tribute above. The 32-plus poems I have created over the years were almost always to pay tribute to someone or to commemorate an event or occasion. I do not remember what inspired this newfound avocation — possibly my memorization of William Shakespeare in college or my lifelong admiration for the poetry of Walt Whitman and Omar Khayyam. I do know it comes easy to me. I just need a few quiet moments to get started, and then it just flows. Here are a few of my favorites.

Ode to Antonio M. Gotto
On the Occasion of his 25th year
with Baylor College of Medicine
1996

There once was a man name Gotto
Who lived by a very strict motto
"You get back what you give
For as long as you live
So for Pete's sake, don't go blotto."

Gotto managed to do it just right
He started out by learning everything in sight
Then he added his bit
To make a better fit
Working at times by moonlight.

He made his first move as a scholar
Rhodes, I think, was his collar
He managed just fine
Never fell out of line
Then moved on with a hoop and a holler.

To med school he came with a leap
At Vanderbilt he made not a peep
In no time at all
While having a ball
The "MD" was his to keep.

Then he and Anita went east
To Mass General no less to feast
On the brains sitting there
In all those prestigious chairs
But intimidated? Not in the least.

Then NIH, Baylor and Cornell
Where his work is chronicled so well
It takes no dim wit
To see in a bit
How his career has careened pell-mell.

Well, I could go on all day
Since there really is so much to say
But you will hear more
From his comrades of yore
While I meander on my merry way.

To Tony and Anita I say
Your friends and colleagues will stay
While we all stand up
And to you raise our cup
For showing us the way every single day.

Ode to William Zoghbi
On the Occasion of his 50th birthday
November 2005

There once was a man from the East
Who was ambitious to say the least
He came here to stay
To work hard, not to play
And found medicine to be his feast.

He dallied long enough
To find love not too tough
To take a new vow
With Huda – a real wow
Together they made the right stuff.

He with echoes, she with genes
By hook or crook or any old means
They made sparks fly
Rose high in the sky
And became the envy of many a dean.

No telling where William's path will lead
His stars are still moving and tough to read
But one thing for sure
His motives are pure
And great things await him, indeed.

So today we salute his 50 years
We are fortunate to be his peers
And as years roll by
We can look at him and sigh
And marvel at his work, over a few beers.

Ode to Don and Mary Louise Chapman
On the Occasion of their 60th anniversary
2007

It's always a pleasure to see
Two people who were meant to be
Paired for life
As husband and wife
Suited to each other to a tee.

Now, sixty years sounds pretty long
But not when life is a song
Mary Lou is a pip
The kids became hip
And in work, you could do no wrong.

So what more could you do
To show you're no schmoo
Why, build a great group
Keep them out of the soup
While building character through and through.

It was Beazley, Peterson and Brook
Who wrote the first part of the book
When Winters showed up
Followed by a couple of pups
Named Spencer and Cashion for a look.

They all liked it so well
They stayed on for a spell
To add some ink
While providing a link
To the story we now can tell.

There were others who came
But never got in the game
For a variety of reasons
Which changed with the seasons
Leaving the scene with no name.

Your friends have heard you say
To keep fresh and alert for the fray
You had to work hard through the day
So at night you could play
Knowing you'd have it no other way.

You've both lead us a merry chase
And kept up such a hectic pace
There are only a few
Still left in the stew
With any stamina to keep up the race.

There is one other claim
When it comes to a name
That bobbles my mind
As one of a kind
And adds to the Chapman fame.

All the Chapmans I know
For several generations or so
Are all called "Doc"
As if by "ad hoc"
A tradition we hope continues to grow.

Now, I'd like to finish this epistle
Knowing it's a bit of a thistle
With a toast to the bride and groom
We've been blessed to have you and to be part of your crew
While you brought your world to full bloom.

Healthcare Reform
A political plea
February 2010

Many people decreed it to be
That healthcare as anyone could see
Needed reforming
A sort of re-borning
To avoid a financial melee.

Major problems were quite visible
That made most people miserable
Like cost and access
Tricky insurance and malpractice
But each issue quite addressable.

Then there's the matter of waste
Not curable just by cut and paste
So look for the source
Not obvious of course
That may require patience not haste.

Because some politicians just don't get it
Their constituents to their great credit
Rose up en masse
Like weeds in the grass
To head off a worsening debit.

So as more people saw through it all
And tea parties slowed it to a stall
Let's think this thing through
So as not to fall into
An uncontrolled financial freefall.

Please look at the problems out there
Try to show us you really do care
Take it step by step
With an eye on the debt
To find benefits that we all may share.

Rather than shake our foundations
Out of sheer and utter frustrations
Take a look at the parts
Readjust it with smarts
Then stand back to laud the creation.

With that thought in mind
Craft reforms of the kind
That look at the mix
To accomplish a fix
To solve this unending old bind.

As a doctor, I want you to know
I believe our profession would show
More trust in the end
If politicians would bend
And think like that sleuth, Hercule Poirot.

He achieved all manner of fame
By listening to all sides of the game
Then melding the ideas
For everyone to see as
A solution that all can acclaim.

So I think we all would agree
That such healthcare reform should be
An open forum for all
Young, old, short, and tall
And quite transparent for all to see.

It's not necessary for all to agree
Expect different opinions to be
Stumbling blocks for some
A trial to overcome
In route to the game-winning tee.

I believe the best leaders today
Are those with attitudes that say
We'll do it somehow
With grace and a bow
The consensus we'll hail with hooray!

Having said all this with vigor and vim
Midst a strong wish for us all to win
To the parties in power
No more of those glowers
We will see if you sink or you swim.

If swimming were to happen indeed
We'd be more than happy to read
That patients come first
Best news, not the worst
That our leaders did, in fact, take the lead.

It just goes to show you all
Common sense wins over a brawl
So it comes as a plea
From my colleagues and me
Make it work for the very long haul.

Ode to Miguel Quiñones
On the Occasion of his receiving the
American Society of Echocardiography Lifetime Achievement Reward
June 2012

We all know a cardiologist named Mike
Who you would instinctively like,
Born with remarkable good humor
With a laugh that goes "karoomer"
He's risen to the top of the dike.

The dike is his world of ultrasound
That Inge Edler long ago found
Was a wonderful way,
As we all now can say,
To study the heart as we gather round.

Dr. Quiñones has for years led the way
In finding new uses most every day
For this valuable tool
In our diagnostic pool
Of services, for which we say Hurray!

It's no wonder he's getting this award
Because by moving this science forward
Cardiologists are now able
To see if the heart is stable
At a cost that most can afford.

So I say three cheers for old ASE
For recognizing the contributions that he,
Dr. Quiñones, known as Mike,
Made climbing his very own dike
And displayed for the whole world to see!

Ode to Jimmy Howell
On the Occasion of his 80th birthday
And 50th year at Baylor College of Medicine
October 2012

Howdy Pardner, my name is Howell
And not yet ready to throw in the towel
Eighty is the age
Still turning the page
While walking the halls on the prowl.

At Baylor, fifty years have passed
In a flash, hard to believe so fast
I paid them my dues
For them all good news
Like money in the bank while I last.

Many patients have become good friends
So they and I hope it never ends
But the truth of the matter
Says the mad Hatter
Really depends on how well one mends.

Mending after one of Howell's jobs
Is as sure as eating corn on the cob
When ripe in the summer
It's never a bummer
And enjoyed by oodles of mobs.

He has been the surgeon's steady Eddie
Always on call and at the ready
For come what may
To this very day
Scalpel in his grip and hand really steady.

He's been known to have a sharp tongue
And more than one resident's been stung
But it's all for the best
As they learn not to jest
With the master at the top of the rung.

So somewhere around now, we can say
This is Dr. Jimmy Frank Howell's Day
Whether eighty or fifty
He's still pretty nifty
So to him we say, "Hip Hip Hooray."

Ode to Richard Wainerdi
On the occasion of his retirement as CEO of the Texas Medical Center
December 2012

Imagine TMC without Wainerdi
There's no telling where we might be
He's livened up the place
While making new space
For all the new players you now see.

For the past years now, twenty-eight
He's managed to add to his plate
New buildings galore
With facades to adore
To house new programs – first rate.

He's managed to keep CEOs in line
While giving them room to opine
Why they should be
Atop their levee
For the whole world to see how they shine.

Adding to this first-rate show
Is the ability always to know
How he should live
And how much to give
So his empire could appropriately grow

We'll always remember Dick with a chuckle
His diplomacy without a brass knuckle
The committees he did chair
Adroitly with flare
Caused dissidents always to buckle.

So to Wainerdi we have only to say
Your twenty-eight years to this day
Have been pretty nice
Plenty of sugar and spice
But you can say you did it, "My Way."

Ode to Dr. Michael E. DeBakey
In whimsical tribute
December 2009

There once was a long-lived man named Mike
Who lived a life like you would like
With Lebanese roots
And family in cahoots
He grew into a strong-minded tike.

His parents and siblings were there
To support, nurture and share
The growth of his mind
Enabling him to find
The skills you'd never have dared.

He read everything in sight
Even the Britannica at night
To open his eyes
As wide as the skies
In an effort to get everything right.

He then left his hometown in LA
Lake Charles, the name, by the way
To seek his good luck
And perhaps make a buck
While finding his life track, as they say.

He plotted his course very clearly
Toward medicine for which he paid dearly
First, college at Tulane
Starting in the fast lane
Combining college and med school together —verily.

In med school his true colors emerged
His talent for new things really surged
A roller pump you could see
Would move blood from you to me
With most complications finally purged.

Then Dr. Alton Ochsner showed him the way
In Old New Orleans by the Bay
To sharpen his skills
With repetitive drills
Into becoming the world's best, day-by-day.

A sojourn to Europe was ahead
Where new skills lay, it was said
After being exposed to the best
He headed back to the West
For a fabulous career stitched by the thread.

One day a call came from Houston
To come see a department to run
Surgery was it name
Most certainly quite lame
And needed a leader to move on.

That's how Dr. Michael E. D.
Came to Baylor and Methodist, you see
With enthusiastic expectation
Tinged with serious trepidation
To build something special for you and me.

The rest of the story is well known
His shadow and influence were strown
Over landscapes widespread
And in publications well read
All of which were truly home grown.

His principles were simple and steadfast
As many found out and were aghast
That he stuck to his line
"Do it right the first time
Or move on and become part of the past."

His creativity led him to try
New techniques and devices by and by
For all parts of the body
Never mind how worn or shoddy
To be fixed before they would die.

Along the way, he taught many a friend
How to properly sew and to mend
Cotton, Dacron or linen
Whether they be young men or young women
And no matter the problem at hand.

His training techniques were severe
Not designed to praise or revere
His persona or style
Though forgotten after awhile
When his trainees learned to persevere.

People from the world came around
To see him on his hallowed ground
Kings, queens, and many of us
Arrived by car, plane, or bus
To seek his judgment and skills deemed so sound.

His fame spread wide to hallowed halls
Presidents and politicians all made their calls
To hear his wise words
To counter the surge
That so often spread nonsense from their stalls.

The Army in the Second World War
Wisely placed him in the Medical Corp
Where with aplomb and some dash
He created the MASH
Thereby saving more lives than before.

After the War came to an end
He found veterans unable to mend
For lack of some places
For those of all races
For first-class doctors to attend.

So he recommended that service hospitals on hand
Be reserved for service veterans so grand
So came about the V.A.
Healing veterans to this day
Still celebrating his stand in the sand.

He lived life hearty and hale
Up before dawn without fail
Elevators were a sin
Walking stairs was for him
Like a ship on the sea in full sail.

His research interests rapidly grew
But organized reference sources were few
So with the help of his pals
And maybe a few gals
The Medical Library of Congress came into view.

These laurels were only a start
Of a mosaic, if you will, as a part
Of a larger grand plan
He envisioned for Man
That would actually replace the heart.

His "firsts" came one after another
Be it vascular, heart, or some other
He never slowed down
Always adorned in his gown
Traveling worldwide – no bother.

One country he visited with acclaim
Was Russia, becoming known by first name
When Boris needed a guide
Michael E. was there to provide
Advice to return him to his main game.

His legacy is there for all to see
No quarter for incompetency
Always do your best
Let Fate do the rest
And you'll be proud of your own legacy.

One special event is duly noted
When Congress unanimously voted
To give him the Gold
In a congressional medal it's told
To honor all things he promoted.

I remember most what he said about people
Keep your goals as high as a steeple
Pay attention to details no matter how small
Your rewards will be there ready to fall
And your reputation will grow exponential.

He could not have foretold what was coming next
His own aorta chose to dissect
But the surgeons who brought
The techniques that he taught
Restored his health to an amazing context.

At age 97 it was a sterling achievement
Postponing the fully expected bereavement
For over two years
Midst high spirits and cheers
He enjoyed accolades and outpouring sentiment.

When finally he left at age ninety-nine
Without any preliminary sign
Done quite abruptly
Without any subtlety
As though he knew it was time.

Now that he's gone what can be said –
That he lived his life as he led
With wisdom and vigor
Creativity and rigor
Sleeping well every night in his bed.

We'll miss him as no other man
As a Christian who lived life with a plan
To help those that he could
Pass on those that he should
As he steadfastly established his brand.

He is as safe now as he can be
From this world's crazy vagaries
He can sit back and relax
Watch the world wane and wax
Content he was all that he could be.

There will not be another of his kind
Combining unique skills with a very sharp mind
That to his very end
He did manage to send
Lessons, which defy most of us to find.

One last thing I might say
As I lay down at night to pray –
As we live it all up
To the brim of our cup
That we do not his rich legacy betray.

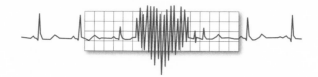

TIMELINE

THE METHODIST HOSPITAL

1908   The Norsworthy Hospital, named for Dr. Oscar Laertius Norsworthy, opens with 30 patients and four stories.

1919   The Methodist Hospital (TMH) is chartered by the Texas Conference of the Texas Methodist Church, South, encompassing the original Norsworthy Hospital.

1923   Sam R. Hay Jr., son of a Methodist Bishop, is hired as first superintendent.

1924   Josie Mooring Roberts is hired as TMH business manager.

        First patients are admitted to TMH on San Jacinto Street in downtown Houston on June 12.

        Methodist Hospital School of Nursing opens with eight students.

        The first Jefferson Davis Hospital opens on Elder Street.

1931   Josie Roberts is named administrator of TMH.

1932   Michael E. DeBakey earns his medical degree at Tulane University School of Medicine.

1933   Michael E. DeBakey earns his masters degree at Tulane University.

1935   Dr. Norsworthy dies.

        Michael E. DeBakey earns his Master of Science degree at Tulane University.

1936   M.D. Anderson Foundation is created with an initial donation of $10,000.

1937   National Cancer Institute Act is passed by Congress, later to be the inspiration for the National Heart Institute.

1938   Michael E. DeBakey becomes 172nd board-certified surgeon in the United States.

The new Jefferson Davis Hospital opens on Allen Parkway.

1939   Walter William Fondren dies. Several months after his death, Mrs. Walter William Fondren is asked to take his place on the TMH board.

M.D. Anderson dies and leaves the bulk of his fortune, $20 million, to the M.D. Anderson Foundation.

1941   Texas Governor Lee O'Daniel signed the bill authorizing a state cancer research hospital and appropriating $500,000 toward the hospital's construction.

1942   In March, the University of Texas (UT) regents accept M.D. Anderson Foundation's offer to name the cancer research hospital for M.D. Anderson and locate it in Houston.

Albert and Mary Lasker Foundation is established.

1943   M.D. Anderson and Baylor University College of Medicine (BUCM) in Dallas sign agreement to bring the medical school to Houston.

BUCM moves to Houston and holds first classes in converted Sears warehouse on Buffalo Drive on July 12, 1943.

Dr. James A. Greene is named chairman of the Department of Medicine at BUCM, where he serves until 1958.

M.D. Anderson Foundation proposes that the cancer hospital site be developed on a tract owned by the City of Houston of more than 134 acres adjoining Hermann Hospital.

A large majority of Houston voters approve the land sale to M.D. Anderson Foundation and endorse the concept of a medical center.

BUCM agreement with Hermann Hospital is established for clinical teaching privileges.

1944   Dr. Don W. Chapman, recognized as the first cardiologist in Houston, arrives in Houston and joins the faculty at BUCM as an instructor in medicine.

Texas Children's Hospital is chartered.

1945   Hugh Roy and Lillie Cullen contribute $1 million to the building campaigns of Baptist Memorial, Hermann Hospital, St. Luke's Episcopal Hospital (SLEH), and TMH.

The Texas Medical Center (TMC) is chartered as a nonprofit corporation.

Land is designated in TMC for TMH to build a new hospital.

1946   Society of Vascular Surgeons is founded, with Drs. Michael E. DeBakey and Alton J. Ochsner as two of the founding members.

1946   In July, Dr. Don W. Chapman performs the first heart catheterization in Houston at Hermann Hospital. Chapman forms the "Dawn Patrol" with voluntary clinical staff to borrow the use of the X-ray facilities before dawn so as not to interfere with established patterns of use.

Dr. Hatch W. Cummings is named chief of internal medicine at TMH, serving in this position until 1970, when a new affiliation agreement with BCM is enacted.

TMC is formally dedicated.

1947   Hugh Roy and Lillie Cullen establish the Cullen Foundation, endowed with more than $80 million in oil properties.

The new Cullen Foundation grants BCM $800,000 to complete initial construction of the new BUCM School in TMC. Named the Roy and Lillie Cullen Building, it opens in fall of 1947, with Dr. Walter H. Moursund as dean.

Residency programs established at TMH in medicine, surgery, obstetrics, neurosurgery, pediatrics, radiology, and pathology through vision of Dr. Cummings.

First classes of BUCM are held in the Cullen Building located in the TMC.

1948   The Fondren Foundation is established by Ella Florence Fondren in honor of Walter W. Fondren, one of the founders of Humble Oil and Refining Company (ExxonMobil).

The Cullen Building at BUCM is officially dedicated.

Ted Bowen becomes assistant administrator at TMH on July 1 and is the hospital's first professionally trained administrator.

National Heart Institute is established with the influence of Mary Lasker.

Mary Lasker is appointed to the National Advisory Heart Council.

In the fall, Dr. Michael Ellis DeBakey moves to Houston to become chairman of the Department of Surgery at BUCM.

1949   First civilian trauma center in United States is established at Jefferson Davis Hospital by Dr. DeBakey.

Dr. Michael Ellis DeBakey joins TMH medical staff.

Groundbreaking for the new TMH in the TMC is held in December.

Dr. Michael E. DeBakey meets Mr. Ben Taub.

Dr. Oscar Creech Jr. joins Dr. DeBakey in the Department of Surgery, serving as head of the peripheral vascular unit until his departure in 1956 to run the Department of Surgery at Tulane University School of Medicine.

The Veterans Administration Hospital becomes BUCM's first affiliated hospital on April 15; Dr. DeBakey is credited with the affiliation.

1949   Jefferson Davis Hospital becomes affiliated with BUCM on August 1 through an arrangement made between Dr. DeBakey and Mr. Ben Taub, chairman of the board of managers at Jefferson Davis (JD).

1950   Dr. George C. Morris Jr. becomes the first surgical resident under Dr. DeBakey, who later says, "he was one of the best surgeons I ever trained." Morris later becomes one of the pioneers in cardiovascular and peripheral vascular surgery.

             TMH signs the first affiliation agreement with BUCM on January 19, and private practice doctors at TMH become voluntary faculty at BUCM.

             Groundbreaking takes place for the M.D. Anderson Hospital in the TMC.

             Dr. Michael E. DeBakey and Mary Lasker meet.

1951   Dr. Denton A. Cooley joins BUCM on June 11, 1951.

             Drs. DeBakey and Cooley are the first in this country to perform successful excision and graft replacement of aneurysms of the aorta and obstructive lesions of the major arteries; surgery is performed at the Jefferson Davis Hospital.

             First homografts are used for aneurysm repair.

             TMH moves to the TMC and opens with 300 beds on November 10, 1951.

             Physicians at TMH successfully treat 30 consecutive patients with mitral stenosis using closed mitral commissurotomy.

             BCM and TMH sign affiliation agreement on October 3, 1951.

             Artist Bruce Hayes creates the mosaic mural on the front of The Methodist Hospital.

             Dr. Cooley performs successful excision of syphilitic aortic aneurysm at Jefferson Davis Hospital.

1952   BUCM signs affiliation agreement with TCH.

             Ten-bed postoperative anesthesia recovery room, the first of its kind in Houston, opens at TMH.

1953   First heart-lung machine is developed by Dr. John H. Gibbon Jr. at Jefferson Hospital in Philadelphia, PA.

             First successful open-heart surgery with Gibbon's heart-lung machine is performed at Jefferson Hospital in Philadelphia, PA.

             Dr. DeBakey performs the first successful carotid endarterectomy, the removal of blockage in carotid artery, thereby establishing the field of surgery for strokes on August 7.

             Dr. Stanley W. Olson is selected dean of BUCM.

             First cardiac catheterization laboratory at TMH opens on sixth floor in the Walter L. Goldston Cardiac Clinic; Dr. Ray K. Skaggs is clinic chief.

             Active staff at TMH rapidly expands to 285.

1953   Emory University-trained Dr. Edward W. Dennis joins BUCM and is named chief of the cardiac clinic at Jefferson Davis (JD); later becomes the principal full-time BUCM cardiologist at TMH.

Dr. DeBakey performs the first successful removal and graft replacement of a syphilitic fusiform aneurysm of the thoracic aorta.

Miss Josie Roberts resigns from TMH on the 29th anniversary of her employment; Ted Bowen succeeds her.

1954   TCH opens in February.

Using his wife's sewing machine, Dr. DeBakey devises Dacron artificial grafts for vascular procedures.

Dr. DeBakey uses the first homemade Dacron graft to repair an abdominal aortic aneurysm.

Dr. DeBakey performs the first successful resection and graft replacement of an aneurysm of the distal aortic arch and upper descending thoracic aorta.

Dr. James K. Alexander is named chief of the cardiology section of the Department of Medicine at BUCM; he begins working at JD and TMH, eventually moving to Ben Taub.

Dr. E. Stanley Crawford joins Dr. DeBakey in the Department of Surgery and becomes internationally known for his innovative surgical techniques in the treatment of complex aortic diseases, particularly Marfan syndrome and aortic dissection.

The M.D. Anderson Hospital and St. Luke's Episcopal Hospital officially open.

Dr. Dan McNamara arrives at TCH to become its first chief of pediatric cardiology.

Dr. Cooley performs the first heart surgery at TCH.

1954-1955. Successful cross circulation between parent and child in 32 children with major congenital cardiac malformations. Clarence Walton Lillehei, University of Minnesota.

1955   Dr. DeBakey is the first to perform a successful resection of an aneurysm of the thoracoabdominal portion of the aorta between the chest and abdomen.

Dr. Edward W. Dennis becomes first full-time BUCM cardiologist at TMH and remains until his death in 1975 at the age of 52.

BUCM affiliated hospital residency program is created.

Cardiorespiratory lab opens on the ninth floor of TMH, with Dr. Edward W. Dennis serving as director.

Dr. Don W. Chapman returns to Houston from two-year service in the U.S. Army.

Dr. Don W. Chapman establishes "The Chapman Group," becoming the "preeminent practicing cardiologist in Houston" and joining the clinical faculty at BUCM with Dr. Paul Peterson, a Baylor graduate.

1955 Dr. DeBakey and colleagues report six cases of aortic dissection treated by surgery.

Drs. DeBakey and Cooley perform 245 aneurysm repairs by July, far surpassing any other series in volume and success.

Drs. DeBakey and Cooley tour Europe and lecture about aneurysm surgery, increasing referrals from around the world.

Dr. John Kirklin perform the first successful open heart surgery at Mayo Clinic using the Mayo modified Gibbon heart-lung machine.

Cooley and colleagues resect a large aortic arch aneurysm that also involves a portion of the descending aorta without the use of cardiopulmonary bypass, first sewing in a temporary graft from the ascending aorta to the distal descending aorta and swinging in two more temporary limbs off that graft, which are anastomosed to the left and right carotid arteries.

1956 Dr. Creech returns to New Orleans to become chairman of the Department of Surgery at Tulane University School of Medicine.

Dr. Stanley Crawford is appointed head of the peripheral vascular unit after Dr. Creech leaves.

First use of the Cooley "coffee pot," a bubble oxygenator similar to Mayo Clinic's Dewall-Lillehei oxygenator, at TMH on April 5.

Dr. John L. Ochsner, son of Alton Ochsner, joins Dr. DeBakey's program at BCM.

Dr. Cooley performs the first open heart surgery with cardiopulmonary bypass at TCH on April 5; by year's end, Cooley performs more open-heart procedures than anyone in the world.

Drs. Cooley and DeBakey are the first to use cardiopulmonary bypass technology to replace the ascending aorta using an aortic allograft.

The Methodist Hospital establishes the first "intense care area" with six beds.

1957 Dr. DeBakey and colleagues, aka "The Houston Group," are the first to resect and replace an aortic arch with a reconstituted aortic arch homograph using cardiopulmonary bypass.

The Cooley "coffee pot" bubble oxygenator is used on 200 patients in TMH, SLEH, and TCH.

Dr. DeBakey establishes experimental machine shop to fabricate innovative mechanical devices for cardiovascular surgery; program is directed toward development of mechanical heart pumps, ventricular assist devices (LVADs), and total artificial heart.

Dr. DeBakey is appointed to National Heart Institute National Heart Advisory Council.

1958 TMH creates a 24-bed general surgery intensive care unit (ICU) next to the second-floor OR; a new 41-bed unit opens in 1963.

1958 BUCM establishes eight internal medicine teaching services at TMH, each with one resident and one intern; rotating residents spend three months in cardiology during their second year.

Cooley has performed more than 310 open-heart operations since 1956, having "almost a monopoly on open-heart surgeries at the time," he later says.

Dr. Jimmy F. Howell becomes a resident at BUCM.

TMH opens a 24-bed cardiovascular ICU, the first of its kind in Houston, in November.

The first patch-graft angioplasty for arterial occlusive disease is successfully performed at TMH.

Dr. DeBakey accepts an invitation from Nikita Khrushchev to visit Russia in December.

Dr. Mason Sones at Cleveland Clinic is the first to visualize a coronary artery.

1959 Dr. Cooley operates on his 120th infant under age one.

Dr. Raymond D. Pruitt, Mayo Clinic's renowned electrocardiographer, joins BUCM as chairman of the Department of Medicine, serving in this position until 1968.

Dr. Arthur C. Beall Jr. becomes an instructor in surgery at BCM, later creating the Beall valve, a prosthetic heart valve that is used worldwide from 1965 until mid-1970.

TMH establishes an eight-bed medical ICU in January.

Professor A. A. Vishnevski, director of the Institute of Surgery in Moscow, visits Houston and TMH on January 20.

Dr. DeBakey receives the AMA Distinguished Service Award.

1960 During the decade, TMH begins to operate at capacity level, converting the solarium into patient rooms.

Dr. Pruitt establishes the cardiology program at TMH under the direction of Dr. Dennis. Training in this program benefits from the large number of patients admitted for cardiovascular surgery.

BUCM and TMH receive a 10-year, $262,500 grant — the first of its kind in the United States — from the National Heart Institute for the country's first Cardiovascular Research Center; later that year, TMH announces the Goldston Cardiovascular Clinical Research Center .

Dr. DeBakey endorses "Medical care for older person," eventually known as Medicare.

Mrs. Fondren breaks her hip and moves into TMH's ninth floor.

Mrs. Fondren, Dr. DeBakey, and Mr. Bowen conceptualize the Fondren-Brown Cardiovascular Research and Training Center.

NIH Cardiovascular Research and Training Center 10-year, $5 million grant is awarded to BCM and TMH.

1961   Goldston Cardiovascular Clinical Research Center opens at TMH, including
a six-bed research ward and laboratories on the 9th floor; Drs. Pruitt and
DeBakey are principal investigators.

Dr. Samuel Kinard, a BUCM graduate trained in cardiology and internal
medicine and working at the University of Colorado, joins Dr. Dennis as full-
time BUCM faculty in cardiology at TMH.

National Library of Medicine is established by Congress and dedicated
December 14, formally opening in early 1962 through the efforts of Dr.
DeBakey.

Dr. John M. Lewis graduates from BUCM in 1955, receives training, and
becomes full-time cardiology staff member with Dr. James K. Alexander
at Jefferson Davis Hospital. He later goes into private practice and joins
voluntary faculty at TMH in 1967.

Dr. H. Edward Garrett from Emory University School of Medicine joins Dr.
DeBakey in the Department of Surgery, personally directing Dr. DeBakey's
clinical service for the next six years.

Dr. Domingo Liotta joins Dr. DeBakey's artificial heart research program at
BUCM.

Dr. Edward Dennis named chairman of the BUCM section of cardiology at
TMH.

Between 1961 and 1965, the TMH cardiology section recruited Dr. Benjamin
McCall of Duke University Medical Center and Dr. John F. Lancaster of Tufts
University.

1962   Dr. C. William Hall joins Dr. Liotta in the BUCM artificial heart research
project.

Dr. Cooley leaves TMH and restricts his practice to SLEH and TCH while
remaining at BUCM.

The Texas Heart Institute (THI) is chartered on August 3.

1963   The first Ben Taub General Hospital opens; Dr. Alexander's clinical and
educational activities in cardiology move to Ben Taub.

TMH opens its west wing with 375 beds, a mosaic mural, and a Fannin Street
entrance; the addition doubles the hospital's capacity to 800 beds.

TMH's new ICU incorporates post-anesthesia recovery; new surgical and
medical ICU opens with 41 beds on second floor.

Doctors at TMH perform the first kidney transplant.

Clifton Webb, Hollywood star, becomes a patient of Dr. DeBakey.

1963 Albert Lasker Award for Clinical Research awarded to Dr. DeBakey.

After successful animal trials, the first ventricular assist device (VAD) is
implanted in a patient with postcardiotomy shock at TMH.

1964   Dr. H. Liston Beazley joins The Chapman Group.

1964 TMH receives $1.73 million grant from NIH for health research facility construction and equipment, to become the Fondren-Brown Building.

Dr. Howell joins Department of Surgery at BUCM as assistant professor; practices at TMH for more than five decades.

Groundbreaking ceremonies for the Fondren-Brown Building take place on October 27.

Dr. DeBakey performs abdominal aortic aneurysm surgery on the Duke of Windsor.

The DeBakey team (Drs. Garrett and Howell) are the first to perform a successful coronary artery bypass graft, although it is not published until 1973.

Dr. DeBakey is awarded NIH grant for artificial heart research.

President Lyndon Johnson announces the "President's Commission on Heart Disease, Cancer, and Stroke" chaired by Dr. DeBakey, with 27 panel members from the fields of medicine, science, philanthropy, and public affairs recommended by Ms. Lasker.

TMH hosts groundbreaking for the cardiovascular and orthopedic centers in the Fondren-Brown Building.

1965 TMH's full-time cardiology faculty is joined by Dr. Manus F. O'Donnell, a graduate of the Medical School of Queens University in Ireland, in October; he practices there for more than 35 years.

Operating at more than capacity, TMH is turning away 50 to 75 patients a day, with a waiting list for those waiting in Houston-area motels; Dr. DeBakey alone has more than 100 hospitalized patients a day.

BUCM cardiologists practicing at TMH include Drs. Ed Dennis, Sam Kinard, Ben McCall, John Lancaster, and Manus O'Donnell.

Coronary angiography is first performed at TMH.

Drs. Sam Henly, Robert Overton, and Don C. Quast form the Surgical Associates.

Dr. H. Edward Garrett performs and publishes the first series of bypass operations to arteries below the knee.

The Methodist Hospital Annex (TMHA) opens; the former Glen Eagle Convalescent Home with 120 beds is connected to the main hospital by a shuttle bus and filled with cardiovascular patients on the first day.

Dr. DeBakey establishes a liaison with Princess Liliane of Belgium (second wife of abdicated King Leopold, III).

Dr. DeBakey performs an aortic valve replacement in the first worldwide live television program on all three national networks via satellite.

Medicare law is established by Congress on July 30 as part of the Social Security Amendment of 1965 and is implemented the following year.

First total artificial heart us implanted in a dog at TMH.

1965 NIH awards $4.5 million to Dr. DeBakey for the Baylor-Rice artificial heart program.

The Heartbeats Band is assembled by Drs. Cooley and Grady Hallman, with Dr. Chapman playing trumpet.

Dr. Jack Roehm, an interventional radiologist trained at the University of Minnesota, is recruited to TMH, ushering in a new era in arterial angiography.

1966 With Dr. John Lancaster as the attending cardiologist, Dr. DeBakey places the first successful partial artificial heart implant, a left VAD, into Marcel DeRudder, who dies five days after the procedure.

DeBakey-trained cardiovascular surgeons Drs. George P. Noon, Edward B. Diethrich, and Charles H. McCollum join BUCM's full-time faculty.

BUCM chairman of medicine, Dr. Raymond D. Pruitt, becomes BUCM dean and chief executive officer after Dean Olson leaves.

Baylor-Rice left VAD is implanted into a Hereford calf.

The NIH general clinical research center grant is awarded to BCM.

Ray C. Fish Foundation pledges $5 million to Texas Heart Institute.

Mr. Ralph Morse becomes Dr. DeBakey's personal photographer.

1967 Dr. Stanley Crawford becomes president of The Methodist Hospital medical staff, 1967-1968.

TMH electrocardiogram department moves to seventh and eighth floors, with Dr. Edward W. Dennis serving as director.

Dr. John Lewis joins BUCM cardiology faculty at TMH.

First human heart transplant is performed by Dr. Christiaan N. Barnard in Cape Town, South Africa.

Dr. Garrett leaves Houston to serve as chairman of the Section of Cardiothoracic Surgery at the University of Tennessee.

SLEH celebrates groundbreaking for an expansion that includes the new Texas Heart Institute facility.

1968 Dr. Cooley performs the first successful heart transplant in the United States at THI on May 2; it was the ninth successful heart transplant worldwide.

Dr. DeBakey performs the first heart transplant at TMH on August 31; it was the 11th in Houston.

Cardiologist Dr. William L. Winters Jr. joins The Chapman Group and TMH as Houston's first trained echocardiographer.

Dr. Pruitt departs BUCM to become dean of the New Mayo Medical School. BUCM's Department of Medicine is without a chairman for two years, with responsibility shared among Drs. Harold Brown, Daniel Jenkins, and Bob Hettig. Dr. Brown eventually becomes acting chairman.

1968   Dr. O'Donnell announces the acquisition of the hospital's first image intensifier in early 1968.

Coronary artery bypass graft (CABG) procedures officially begin at TMH. By October 1970, Drs. Morris, Crawford, Howell, DeBakey, and DeBakey Surgical Associates have performed more than 314 procedures.

Dr. DeBakey becomes president and chief executive officer at BUCM.

The Fondren-Brown Building opens. The Fondren side is a seven floor, 165,000-square-foot building with the capacity to add an additional six floors; 42% is devoted to research/training in both orthopedic and CV research, with 50 beds for teaching / research. The Brown side has five floors and 108,000 square feet with the capacity to add four additional floors; 42% of the building is devoted to CV research/training, with eight specialty ORs with central monitoring and computer system and labs.

Dr. DeBakey teams with Drs. Ted Diethrich and John Liddicoat at TMH to perform the world's first multiple organ transplants of a heart, lung, and two kidneys from one donor patient to four recipient patients.

The Fondren-Brown Building's third-floor Fondren ICU opens to meet the needs of 50 cardiovascular patients. Also included is the special organ transplant unit to allow maximum isolation and the observance of strict sterile technique.

Baylor University releases BUCM from Baptist Convention control; once severed from denominational ties, the school becomes known as Baylor College of Medicine (BCM).

Drs. George Noon and Arthur Beall perform the first lung transplant at TMH for a patient with emphysema.

1969   BUCM becomes a freestanding institution, named Baylor College of Medicine (BCM), with Dr. DeBakey named president and L.F. McCollum named chairman; the college seeks and receives state funding to begin in 1971.

The first cardiac ultrasound laboratory in the southwest is established by Dr. William L. Winters Jr. in the Fondren-Brown Building basement; Ms. Jean Gaffney volunteers to learn technique.

Drs. Cooley and Liotta from the Texas Heart Institute are the first to implant a total artificial heart in patient Haskell Karp.

Dr. DeBakey is awarded the Presidential Medal of Freedom by President Lyndon Johnson on January 20.

Dr. Cooley resigns from BCM faculty.

1970   The Medical Center Cardiovascular Research Foundation is established to support research of The Chapman Group.

Dr. Henry D. McIntosh from Duke University is named chair of the Department of Medicine at BCM, endowed by the Bob and Vivian Smith Foundation.

1970   TMH and BCM sign a new affiliation agreement, with the provision that the newly selected chairs of BCM's clinical departments will become chiefs of clinical services at TMH except for general surgery, which is grandfathered to Dr. John Overstreet.

Dr. Kinsman (Ted) E. Wright Jr. joins the full-time faculty at TMH and establishes a cardiology diagnostic laboratory using noninvasive techniques for diagnosing cardiac problems.

Dr. DeBakey stops heart transplants after performing his 12th transplant (a predetermined number) because of rejection problems.

BCM launches new curriculum, in which the period of education and training to quality for a medical degree is shortened to 34 months over a three-year period, with six weeks each teaching in a public hospital and in TMH.

Dr. Mark Entman is recruited from Duke and begins developing a laboratory research program at BCM that includes Dr. Howard K. Thompson as chief of computer sciences and Dr. C. Thomas Caskey as chief of molecular and human genetics.

Dr. Miguel Quiñones, after residency training at Columbia University, comes to BCM for fellowship training in cardiology, joining Dr. Alexander at Ben Taub.

Dr. McIntosh establishes a cardiology section at BCM and instigates an expanded teaching program in cardiology at TMH with greater involvement of voluntary faculty members.

Dr. Ted Diethrich leaves BCM to establish the Arizona Heart Institute in Phoenix, taking Dr. Sam Kinard with him.

The graduate-level training program (with interns, residents, and fellows) in BCM's Department of Medicine grows in numbers and quality, reaching 86 trainees by 1971 and 185 trainees by 1977.

The Chapman group continues to grow to include Drs. Chapman, H. Liston Beazley, W. Richard Cashion, James Costin (for one year only), Mark J. Hausknecht, David A. Samuels, William H. Spencer, and William L. Winters Jr.

A new medical ICU opens on the 2nd floor of TMH's Fondren building.

1971   Dr. Antonio M. Gotto joins BCM as the founder and chief of the newly established section on atherosclerosis and lipoprotein research and replaces Dr. Joseph Merrill as scientific director of the cardiovascular research center at TMH.

Mr. Larry Mathis begins his career at TMH as an administrative resident, earning multiple promotions.

1972   BCM's entering class expands to 168 students from the previous 84 students in 1968 (before state funding).

1972   Cardiovascular pathologist Dr. Jack L. Titus is recruited to become chairman of the Department of Pathology at BCM and TMH. He moves to Minnesota in 1987 where he remains until his death June 15, 2011.

Dr. Albert E. Raizner is named director of the peripheral circulation research laboratory at BCM, located at the VA Medical Center, where he serves in that capacity until 1974.

The National Heart and Lung Institute (NHLI) establishes the national high blood pressure education program.

1973   Dr. Gotto recruits Drs. O. David Taunton, Joel D. Morrisett, and Ellison Wittels to join him at BCM and TMH.

1974   TMH and BCM are designated the nation's first National Heart and Blood Vessel Research and Demonstration Center with a $13.3 million grant from the NHLBI, with Dr. Gotto as the scientific director and Dr. DeBakey as the medical director.

Dr. McIntosh serves as president of the American College of Cardiology (ACC).

TMH opens the pacemaker evaluation clinic, an extension of the cardiology diagnostic laboratory, with Dr. Kinsman E. Wright as director.

Dr. McIntosh recruits research cardiologists Drs. James C. Cole and Henry G. Hanley and clinical cardiologist Dr. Assad Rizk.

Cardiovascular recovery room opens on 3rd floor of Fondren building with 10 beds, and cardiology residents receive training in CCU with pulmonary specialists.

Dr. Albert E. Raizner is named director of the cardiac catheterization laboratory at the VA Medical Center, serving there until 1979.

1975   Dr. Edward W. Dennis, chief of cardiology at TM, unexpectedly dies in August at the age of 52. Dr. O'Donnell becomes interim director of catheterization labs at TMH.

1975   Dr. Gerald Lawrie joins Dr. DeBakey's surgical team.

1976   Dr. McIntosh resigns as chairman of medicine at BCM after developing the general medicine residency program to national rank, but he remains in cardiology at BCM until 1977.

Mrs. Fondren takes up permanent residence at TMH.

1977   Dr. Gotto is named chairman of BCM's Department of Medicine and chief of internal medicine at TMH, serving until 1997; Dr. Edward Lynch is appointed associate chairman.

Dr. Richard R. Miller is named chief of BCM's cardiology section and chief of the cardiology service at TMH. He expands the clinical research program and serves in this position until he leaves in 1981.

Mr. Ron Girotto arrives in Houston to become the administrator for Dr. Bobby Alford in the ENT department at TMH.

1977   BCM and TMH jointly open the Neurosensory Center of Houston.

Dr. Raizner establishes the Interventional Cardiology Associates.

TMH's peripheral vascular laboratory opens in the Brown Building, with Drs. Noon and McCollum serving as directors.

TMH opens the Alkek Tower, adding five additional floors to the Brown building.

Dr. Entman is named chief of the newly established cardiovascular sciences section of the BCM Department of Medicine.

The Chapman group opens the first nuclear stress test laboratory in Houston, run by Drs. C. James Costin and Richard Cashion; it moves to TMH soon after.

Dr. Raizner is named co-chief of the cardiology section at the VA Medical Center.

The Living Heart, written by Drs. DeBakey and Gotto, is published.

Dr. Quiñones returns from his tour of duty in the U.S. Armed Forces and joins the BCM faculty at TMH, serving as codirector of the TMH-BCM echo lab with Dr. Wright; together they develop clinical and research activities in echocardiography at TMH.

As chairman of the Lasker Award committee in New York, Dr. DeBakey honors Drs. Inge G. Elder and C. Hellmuth Hertz with the Lasker Award for Clinical Medical Research for launching echocardiography, a noninvasive diagnostic technique to detect heart disorders using ultrasound.

Dr. Kinsman Wright leaves BCM for Chattanooga, Tennessee, to establish the Chattanooga Heart Clinic.

The Michael E. DeBakey International Cardiovascular Surgical Society is founded, later becoming the Michael E. DeBakey International Surgical Society.

1978   Dr. Craig M. Pratt joins the BCM faculty at TMH and eventually becomes director of the CCU and director of research at the Methodist DeBakey Heart Center.

TMH participates as one of the 37 investigators in the first major clinical trial for beta-blockers sponsored by NHLBI: The Beta-Blocker Heart Attack Trial (BHAT).

Dr. Andreas Gruentzig presents a talk in November on percutaneous transluminal coronary angioplasty at the American Heart Association meeting in Dallas, Texas.

Dr. Mario S. Verani moves from the Houston V.A. Medical Center to join Dr. Cashion in TMH's new nuclear stress lab.

Houston Cardiology Society is founded.

Nuclear cardiologist Dr. Lawrence A. Reduto is recruited from Yale-New Haven Hospital.

1979   A six-floor addition opens in the Fondren building, housing new catheterization labs, noninvasive labs, a new CCU, offices, and beds for cardiology and pulmonary patients.

Dr. DeBakey steps down as president of BCM and is named chancellor, with Dr. William T. Butler taking his place as BCM president.

The bronze bust of Dr. DeBakey, commissioned by Princess Liliane of Belgium, is dedicated at TMH.

The NHLBI renews a four-year grant of $3,928,900 to the Medicine Lipid Research Clinic, located on the seventh floor of the Fondren building.

The North American Society of Pacing and Electrophysiology is established, with Dr. Spencer serving as an early member.

Dr. Raizner is named director of TMH's cardiac catheterization laboratories, where he will serve until 2002.

The newly combined echocardiography lab opens on the Fondren Building's 9th floor under the direction of Drs. Winters and Quiñones.

Dr. James B. Young, a BCM graduate who trained in cardiology at BCM, joins the faculty and develops a research and clinical program in heart failure. After achieving national prominence, he is recruited by the Cleveland Clinic in 1995.

Dr. Christopher R.C. Wyndham is recruited to BCM and TMH as head of the new cardiac electrophysiology laboratory.

The Chapman group becomes the first tenants of Scurlock Tower on December 30, 1979.

Dr. Cashion attends/teaches a basic science course on nuclear medicine at the Bethesda U.S. Naval Hospital.

1980   Dr. William L. Winters Jr. is elected president of TMH medical staff for a two-year term.

The Wiess Circulator Dynamics Laboratory opens with three cath labs on the 10th floor of the Fondren Building. Under the medical direction of Dr. Raizner, the center performs 4,000 procedures. (the original copy reads "Three cath rooms (4,000 procedures in 1979)."

Angioplasty is first performed at TMH in March by Drs. Raizner, Winters, and John Lewis.

TMH bed capacity grows to 1,218.

TMH opens the Scurlock Tower, a Total Health Care Center devoted to the provision of high-quality ambulatory and preventive care. BCM's Department of Medicine opens its first clinic.

TMH begins cardiology teaching service, with cardiology A run by BCM, cardiology B run by The Chapman group, and cardiology C run by Dr. William R. Gaston.

1980   Drs. Nadim Zacca, Raizner, and Noon perform first rotational atherectomy at TMH using a diamond- tipped file to wear down arterial plaque.

Dr. DeBakey and TMH surgical team perform a splenectomy on the Shah of Iran in Cairo, Egypt, on March 23.

Dr. William H. Spencer is the first at TMH to implant the Cordis dual-chamber pacemaker in the early '80s.

1981   Chez Eddy Restaurant opens in Scurlock Tower.

1982   TMH receives additional three-year grant of $9.2 million from the NIH to support the National Research and Demonstration Center.

Dr. Cooley resumes heart transplantation efforts at TCH and THI at SLEH after anti-rejection drug cyclosporine becomes available.

Ted Bowen resigns as president of TMH due to poor health.

Ella F. Fondren dies at age 101 after living in TMH for the last five years of her life.

Dr. Richard Miller resigns as chief of cardiology; Dr. Quiñones serves as acting chief.

Dr. Robert Roberts is named chief of cardiology at BCM and TMH and serves for the next 20 years; by 1982 there are 10-12 cardiologists on the BCM full-time staff and 20-plus in private practice.

BCM and TMH begin a five-year cardiology training program that integrates training in clinical cardiology and research under the direction of Dr. Roberts.

1983   Mr. Larry Mathis is named president of TMH.

Government initiates payment for "diagnosis-related groups," or DRGs.

TMH establishes a one-year elective training in echocardiography.

TMH establishes a one-year elective training in interventional cardiology.

1984   As part of the thrombolysis in myocardial infarction trial, TMH physicians are among the first to administer clot-dissolving drugs directly to the coronary artery to treat heart attack patients.

TMH helicopter service is established.

Anti-rejection drug cyclosporine receives FDA approval.

Drs. DeBakey and Noon resume heart transplants at TMH.

Multiorgan transplant center is established at TMH and BCM under the direction of Dr. Young, who is clinical coordinator and scientific director.

Texas Heart Institute forms Cardiovascular Care Providers, which establishes a bundled payment plan for bypass surgery.

Dr. Raizner first articulates the need for a unifying vision to recognize the accomplishments of many components of TMH cardiovascular community.

Dr. Gotto assumes presidency of the American Heart Association.

1984   TMH radiologist Dr. Jack Roehm develops inferior vena cava
             "Bird's nest filter."

1985   NHLBI launches the National Cholesterol Education Program (NCEP) in
             November.

             Dr. Stanley Crawford and son, Dr. John L. Crawford II, publish *Diseases of the
             Aorta and an Atlas of Angiographic Pathology and Surgical Techniques,*

             TMH creates the Michael E. DeBakey Heart Center, while Dr. DeBakey raises
             $5 million to establish the Michael E. DeBakey Heart Center Foundation,
             which continues to support the center to this day.

             Dr. Gotto is named scientific director of the Michael E. DeBakey Heart Center
             at BCM and TMH.

             The Living Heart Diet is published 1985, with Drs. Gotto, DeBakey, Foreyt and
             nutritionist Lynn Scott serving as coauthors.

             A mobile cath Lab is established by The Chapman group.

             The Chapman group establishes a satellite office at Rosewood Hospital
             in Houston, Polly Ryon Hospital in Richmond, and in Baytown and
             Jasper, Texas.

             Physicians at TMH perform the first heart-lung transplant in Texas and one of
             the first in the country.

             Dr. William A. Zoghbi joins BCM cardiology faculty at TMH and later
             becomes director of the echo lab.

             TMH is one of three institutions to simultaneously discover that radiation
             immediately following angioplasty dramatically reduces restenosis, with Dr.
             Raizner being the first to test this in patients.

             Dr. Chapman receives the first Laureate Award for the Texas Chapter of the
             American College of Physicians.

             Dr. Hartwell Whisennand performs the first liver transplant at TMH.

1986   TMH establishes the annual Richard Van Reet Award for the outstanding
             cardiology fellow.

             TMH establishes the Center for Research in Cardiovascular Interventions,
             naming Dr. Raizner its executive director. Drs. Raizner and Steven Minor form
             Interventional Cardiology Associates, later joined by Drs. Clement DeFelice,
             Gopi Shah, and Michael Raizner (son of Dr. Al Raizner).

1987   The American Heart Association establishes the Bugher Training Program in
             Molecular Biology of the Cardiovascular System, naming Dr. Robert Roberts
             the principal investigator.

             The National Heart, Lung and Blood Institute awards a $14 million grant to
             form the National Research and Demonstration Center at BCM and TMH – a
             revival of the defunct super center that ended in 1982.

             TMH recognized as a Medicare-designated heart transplant center in Texas,
             one of the first seven in the country.

1987   Dr. Pratt serves as chairman of the U.S. Food and Drug Administration's
        Cardiovascular and Renal Drugs Advisory Committee through 1993.

        Dr. John J. Mahmarian joins BCM and TMH in nuclear cardiology after
        completing training at BCM.

        Dr. Neal S. Kleiman joins BCM full-time cardiology faculty at TMH.

        Dr. DeBakey receives the National Medal of Science from President Ronald
        Reagan.

1988   TMH opens Smith Tower to provide additional outpatient clinical space;
        TMH internal medicine service, including cardiology, moves offices and clinics
        to Smith Tower.

        Drs. Raizner, Minor, and Kleiman perform the country's second implantation
        of a stent to reinforce the artery wall during angioplasty.

        Dr. Jack Titus retires and Dr. Michael W. Lieberman is named chairman of the
        Department of Pathology at BCM and chief of pathology at TMH.

1989   The new Ben Taub General Hospital opens.

        Dunn Tower is constructed adjacent to TMH and brings total bed capacity to
        1,527, making TMH the largest private teaching hospital in the country.

        Dr. Kleiman becomes assistant director of TMH catheterization laboratories.

1990   Dr. Winters is named president of the ACC.

        The Health Care Financing Administration starts the Heart Bypass Center
        Demonstration Project, with TMH being one of seven participating hospitals
        in the country.

1991   Drs. Roberts and Pratt chair the ACC's 1991 Scientific Session.

        The new Houston Veterans Affairs Medical Center opens in June; with 1,000
        beds, it is the second largest federal building in the United States, exceeded
        only by the Pentagon.

        Dr. Inge Edler receives the ACC Distinguished Fellowship Award from ACC
        President William L. Winters Jr.

        Dr. Winters becomes the ACC representative of the AMA's newly formed
        Specialty Society Relative Value Scale Update Committee.

        The *Chez Eddy Living Heart Cookbook* is published.

        Dr. Winters is named chair of the newly established John S. Dunn Sr.
        Endowment for Cardiovascular Research and Education.

1992   Dr. Spencer is named head of the hospital's pacemaker clinic, serving until
        2000.

        The William L. Winters Jr., M.D., Annual Lectureship is established at TMH
        and BCM, with Dr. Francis Klocke as the first lecturer.

        Dr. E. Stanley Crawford dies on October 27.

1993   Dr. DeBakey retires as chairman of the BCM Department of Surgery in January.

Chez Eddy restaurant closes in September.

Dr. John W. Overstreet steps down as chief of the surgery department at TMH.

1994   BCM celebrates its 50th anniversary.

Drs. Winters and Spencer join the BCM cardiology full-time faculty at TMH.

Dr. Spencer starts interatrial septal pacing research.

BCM establishes the Don W. Chapman Chair in Cardiology and appoints Dr. Roberts as the first chair.

Drs. Gaston and John Lewis join full-time cardiology faculty at TMH.

Elected Department Deputy Chair Program is initiated by volunteer BCM faculty, which elects Dr. Winters as the first deputy chair of the Department of Medicine.

Scandinavian Simvastatin Survival Study commences.

TMH discusses possible merger with SLEH.

Dr. John C. Baldwin is appointed new chair of BCM Department of Surgery in July, replacing Dr. DeBakey.

Dr. Javier La Fuente joins cardiovascular surgery department at BCM.

Dr. Antonio Pacifico establishes the Texas Arrhythmia Institute.

1995   Dr. Mahesh K. Ramchandani joins cardiovascular surgery department at BCM.

1996   Dr. Ralph D. Feigin is named president of BCM.

Dr. George Cooper Morris Jr. dies.

Dr. Henry D. McIntosh receives the ACC Distinguished Service Award.

TMH and SLEH abandon merger plans.

Dr. Spencer introduces echo-guided alcohol ablation procedure at TMH to treat hypertrophic cardiomyopathy.

TMH secures its first HMO contract with HMO-CIGNA Healthcare in March.

Dr. Gotto leaves BCM to become dean of Cornell Medical College in New York; Dr. Andrew I. Schafer is appointed interim chair of the Department of Medicine.

Dr. DeBakey consults with President Boris N. Yeltsin about coronary bypass.

TMH joins 39 additional managed care plans by September, covering 2.5 million people.

The BCM /Methodist Primary Care Associates is formed.

Mr. Larry Mathis retires from TMH after serving as CEO for 13 years.

1996   TMH becomes The Methodist Health Care System, embracing TMH, Diagnostic Hospital, San Jacinto Methodist Hospital, and others in the future.

1997   Henry Pownall, Ph.D., is named chief of the section of atherosclerosis and lipoprotein research at BCM.

Texas Surgical Associates is founded.

The *New Living Heart*, authored by Drs. DeBakey and Gotto, is published.

Peter W. Butler is named CEO of TMH in September.

Upon Dr. Overstreet's retirement, TMH establishes the John W. Overstreet Award, with the first award going to Dr. Juan Olivero in 1998 and the second year to Dr. William L. Winters Jr. in 1999.

1998   Drs. Chapman and Winters are recognized for their 15-plus years of outstanding service to the ACC and become two of the first four fellows designated to receive the newly inaugurated Master of the American College of Cardiology award (MACC). The ACC announces it will limit the number of subsequent Master designations to four each year.

Dr. Roberts receives the ACC Distinguished Scientist Award.

Debra Feigin Sukin joins the TMH administrative staff.

Dr. Raizner and TMH colleagues participate in the Multi-Center Coronary Stent Trial.

BCM salutes Dr. DeBakey for 50 years of service.

Dr. Schafer is named chairman of the BCM Department of Medicine and serves until 2001.

Dr. Michael Reardon performs the first successful autotransplant for cardiac malignancy at TMH.

Dr. Gotto and colleagues at Weill Cornell Medical College participate in the Air Force/Texas Coronary Atherosclerosis Prevention Study.

1999   Mr. Ron Girotto retires as COO, and Dr. Lynn M. Schroth officially replaces him.

TMH joins University HealthService Consortium.

Ted Bowen dies on September 29.

2000   Dr. Joseph Coselli performs his 1,600th thoracoabdominal aortic aneurysm repair procedure at TMH, more than any other surgeon in the world; he leaves TMH in 2004 to join Dr. Cooley at THI.

Dr. Matthias Loebe joins the cardiovascular surgery department at BCM.

The MicroMed DeBakey Ventricular Assist Device is implanted for the first time in the United States.

The Winters Center for Heart Failure Research is established at BCM and TMH.

2000   Dr. Spencer is named Distinguished Medical Alumnus of Duke University Medical Center.

Dr. Raizner is named medical director of the Methodist DeBakey Heart Center (MDHC).

2001   Peter Butler resigns as CEO of TMH.

Ron Girotto returns as CEO of TMH on September 25.

TMH initiates discussions on plans for a north campus building that would house the cardiovascular and neurological service lines, including the MDHC.

Mary and Gordon Cain provide a $5 million grant to the Winters Center for Heart Failure Research.

Dr. Douglas L. Mann is named the Mary and Gordon Cain Chair of Internal Medicine at BCM and serves until 2005.

Dr. Eric K. Peden joins the cardiovascular surgery department at BCM.

Dr. Guillermo Torre-Amione begins clinical trial with immune modulation therapy (IMT), eventually leading to European approval.

Methodist DeBakey Heart Center is officially named and dedicated at TMH on February 19. Affiliated with BCM, it consists of 10 operating rooms, 8 cath labs, 154 acute-care beds, and 30 beds for transplant candidates.

Interventional cardiologist Dr. Clement A. DeFelice initiates the transcatheter procedure to close ostium secundum atrial septal defects at TMH.

Dr. Raizner develops "brachytherapy" to treat in-stent stenosis.

Dr. Mario S. Verani dies on October 30.

2002   The John S. Dunn Sr. Endowment establishes the chair in echocardiography at BCM, with Dr. William Zoghbi named to that position; it later becomes the William L. Winters Jr. Chair in Imaging after the separation of BCM and TMH.

Dr. Alan B. Lumsden joins the BCM Department of Surgery.

All aspects of TMH integrated health delivery system are discontinued in May.

Dr. McIntosh receives the ACC International Service Award.

The first Mario S. Verani Annual Lecture features Dr. George A. Beller.

Dr. Arthur C. Beall Jr. dies on December 8.

2003   Dr. Peter Traber is named president of BCM.

Dr. Kleiman opens one of the first stereotactic cardiac catheterization labs in the MDHC.

Dr. Quiñones is named medical director of the MDHC, succeeding Dr. Raizner.

2004   TMH board approves the building of a research institute, a new outpatient center, and a new 400-bed patient tower (North campus).

2004   TMH Physician Organization is formed on July 1.

Dr. Lieberman resigns as BCM pathology chairman to become TMH pathology chairman and director of the research institute.

Dr. Stephen B. Greenberg is named chairman of the Department of Medicine at BCM and serves until 2007.

Dr. Matthias Loebe performs the nation's first percutaneous implantation of a left ventricular assist device (LVAD) at MDHC.

The VA Medical Center is renamed the Michael E. DeBakey VA Medical Center.

MDHC begins publishing the *Methodist DeBakey Cardiovascular Journal*, a peer-reviewed quarterly publication.

Dr. Roberts leaves BCM and TMH to assume role of president, CEO, and chief scientific officer of the University of Ottawa Heart Institute; at his departure, there remains 46 full-time cardiology faculty at BCM, of which 11 are at TMH.

Dr. Zoghbi serves as interim chairman of the BCM cardiology section.

BCM and TMH end their 50-year-long affiliation on April 21.

TMH announces its affiliation with Weill Cornell Medical College in New York, where Dr. Gotto serves as dean and provost.

TMH and the University of Houston form a "long term agreement to expand health science and medical education programs as well as enhancing health care for the community," as stated in a memorandum from Mr. Girotto to the medical staff on October 12.

2005   Dr. Douglas L. Mann is named chief of the section of cardiology at BCM and SLEH/Texas Heart Institute and the Don W. Chapman Chair of Cardiology.

All BCM fellows and residents are abruptly removed from TMH on August 31.

Eleven cardiologists resign from BCM to form the Department of Cardiology at TMH on August 31.

Dr. Winters receives Houston's Most Fascinating Award from Friends of the Texas Medical Center Library.

Dr. Quiñones is named chief of the new Department of Cardiology at TMH.

Dr. Raizner is elected to deputy chairman of the Department of Cardiology at TMH.

TMH establishes an anesthesiology department, with Dr. Joseph J. Naples serving as chairman.

TMH becomes the first hospital in Texas to be recognized by the American Heart Association and the American Stroke Association in their "Get with the Guidelines" Program, which measures and identifies hospitals that meet high-quality measures for treating heart disease.

2005   Drs. Lumsden and Reardon perform the country's first hybrid vascular procedure at TMH to repair a large aneurysm of the aortic arch, combining a catheter stent with a surgical intervention.

2006   Dr. Christie M. Ballantyne is named chief of the section of atherosclerosis and vascular medicine, which was previously named the section of atherosclerosis and lipoprotein research at BCM and TMH.

TMH Institute of Education is established, with Dr. Winters serving as chairman.

Dr. Winters receives the Neuhaus Institute of Learning "ICON" Award.

TMH becomes affiliated with the University of Texas Medical Branch in Galveston's cardiology training program, which is ACGME approved.

Dr. DeBakey undergoes a successful surgical treatment in January for an acute type I aortic dissection by Dr. Noon.

The inaugural TMH Humanitarian Award is presented to heart surgeon Dr. Rafael Espada for his work in Guatemala and Houston.

Dr. Jean Bismuth joins the MDHC surgery department.

2007   Drs. Miguel Valderrabano, Stephen Little, and Jerry Estep join the MDHC Department of Cardiology; Brian Bruckner, the MDHC Surgery Department.

Dr. David Tweardy, chief of the infectious disease section, begins serving as interim chair of the Department of Medicine at BCM in September.

Dr. Gerald Lawrie performs the world's first "American Correction" mitral valve repair using the da Vinci surgical robot at the MDHC.

Dr. Roberts receives the Master of the ACC award.

Dr. Michael Schneider leaves BCM to become chairman of cardiology at the Imperial College of London.

Dr. Chapman dies on May 3.

After three decades in cardiovascular surgery at BCM and TMH, Dr. Espada gives up his practice to seek the office of vice president of Guatemala. He and running mate Alvaro Colom win the election with nearly 53 percent of the vote.

2008   Methodist DeBakey Heart Center is renamed the Methodist DeBakey Heart & Vascular Center (MDHVC) at TMH.

Cardiologists Su Min Chang and Dipan J. Shah and cardiovascular surgeon Mark G. Davies join the MDHVC.

Dr. Robert F. Todd is named chair of the Department of Medicine at BCM in September.

Dr. Lumsden is named chair of TMH's department of cardiovascular surgery.

Dr. Nadim Nasir replaces Dr. Raizner as the elected deputy chairman of cardiology at TMH.

2008   Dr. Winters receives the Wellsprings Medical Legend Award.

Dr. DeBakey receives the Congressional Gold Medal from President George W. Bush on April 23.

MDHVC begins groundbreaking stem cell research for treating cardiac and vascular diseases.

MDHVC hosts "Pumps & Pipes," a unique conference designed to cultivate unique research opportunities between Houston's two largest industries, medicine and energy.

MDHVC teams with the Houston Texans and the American Red Cross to train thousands of Houstonians in CPR and automated external defibrillator (AED) use.

MDHVC is one of the first to repair a leak surrounding a patient's prosthetic mitral valve with a transcatheter technique that employs three-dimensional echocardiography.

Dr. DeBakey dies on July 11.

The first Michael E. DeBakey lectureship features Dr. Bobby Alford on January 16.

2009   Dr. James K. Alexander dies on March 29.

Dr. Ballantyne is named interim chief, section of cardiology, Department of Medicine, at BCM.

Dr. Davies is appointed vice chairman of the cardiovascular surgery department at TMH.

Dr. Lumsden is named medical director of the MDHVC.

Dr. Hosam F. El Sayed joins the MDHVC surgery department.

MDHVC opens a new multidisciplinary valve clinic for patients with complex cardiac valve disease.

The inaugural Leading Hearts Gala is held on October 24, benefitting the MDHVC and raising more than $1.1 million.

2010   Dr. Manus O'Donnell dies on March 22.

Dr. Zoghbi becomes president of the American Society of Echocardiography (ASE).

The MDHVC opens a new multidisciplinary aortic network dedicated to patients across Houston with aortic disease.

The George P. Noon, MD, Award is established at TMH.

Dr. Lumsden is appointed as the Walter W. Fondren III Distinguished Endowed Chair and medical director of the MDHVC.

Drs. George Schroth, Faisal Nabi, Amish Dave, and Sanjay Kunapuli join MDHVC's Department of Cardiology.

Dr. Lewis dies on January 13.

2010   Dr. Gaston dies on March 1.

2011   Dr. Ballantyne is named chief, section of cardiology, Department of Medicine, at BCM. Continues to serve as chief of the section of cardiovascular research and chief of the division of atherosclerosis and vascular medicine at BCM.

The Cardiovascular Education Fund is established in the name of Dr. Don W. Chapman as a gift from the William L. Winters family.

MDHVC is ranked No. 19 in the country in the *U.S. News & World Report* annual Best Hospitals issue.

Dr. Winters receives the first George P. Noon, MD, Award.

MDHVC launches a first-of-its-kind national center for comprehensive continuing medical education in cardiovascular and vascular disease, called the DeBakey Institute for Cardiovascular Education and Training (DICET).

The Methodist Hospital announced in June that the 2012 groundbreaking plans for the North Campus were being placed on hold due to the uncertainty of health care reform and the economy.

Dr. Mahmarian becomes president of American Nuclear Cardiology Society.

TMH welcomes the first class of four cardiology fellows in its new ACGME-approved cardiology training program.

Dr. Winters receives the Laureate Award from the American College of Physicians' South Texas Chapter.

2012   Dr. Quiñones receives the MACC award.

Dr. Zoghbi receives the MACC award and becomes president of the ACC.

Dr. Quiñones receives the Lifetime Achievement Award of the ASE.

Dr. C. Huie Lin joins the MDHVC.

Dr. Barry Trachtenberg joins the MDHVC.

Mrs. Don W. Chapman establishes the MDHVC eLibrary in the name of Dr. Winters.

As ACC president, Dr. Zoghbi is selected to participate in the 8,000-mile Olympic Torch Relay as one of the torchbearers carrying the flame across the United Kingdom in the 70-day lead-up to the summer Olympic opening ceremonies.

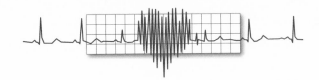

MICHAEL ELLIS DEBAKEY, MD
Selected Major Awards and Honors

2000s

- Congressional Gold Medal (2008)
- Lasker Clinical Medical Research Award renamed as the Lasker DeBakey Clinical Medical Research Award (2007)
- History Making Texan Award, the Texas State History Museum Foundation (2006)
- The Association of American Medical Colleges David E. Rogers Award (2004)
- Veterans Affairs Medical Center named in DeBakey's honor (2004)
- American Heart Association Lifetime Achievement Award (2003)
- Lomonosov Large Gold Medal, Russian Academy of Sciences (2003)
- The Ben Taub Humanitarian Award (2003)
- Medal of Merit, International Academy of Cardiovascular Sciences (2002)
- MUSC "Lindbergh-Carrel Prize" (2002)
- International Academy of Cardiovascular Sciences Medal for Distinguished Achievements in Cardiovascular Sciences (2002)
- NASA Invention of the Year Award (2001)
- Houston Hall of Fame (2001)
- Villanova University Mendel Medal Award (2001)

- Library of Congress Bicentennial Living Legend Award (2000)
- American Philosophical Society Jonathan Rhoads Medal (2000)
- American Medical Association Virtual Mentor Award (2000)

1990s

- Lifetime Achievement Award for Science and Technology from Children Uniting Nations (1999)
- Texas Senate and House of Representatives, Adoption of Resolutions honoring Dr. DeBakey for 50 years of medical practice in Texas (1999)
- Russian Academy of Sciences Foreign Member (1999)
- John P. McGovern Compleat Physician Award (1999)
- Research!America's Lifetime Achievement Award (1998)
- Karolinska Institute's Honorary Degree of Doctor of Medicine and the title "Foreign Adjunct Professor" (1997)
- Russian Military Medical Academy, Boris Petrovsky International Surgeons Award and First Laureate of the Boris Petrovsky Gold Medal (1997)
- Premio Giuseppe Corradi Award for Surgery and Scientific Research (1997)
- Common Wealth Award, Sigma Xi
- Health Care Hall of Fame (1996)
- Women's International Center Samaritan Living Legacy Award (1994)
- Giovanni Lorenzini Foundation Prize for the Advancement of Biomedical Science (1994)
- Texas Society for Biomedical Research Distinguished Service Award (1994)
- American Heart Association Lifetime Achievement Award (1994)
- Foundation for Biomedical Research Lifetime Achievement Award (1991)
- American College of Healthcare Executives Honorary Fellow (1990)
- American Legion Distinguished Service Award (1990)
- The Michael DeBakey Medal, American Society of Mechanical Engineers (1990)
- William Procter Prize for Scientific Achievement, Sigma Xi

1980s

- The Michael DeBakey Medal, American Society of Mechanical Engineers (1989)

- Association of American Medical Colleges Special Recognition Award (1988)

- Academy of Surgical Research Markowitz Award (1988)

- National Medal of Science (1987)

- Theodore E. Cummings Memorial Prize for Outstanding Contributions in Cardiovascular Disease (1987)

- First President of the Association of International Vascular Surgeons (1983)

- Institute of Medicine of the National Academy of Sciences (1982)

- Chair of the Board of Governors, Foundation for Biomedical Research (1981)

- American Surgical Association Distinguished Service Award (1981)

- Veterans of Foreign Wars Commander-in-Chief's Medal and Citation (1980)

- Merit Order of the Republic of Egypt, First Class (1980)

- Independence of Jordan Medal (1980)

1970s

- Texas Scientist of the Year, Texas Academy of Science (1979)

- Michael E. DeBakey International Cardiovascular Surgical Society formed by DeBakey's former students; name was later changed to the Michael E. DeBakey International Surgical Society to include more of his surgical residents and trainees (1976)

- U.S.S.R. Academy of Science 50th Anniversary Jubilee Medal (1973)

1960s

- Presidential Medal of Freedom with Distinction (1969)

- Eleanor Roosevelt Humanities Award (1969)

- American Heart Association Gold Heart Award (1968)

- Prix International Dag Hammarskjold Great Collar with Golden Medal (1967)

- American Medical Association Billings Gold Medal Exhibit Award (1967)

- Medical World News Doctor of the Year (1965)

- Albert Lasker Award for Clinical Medical Research (1963)

1950s

- American Medical Association Distinguished Service Award (1959)
- Leriche Award (1959)
- International Society of Surgery Distinguished Service Award (1958)
- American Medical Association Hektoen Gold Medal Award (1954 and 1970)
- Rudolph Matas Award in Vascular Surgery (1954)

1940s

- Task Force on Medical Services of the Hoover Commission on Organization of the Executive Branch of the Government (1949)
- Legion of Merit, United States Army (1945)

Additional Honors

- Tulane Medical Alumni Association
- International Health and Medical Film Festival
- International College of Angiology
- Encyclopedia Britannica
- Lifetime Achievement Awards from the Academy of Medical Films

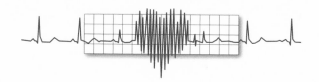

ENDNOTES

Chapter 1: Perseverance, 1948

1. Carter BN, DeBakey ME. War wounds of the extremities. *Bull Am Coll Surg.* 1944;29: 117-121.
2. DeBakey ME, Simeone FA. Battle injuries of the arteries in World War II: an analysis of 2471 cases. *Am Surg.* 1946;123: 534-579.
3. Ochsner AJ, Dixon L, DeBakey ME. Primary bronchoiogenic carcinoma. *Chest.* Official Publication of the American College of Chest Physicians. 1945;11; 97-129.
4. Tulane University Health Sciences Center Rudolph Matas Library; History and Archives. The Sixth Charity Rises. www.tulane.edu/~matas/historical/charity/charity7.htm. Accessed August 29, 2013.
5. Ochsner A, DeBakey ME. Primary pulmonary malignancy: Treatment by total pneumonectomy; analysis of collected cases and presentation of 7 personal cases. *Surg Gyn Obstet.* 1939;68:435-451.
6. DeBakey ME. Historical perspectives of the American Association for Thoracic Surgery: Alton Ochsner, MD (1896-1981). *J Thorac Cardiovasc Surg.* 2005;130(3): 875.
7. DeBakey ME. A conversation with the editor, Interview with William C. Roberts. *Am J Cardiol.* 1997;79(7): 929-950.
8. Gillentine WH, DeBakey ME. New method of syringe transfusion. *New Orleans Med Surg J.* 1934;87: 386-389.
9. McCollum CH. The distinguished service award medal for the Society of Vascular Surgery, 1999: Michael Ellis DeBakey, MD. *J Vasc Surg.* 2000;31(2): 406-409.
10. DeBakey ME. A simple continuous-flow blood transfusion instrument. *New Orleans Med Surg J.* 1934;87: 386-389.
11. DeBakey ME. John Gibbon and the heart-lung machine: a personal encounter and his import for cardiovascular surgery. *Ann Thorac Surg.* 2003;76: S2188-2194.
12. Miller BJ, Gibbon JH, Gibbon MH. Recent advances in the development of a mechanical heart and lung apparatus. *Ann Surg.* 1951;134: 694.
13. Wilds J, Harkey I. *Alton Ochsner, Surgeon of the South.* Baton Rouge and London: Louisiana State University Press; 1990.
14. Ochsner A, DeBakey M. Subphrenic abscess: a collective review and an analysis of 3,608 collected and personal cases. *Int Abstr Surg.* 1938;66: 426-438.

15. DeBakey ME. Kismet or assidiuty? *Surgery.* 2005;137(2): 255-256.
16. Outlaw WN. Soldier, Surgeon, Statesman. *Vanguard, U.S. Department of Veterans Affairs.* 2008;May/June: 20-21.
17. King B, Jatoi I. The Mobile Army Surgical Hospital (MASH): A Military and Surgical Legacy. *J Nat'l Med Assoc.* 2005;97(5): 648-656.
18. Carter BN, DeBakey ME. Current observations on war wounds of the chest. *J Thorac Surg.* 1944;13: 271-293.
19. DeBakey ME, Carter BN. Current considerations on war wounds of the chest. *Am Surg.* 1945;121:545-563.
20. Surgeon general praises record of army physicians. *Associated Press.* 1944 Oct 7.
21. DeBakey, Michael Ellis (Methodist DeBakey Heart & Vascular Center, The Methodist Hospital, Houston, TX). Conversation with: William L. Winters Jr. (Methodist DeBakey Heart & Vascular Center, The Methodist Hospital, Houston, TX). 2007 Dec 20.
22. DeBakey ME. History, the torch that illuminates: lessons from military medicine. *Military Medicine.* 1996;161: 711-716.
23. Bradley ON, Blair C. *A General's Life, An Autobiography by General of the Army Omar N. Bradley.* New York, NY: Simon & Shuster; 1983.
24. Roosevelt E. My Day. *United Feature Syndicate, Inc.* 1945 May 22.
25. U.S. Department of Veterans Affairs. *Policy Memorandum No. 2: Policy in association of veterans' hospitals with medical schools.* U.S. Department of Veterans Affairs. www.va.gov/oaa/Archive/PolicyMemo2.pdf. Accessed 2013 Sep 3.
26. Berkowitz ED, Santangelo MJ. *The Medical Follow-up Agency, The First Fifty Years 1946–1996.* Washington, D.C.: National Academy Press; 1999.
27. McComb, David. *Oral History Interview of Michael E. DeBakey from the Lyndon Baines Johnson Library.* Bethesda, MD: National Library of Medicine; 1969.
28. DeBakey ME. Military surgery in World War II: a backward glance and a forward look. *N Engl J Med.* 1947;236: 341-350.
29. Stoney WS. *Pioneers of Cardiac Surgery.* Nashville, TN: Vanderbilt University Press; 2008.
30. Baylor Names Chairman of Surgery Unit. *Houston Chronicle.* 1948 Jul 21.
31. Moursund WH. *A History of Baylor University College of Medicine, 1900-1953.* Houston, TX: Gulf Printing Company; 1956.
32. Jones RC. History of the Department of Surgery at Baylor Medical Center. *Proc (Bayl Univ Med Cent).* 2004;17(2): 130–167.
33. Truman HS. Annual Budget Message to the Congress: Fiscal Year 1950. The American Presidency Project. www.presidency.ucsb.edu/ws/?pid=13434. Accessed 2013 Sep 3.
34. Magnuson PB. *Ring the Night Bell, the autobiography of a surgeon.* Boston, MA: Little, Brown & Company; 1960.
35. Black HS, Cunningham GR. *A Brief History Of The Houston Veterans Hospital And Its Research Program 1949 – 2003.* Houston, TX: Homer S. Black, Ph.D.; 2005. http://www.homersblack.com/VA%20History%20Pamphlet.htm. Accessed 2013 Sep 3.

Chapter 2: Deliberate Decisions by Strong Women, 1924-1929

1. Chapman BT. Early business leaders gave gifts of life to Methodist Hospital. *Houston Business Journal.* March 7, 2008.
2. Brown PH, Broeske PH. *Howard Hughes: The Untold Story.* Cambridge, MA: Da Capo Press; 2004:6.
3. Advertisement for Norsworthy Hospital. Medical Insurance and Health Conservation. 1910; 19(9): XVI.
4. Carroll BH. *Standard History of Houston Texas from a Study of the Original Sources.* Knoxville, TN: H. W. Crew & Co.; 1912:136.
5. The Bell Home Helped Shape Houston's History. *Midtown Paper, a publication of Midtown Management District.* 2007 2nd Qtr.

6. Speer, James B. (The Methodist Hospital History Project, The Methodist Hospital Archives at The John P. McGovern Historical Collections and Research Center in the Texas Medical Center Library, Houston, TX). Interview with: Mrs. Josie Mooring Roberts (The Methodist Hospital, Houston,TX). 1975 Mar.

7. Sibley MM. *The Methodist Hospital of Houston, Serving the World*. Austin, TX: Texas State Historical Association; 1989:43.

8. Sibley MM. *The Methodist Hospital of Houston, Serving the World*. Austin, TX: Texas State Historical Association; 1989:44.

9. Sibley MM. *The Methodist Hospital of Houston, Serving the World*. Austin, TX: Texas State Historical Association; 1989:73.

10. Cornerstone Laid For New Hospital. *Houston Post*. June 1, 1950.

11. Sibley MM. *The Methodist Hospital of Houston, Serving the World*. Austin, TX: Texas State Historical Association; 1989:77.

12. H.R. Cullens Give $1,000,000 for New Methodist Hospital. *Houston Post*. March 4, 1945.

13. Speer, James B. (The Methodist Hospital History Project, The Methodist Hospital Archives at The John P. McGovern Historical Collections and Research Center in the Texas Medical Center Library, Houston, TX). Interview with: Ted Bowen (The Methodist Hospital, Houston TX). 1978 Dec.

14. Bowen T. The Methodist Hospital, Houston, Texas: Its Past, Present, and Future. Speech to the medical staff at The Methodist Hospital. 1965 Nov 1: Houston, TX.

15. Houston Hospital Makes Record And Confronts Future With Hope. *The Southwestern Advocate*. November 11, 1948

16. Fuermann G. *Houston: Land of the Big Rich*. Garden City, NY: Doubleday & Company, Inc.; 1951:198.

17. Hurt H III. *A Trust Corrupted, A City Betrayed, Part One. Texas Monthly*. 1986;14(2):178.

18. Sibley MM. *The Methodist Hospital of Houston, Serving the World*. Austin, TX: Texas State Historical Association; 1989:88.

19. Speer, James B. (The Methodist Hospital History Project, The Methodist Hospital Archives at The John P. McGovern Historical Collections and Research Center in the Texas Medical Center Library, Houston, TX). Interview with: Mrs. W. W. Fondren (Philanthropist, Houston, TX). 1975 Mar.

20. Guide to Walter W. and Ella F. Fondren Papers, 1838-1973, MS 390. Rice University Fondren Library website. http://library.rice.edu/collections/WRC/finding-aids/manuscripts/0390. Accessed September 4, 2013.

21. Lynch EC. Evolution of Baylor Medicine Training: 1943 to 2000. First Annual Department of Medicine Resident Colloquium. Baylor College of Medicine, Houston, TX. 2001 Mar 10.

22. DeBakey ME. A conversation with the editor, Interview with William C. Roberts. *Am J Cardiol*. 1997;79(7): 929-50.

23. Sibley MM. *The Methodist Hospital of Houston, Serving the World*. Austin, TX: Texas State Historical Association; 1989:114.

Chapter 3: Assembling the Team, 1943-1950

1. Who's Who – Ben Taub (1889-1982). Houston History website. http://www.houstonhistory.com/citizens/whoswho/business/history22hof.htm. Accessed September 5, 2013.

2. DeBakey, Michael Ellis (Methodist DeBakey Heart & Vascular Center, The Methodist Hospital, Houston, TX). Interview with: William L. Winters Jr. (Methodist DeBakey Heart & Vascular Center, The Methodist Hospital, Houston, TX). 2007 Dec 20.

3. Thompson T. *Hearts; of surgeons and transplants, miracles and disasters along the cardiac frontier*. New York, NY: The McCall Publishing Company; 1971:11.

4. Thompson T. *Hearts; of surgeons and transplants, miracles and disasters along the cardiac frontier*. New York, NY: The McCall Publishing Company; 1971:12.

5.   Chapman DW, ed. *Heart, Helicopters, and Houston (Fifty Golden Years of Heart Disease as seen by an Insider)*. Austin, TX: Nortex Press; 1996:52.

6.   Moursund WH Sr., ed. *A History of Baylor University College of Medicine, 1900-1953*. Houston, TX: Gulf Printing Company; 1956:168.

7.   DeBakey ME. Michael Ellis DeBakey: a conversation with the editor. Interview by William C. Roberts. *Am J Cardiol*. 1997;79(7): 929-950.

8.   Chapman DW, ed. *Heart, Helicopters, and Houston (Fifty Golden Years of Heart Disease as seen by an Insider)*. Austin, TX: Nortex Press; 1996:53.

9.   Forssman W. Die Sondierung des rechten Herzens. *Wien Klin Wschr*. 1929;8: 2085-2087.

10.   Cournand A, Ranges HA. Catheterization of the right auricle. *Proc Soc Exp Biol Med*. 1941;46:462-466.

11.   Dexter L, Haynes FW, Burwell CS, et al. Studies of congenital heart disease; the pressure and oxygen content of blood in the right auricle, right ventricle, and pulmonary artery in control patients, with observations on the oxygen saturation and source of pulmonary capillary blood. *J Clin Invest*. 1947 May;26(3):554-60.

12.   Chapman, Don (The Methodist Hospital, Houston, TX). Conversation with: William L. Winters Jr. (Methodist DeBakey Heart & Vascular Center, The Methodist Hospital, Houston, TX). 2006 Jan 25.

13.   Gross RE, Hubbard JP. Surgical litigation of a patent ductus arteriosus. Report of a first successful case. *J Am Med Assoc*. 1939;112:729-731.

14.   Crafoord C, Nylin G. Congenital coarctation of the aorta and its surgical treatment. *J Thorac Surg*. 1945;14: 347-61.

15.   Blalock A, Taussig HB. The surgical treatment of malformations of the heart in which there is pulmonary stenosis or pulmonary atresia. J Am Med Assoc. 1945;128: 189-202.

16.   Chapman, Don (The Methodist Hospital, Houston, TX). Conversation with: William L. Winters Jr. (Methodist DeBakey Heart & Vascular Center, The Methodist Hospital, Houston, TX). 2004 Feb 4.

17.   Chapman DW, Gugle LJ. Intravenous catheterization of the heart in the diagnosis of congenital heart disease. J Lab Clin Med. 1948;33(11): 1489.

18.   Chapman DW, ed. *Heart, Helicopters, and Houston (Fifty Golden Years of Heart Disease as seen by an Insider)*. Austin, TX: Nortex Press; 1996:73.

19.   Chapman DW, Earle DM, Gugle LJ, Huggins RA, Zimdahl W. Intravenous catheterization of the heart in suspected congenital heart disease; report of 72 cases. *Arch Intern Med* (Chic). 1949;84(4): 640-59.

20.   Surgeon tells of new relief from artery hardening. *Houston Chronicle*. January 15, 1949.

21.   DeBakey ME, Ochsner A. Critical evaluation of sympathectomy in peripheral vascular disease. *Wis Med J*. 1949;48: 689-698.

22.   Leahy J. Homicide rate on track to be worst in a decade. *Houston Chronicle*. October 21, 2006.

23.   DeBakey ME, Amsparker WH. Acute arterial injuries. *Surg Clin North Am*. 1949;29: 1513-1522.

24.   Johnson M. Baylor, helped by the Army, studies blood vessels. *Houston Post*. February 14, 1949.

25.   Cearnal L. Dr. Michael DeBakey's contributions to emergency care and trauma care. *Ann Emerg Med*. 2009;53(1): 10A.

26.   DeBakey LA. Tribute: Oscar Creech Jr., M.D., 1916-1967. *Arch Surg*. 1968;96: 483-484.

27.   Affiliation agreement between the trustees of Baylor University and the trustees of The Methodist Hospital located in the City of Houston and Harris County, Texas. Xerox copy of original document dated October 3, 1950.

28.   Sibley MM. *The Methodist Hospital of Houston, Serving the World*. Austin, TX: Texas State Historical Association; 1989:112.

29.   Affiliation agreement between the trustees of Baylor University and the trustees of The Methodist Hospital located in the City of Houston and Harris County, Texas. Xerox copy of original document dated October 3, 1950.

30.   Brunicardi FC. Residency Program at Michael E. DeBakey Department of Surgery, Baylor College of Medicine. *Arch Surg*. 2003;138: 582-584.

31. George C. Morris Jr., M.D. The Michael E. DeBakey Department of Surgery, Baylor College of Medicine website. http://www.bcm.edu/surgery/index.cfm?pmid=15110. Updated June 7, 2012. Accessed September 6, 2013.

32. Minetree H. *Cooley: The Career of a Great Heart Surgeon*. New York, NY: Harper & Row, Publishers, Inc.; 1973:126.

33. Lord Brock – cardiac surgery. British Cardiovascular Society website. http://www.bcs.com/pages/Lord%20Brock_cardiac_surgery.asp. Accessed September 6, 2013.

34. Minetree H. *Cooley: The Career of a Great Heart Surgeon*. New York, NY: Harper & Row, Publishers, Inc.; 1973:111.

35. Maxwell, Zella (Texas Children's Hospital History Project, Texas Children's Hospital Archives, The John P. McGovern Historical Collections and Research Center in The Texas Medical Center Library Houston, TX). Interview with: Denton A. Cooley (Texas Heart Institute, Houston, TX). 1979 Jul.

36. Livesay JJ, Messner GN, Vaughn WK. Milestones in the treatment of aortic aneurysm, Denton A. Cooley, M.D., and the Texas Heart Institute. *Tex Heart I J*. 2005;32(2):131-135.

37. Minetree H. *Cooley: The Career of a Great Heart Surgeon*. New York, NY: Harper & Row, Publishers, Inc.; 1973:108.

38. Minetree H. *Cooley: The Career of a Great Heart Surgeon*. New York, NY: Harper & Row, Publishers, Inc.; 1973:117.

39. Minetree H. *Cooley: The Career of a Great Heart Surgeon*. New York, NY: Harper & Row, Publishers, Inc.; 1973:122.

40. Combs CN. Aneurysm of the aorta; report of case. *Ill Med J*. 1910;18:650-652.

41. Hunt CL. Syphilitic cardiovascular disease. Can Med Assoc J. 1952;66:324-328.

42. Bahnson HT. Consideration in the excision of aortic aneurysms. *Ann Surg*. 1953;138(3):377-386.

43. Cooley DA, DeBakey ME. Surgical considerations of intrathoracic aneurysms of the aorta and great vessels. *Ann Surg*. 1952;135:660-680.

44. Minetree H. *Cooley: The Career of a Great Heart Surgeon*. New York, NY: Harper & Row, Publishers, Inc.; 1973:128.

45. Cooley DA. Early development of surgical treatment for aortic aneurysms, personal recollections. Tex Heart I J. 2001;28(3):197-199.

46. Cooley DA, DeBakey ME, Chapman DW. The surgical treatment of mitral stenosis by commissurotomy: report of fifty cases. Am J Surg. 1953;19(2):165-173.

47. Cooley DA, DeBakey ME, Skaggs RH, Chapman DW. Surgical treatment of mitral and aortic valve stenosis: results of 115 valvotomies. *Surg Med*. 1954;50:19-26.

Chapter 4: Inside the Beating Heart, 1949-1956

1. Sibley MM. *The Methodist Hospital of Houston, Serving the World*. Austin, TX: Texas State Historical Association; 1989:133

2. Speer, James B. (The Methodist Hospital History Project, The Methodist Hospital Archives at The John P. McGovern Historical Collections and Research Center in the Texas Medical Center Library, Houston, TX). Interview with: Mr. and Mrs. Ted Bowen (The Methodist Hospital, Houston TX). 1978 Dec.

3. Mrs. Roberts to Quit At Hospital. *Houston Post*. December 30, 1952.

4. Methodist Hospital Has Modern Gadgets. *Houston Chronicle*. November 9, 1951.

5. Hospital Progresses Under Woman Leader. *Houston Chronicle*. November 11, 1951.

6. Sibley MM. *The Methodist Hospital of Houston, Serving the World*. Austin, TX: Texas State Historical Association;132

7. Speer, James B (The Methodist Hospital History Project, The Methodist Hospital Archives at The John P. McGovern Historical Collections and Research Center in the Texas Medical Center Library, Houston, TX). Interview with: Mrs. Josie Mooring Roberts (The Methodist Hospital, Houston, TX). 1975 Mar.

8. Blackburn L. Meet Methodist's Ted Bowen, Youngest Head of a Big Hospital in Texas. *Houston Press*. February 27, 1953.

9. DeBakey ME, Cooley DA. Surgical treatment of aneurysm of abdominal aorta by resection and restoration of continuity with homograft surgery. Surg Gynecol Obstet. 1953;47:257-266.

10. DeBakey ME, Creech O Jr, Cooley DA. Occlusive disease of the aorta and its treatment by resection and homograft replacement. Am Surg. 1954;140:290-310.

11. Morse CFJ. Dead Man's Arteries Save Life of Wethersfield Man. *Hartford Courant*. July 8, 1955.

12. Associated Press. Rare Operation Patches Aorta With Accident Victim's Artery. *Toledo Blade*. November 18, 1952.

13. Gibbon JH. Application of a mechanical heart and lung apparatus to cardiac surgery. *Minn Med*. 1954;37:171-185.

14. Operation Success, Hospital Reports. UPI. The Methodist Hospital Archives at The John P. McGovern Historical Collections and Research Center in the Texas Medical Center Library. March 2, 1952

15. Gibbon JH, Hill JD. Part 1: the development of the first successful heart-lung machine. *Ann Thorac Surg*. 1982;34:337-341.

16. Cohn LH. Fifty years of open heart surgery. *Circulation*. 2003;107: 2168-2170.

17. Medicine: Sheriff's Graft. *Time*. June 29, 1953.

18. DeBakey ME, Cooley DA. Successful resection of aneurysm of thoracic aorta and replacement by graft. *J Am Med Assoc*. 1953;152(8): 673-676.

19. DeBakey ME. Michael Ellis DeBakey: a conversation with the editor. Interview by William C. Roberts. *Am J Cardiol*. 1997;79(7): 929-950.

20. Two Men Recovering After Unusual Surgery. *Houston Chronicle*. March 8, 1953.

21. DeBakey ME. Successful carotid endarterectomy for cerebrovascular insufficiency, nineteen-year follow-up. *J Am Med Assoc*. 1975;233(10): 1083-1085.

22. Chapman DW. *Heart, Helicopters, and Houston (Fifty Golden Years of Heart Disease as seen by an Insider)*. Austin, TX: Nortex Press; 1996:52.

23. The Methodist Hospital Medical Staff News Notes. *The Methodist Hospital Medical Staff News*. The Methodist Hospital Archives at The John P. McGovern Historical Collections and Research Center in the Texas Medical Center Library. 1954;1(7).

24. Chapman DW, Skaggs RH, Johnson IM, Mills LC, Cooley DA. Venous catheterization of the heart in selection of patients for mitral commissurotomy. *South Med J*. 1953;46(4): 343-347.

25. Chapman DW, Skaggs RH, Johnson IM, Mills LC, Cooley DA. Clinical selection and preoperative preparation of patients with mitral stenosis for surgical treatment (commissurotomy). *South Med J*. 1953;46(5): 439-442.

26. Maxwell, Zella (Texas Children's Hospital History Project, Texas Children's Hospital Archives, The John P. McGovern Historical Collections and Research Center in the Texas Medical Center Library Houston, TX). Interview with: Denton A. Cooley (Texas Heart Institute, Houston, TX). 1979 Jul.

27. DeBakey ME, Crawford ES, Cooley DA, Morris GC Jr. Successful resection of fusiform aneurysm of aortic arch with replacement by homograft. *Surg Gynecol Obstet*. 1957;105(6): 657-664.

28. DeBakey ME, Creech O Jr, Morris GC Jr. Aneurysm of thoracoabdominal aorta involving the celiac, superior mesenteric, and renal arteries; report of four cases treated by resection and homograft replacement. Ann Surg. 1956;144(4): 549-573.

29. DeBakey ME. Successful resection of aneurysm of distal aortic arch and replacement by graft. *J Am Med Assoc*. 1954;155(16): 1398-1403.

30. Cooley DA, DeBakey ME. Resection of entire ascending aorta in fusiform aneurysm using cardiac bypass. *J Am Med Assoc*. 1956;162(12): 1158-1159.

31. DeBakey ME, Cooley DA. Treatment of aneurysms of the aorta by resection and restoration of continuity with aortic homograft. *Angiology*. 1954;5(3): 251-254.

32. DeBakey ME, Blaisdell FW. The Society for Vascular Surgery: As I remember–An interview with Dr. Michael E. DeBakey. *J Vasc Surg*. 1996;23:1031-1034.

33. DeBakey ME, Cooley DA, Crawford ES, Morris GC Jr. Clinical applications of a new flexible knitted Dacron arterial substitute. *Arch Surg*. 1958;77:713-724.

34.   Crawford ES, DeBakey ME, Cooley DA. Clinical use of synthetic arterial substitutes in three hundred and seventeen patients. *Arch Surg.* 1958;76(2)L261-270.

35.   Kambic HE, Kantrowitz A, Sung P. STP 898: Vascular graft update: safety and performance. STP 898: West Conshohocken, PA: ASTM *International*; 1986:17.

36.   Ernst CB. In Memoriam, E. Stanley Crawford, 1922-1992. *J Vasc Surg.* 1993;17: 618-619.

37.   10 Million Watch TV Heart Surgery. *United Press.* December 4, 1954.

38.   DeBakey ME. The National Library of Medicine, Evolution of a Premier Information Center. *J Am Med Assoc.* 1991;266(9): 1252-1258.

39.   Miles WD. A History Of The National Library Of Medicine: The Nation's Treasury of Medical Knowledge. National Library of Medicine website. http://www.nlm.nih.gov/hmd/manuscripts/miles/miles.html, Updated January 18, 2012. Accessed September7, 2013.

40.   Rettig RA, *Cancer Crusade: The Story of the National Cancer Act of 1971.* Bloomington, IN: iUniverse Publishing; 2005:26.

41.   Drew EB. The Health Syndicate/Washington's Noble Conspirators. *The Atlantic Monthly.* December 1967, pages 75-82.

42.   The Mary Lasker Papers: Mary Lasker and the Growth of the National Institutes of Health. Profiles in Science, National Library of Medicine website. http://profiles.nlm.nih.gov/ps/retrieve/Narrative/TL/p-nid/200. Accessed September 7, 2013.

43.   Neen Hunt, Mary Woodward Lasker: First Lady of Medical Research. National Library of Medicine website. http://profiles.nlm.nih.gov/ps/retrieve/ResourceMetadata/TLBBMP. Updated December 13, 2007. Accessed September 7, 2013.

44.   Brozan N. Woman In The News: Mary Lasker; Lobbyist On A National Scale. *New York Times.* November 21, 1985.

45.   DeBakey ME. *Oral History Interview of Michael E. DeBakey from the Lyndon Baines Johnson Library.* Bethesda, MD: National Library of Medicine; 1969.

46.   Cohen RM. An Interview with Michael DeBakey. *Lasker Luminaries.* New York, NY: Albert and Mary Lasker Foundation; 2000.

47.   Collins HA, Harberg FJ, Soltero LR, McNamara DG, Cooley DA. Cardiac surgery in the newborn. *Surgery.* 1959;45: 506-519.

48.   Cooley DA. Early development of congenital heart surgery: open heart surgeries. *Ann Thorac Surg.* 1997:64(5):1544-1548.

49.   Lillehei CW, Varco RL, Cohen M, Warden HE, Patton C, Moller JH, The first open-heart repairs of ventricular septal defect, atrioventricular communis, and tetralogy of Fallot using extracorporeal circulation by cross-circulation: a 30-year follow-up. *Ann Thorac Surg.* 1986:1:4-21.

50.   Fedak PW. Open hearts: the origins of direct vision intracardiac surgery. *Tex Heart Inst J.* 1998;25(2):100-111.

51.   Lillehei CW, Cohen M, Warden HE, Varco RL. The direct-vision intracardiac correction of congenital anomalies by controlled cross circulation, results in thirty-two patients with ventricular septal defects, tetralogy of Fallot, and atrioventricularis communis defects. *Surgery.* 1955;38(1):11-29.

52.   Stoney WS. Historical perspectives in cardiology, evolution of cardiopulmonary bypass. *Circulation.* 2009;119: 2944-2853.

53.   DeWall RA, Gott VI, Lillehei CW, Read RC, Varco RI, Warden HF. Total body perfusion for open cardiotomy utilizing the bubble oxygenator: Physiologic responses in man. *J Thorac Cardiovasc Surg.* 1956;32: 591-603.

54.   Cooley DA. Recollections of early development and later trends in cardiac surgery. J Thorac Cardiovasc Surg. 1989;98(5 pt 2): 817-21..

55.   Minetree H. *Cooley: The Career of a Great Heart Surgeon.* New York, NY: Harper & Row, Publishers, Inc.; 1973:133

56.   Medicine: Surgery In the Heart. *Time.* April 30, 1956.

57.   Cooley DA. Recollections of early development and later trends in cardiac surgery. J Thorac Cardiovasc Surg. 1989;98(5 pt 2): 817-21.

Chapter 5: The Power of Persuasion, 1956-1960

1. Speer, James B. (The Methodist Hospital History Project, The Methodist Hospital Archives at The John P. McGovern Historical Collections and Research Center in the Texas Medical Center Library, Houston, TX). Interview with: Mr. and Mrs. Ted Bowen (The Methodist Hospital, Houston TX). 1978 Dec.

2. Winters Jr., William L. (Methodist DeBakey Heart & Vascular Center, The Methodist Hospital, Houston, TX). Interview with: Michael Ellis DeBakey (Methodist DeBakey Heart & Vascular Center, The Methodist Hospital, Houston, TX). 2007 Dec.

3. Maxwell, Zella (Texas Children's Hospital History Project, Texas Children's Hospital Archives, The John P. McGovern Historical Collections and Research Center in The Texas Medical Center Library Houston, TX). Interview with: Denton A. Cooley (Texas Heart Institute, Houston, TX). 1979 Jul.

4. Takach TJ, Ott DA. Congenital heart surgery in Houston, the early years. *Tex Heart I J.* 1997;24(3): 233-237.

5. Goor DA. *The Genius of C. Walton Lillehei and the True History of Open Heart Surgery.* New York, NY: Vantage Press; 2007:40.

6. Cooley DA, DeBakey ME, Morris GC Jr. Controlled extracorporeal circulation in surgical treatment of aortic aneurysm. *Ann Surg.* 1957;146(3): 473-485.

7. DeBakey ME. The odyssey of the artificial heart. *Artif Organs.* 2000;24(6): 405-411.

8. DeBakey ME. Development of mechanical heart devices. *Ann Thorac Surg.* 2005;79;S2228-31.

9. Stoney WS. *Pioneers in Cardiac Surgery.* Nashville, TN: Vanderbilt University Press; 2008:393.

10. DeBakey ME. A conversation with the editor, Interview with William C. Roberts. *Am J Cardiol.* 1997;79(7): 929-50.

11. Sibley MM. *The Methodist Hospital of Houston, Serving the World.* Austin, TX: Texas State Historical Association; 1989:149.

12. Wilburn G. Methodist Hospital will add 59 rooms. *Houston Chronicle.* September 7, 1958.

13. 24-bed unit ready at Methodist Hospital. *Houston Chronicle.* November 18, 1958/

14. Operating rooms play vital role in development of surgical procedures. *The Journal,* a publication of The Methodist Hospital, Houston. June 6, 1963.

15. DeBakey ME, Crawford ES, Morris GC, Cooley DA. Patch graft angioplasty in vascular surgery. *J Cardiovasc Surg.* 1962;3: 106-141.

16. Cooley DA, DeBakey ME, Crawford ES, Morris GC Jr. Surgery of the aorta and major arteries: experience with more than 2700 cases. *Medicine of Japan in 1959.* Tokyo, Proc. 15th Gen Assembly of Japan Med Cong. 1959;4: 491-494/

17. DeBakey ME. Presidential address: changing concepts in thoracic vascular surgery. *J Thorac Cardiovasc Surg.* 1959;38: 145-165.

18. Morris GC Jr, Cooley DA, DeBakey ME, Crawford ES. Coarctation of the aorta with particular emphasis upon improved techniques of surgical repair. *J Thorac Cardiovasc Surg.* 1960;40: 705-722.

19. DeBakey ME. Changing concepts in vascular surgery. *J Cardiovasc Surg.* 1960;1: 3-44.

20. Crawford ES, DeBakey ME. Arteriography in diagnosis and treatment of atherosclerotic occlusive vascular lesions. *Heart Bull.* 1959;8: 8-12.

21. Beall AC, Morris GC Jr, Crawford ES, Cooley DA, DeBakey ME. Translumbar aortography: re-evaluation. *Surgery.* 1961;49: 772-778.

22. DeBakey ME, Lawrie GM, Glaeser DH. Patterns of atherosclerosis and their surgical significance. *Am Surg.* 1985;201: 115-131.

23. Heart operation details released. *Houston Chronicle.* September 15, 1958.

24. Watson J. Four Houston specialists to speak at heart congress. *Houston Post.* September 15, 1958.

25. Cooley DA, Collins HA, Morris GC Jr, Soltero-Harrington LR, Harberg FJ. The pump oxygenator in cardiovascular surgery: observations based on 450 cases. *Am Surg.* 1958;24: 870-882.

26. Cooley DA, Morris GC Jr, Altar S. Cardiac myxoma: surgical treatment in four cases. *Arch Surg.* 1959;78: 410-417.

27. Morris GC Jr, Cooley DA, Crawford ES, Berry WB, DeBakey ME. Renal revascularization for hypertensions: clinical and physiologic studies in 32 cases. *Surgery*. 1960;48: 95-110.

28. Morris GC Jr, DeBakey ME, Cooley DA, Crawford ES. Surgical treatment of renal hypertension. *Am Surg*. 1960;151: 854-866.

29. Morris GC Jr, Edwards W, Cooley DA, Crawford ES, DeBakey ME. Surgical importance of profunda femoris artery: Analysis of 102 cases with combined aortoiliac and femoropopliteal occlusive disease treated by revascularization of deep femoral artery. *Arch Surg*. 1961;82: 32-37.

30. Neelakandhan KS. The challenge of aortic aneurysms. *India J Thorac Cardiovasc Surg*. 1995;11(1): 1-6.

31. Lemann N. Super medicine. *Texas Monthly*. April 1979.

32. Baylor surgery chief to address Russian doctors. *Houston Post*. December 11, 1958.

33. Wilburn G. Soviet visitor lauds local doctors' work. *Houston Chronicle*. January 20, 1959.

34. Brenner Drew E. The health syndicate/Washington's noble conspirators. *Atlantic Monthly*. December 1967;200: 75-82.

35. Rusk HA. The medical care issue, democrats' platform commits the party to social security plan in campaign. *The New York Times*. July 17, 1960.

36. Federal Support of Medical Research: Report of the Committee of Consultants on Medical Research to the Subcommittee on Departments of Labor and Health, Education, and Welfare of the Committee on Appropriations, United States Senate, 86th Congress, Second Session, May 1960. Washington, D.C.: U.S. Government Printing Office; 1960.

37. DeBakey ME, Crawford ES, Cooley DA, Morris GC Jr. Surgical considerations of occlusive disease of innominate, carotid, subclavian and vertebral arteries. *Ann Surg*. 1961;154(4): 698–725.

38. Crawford ES, DeBakey ME, Fields ME, Morris GS Jr, Cooley DA. Surgical consideration in the treatment of cerebral arterial insufficiency. *Post Grad Med*. 1959;26: 227-237.

39. Woolley JT, Peters G. Democratic Party Platform, July 11, 1960. The American Presidency Project website. http://www.presidency.ucsb.edu/ws/?pid=29602. Accessed September 11, 2013.

40. DeBakey ME. The role of government in health care: a societal issue. Talk presented at: Rice University President's Lecture; April 15, 2005; Houston, Texas.

41. Baylor gets $262,000 grant for first cardio vascular center. *Houston Chronicle*. October 2, 1960.

42. DeBakey ME. The centers of excellence concept. *J Methodist DeBakey Heart Center*. 2004;1(1): 1.

Chapter 6: The Lasker Connection, 1960-1964

1. Sibley MM. *The Methodist Hospital of Houston, Serving the World*. Austin, TX: Texas State Historical Association; 1989:170.

2. Speer, James B. (The Methodist Hospital History Project, The Methodist Hospital Archives at The John P. McGovern Historical Collections and Research Center in the Texas Medical Center Library, Houston, TX). Interview with: Ted Bowen (The Methodist Hospital, Houston TX). 1978 Dec.

3. Speer, James B. (The Methodist Hospital History Project, The Methodist Hospital Archives at The John P. McGovern Historical Collections and Research Center in the Texas Medical Center Library, Houston, TX). Interview with: Mrs. W. W. Fondren (Philanthropist, Houston, TX). 1975 Mar.

4. Parish, Betsy (Writer). Interview with: Manus F. O'Donnell, M.D. (Methodist DeBakey Heart & Vascular Center, The Methodist Hospital, Houston, TX). 2009 Aug.

5. Sones FM, Shirey EK. Cine coronary arteriography. *MOD CON Cardiovasc Dis*. 1962;31: 733-738.

6. DeBakey ME. Research Related to Surgical Treatment of Aortic and Peripheral Vascular Disease. *Circulation*. 1979;60(7): 1619-1635.

7. Starr A, Edwards ML. Mitral Replacement: Clinical Experience with a ball-valve prosthesis. *Ann Surg*. 1961;154: 726-740.

8. Lefrak EA, Starr A. Starr Edwards Ball Valve. In: Lefrak EA, ed. *Cardiac Valve Prosthesis*. New York, NY: Appleton-Century-Crofts; 1979:67-117.

9. Beall AC Jr, Bricker DL, Cooley DA, DeBakey ME. The use of valve replacement in the management of patients with acquired valvular heart disease. *Am J Surg*. 1965;110: 831-844.

10. Beall AC Jr, Morris GC Jr, Cooley DA, DeBakey ME. Homotransplantation of the aortic valve. *J Thorac Cardiovasc Surg*. 1961;42: 497-506.

11. Winters WL Jr. Tribute to Arthur C. Beall Jr. *Methodist DeBakey Cardiovasc J*. 2012;8:2: 58.

12. Cooley DA, Beall AC Jr, Grondin P. Open-heart operations with disposable oxygenators, 5 percent dextrose prime, and normothermia. *Surgery*. 1962;52: 713-719.

13. Lefrak EA, Starr A. Starr Edwards Ball Valve. In: Lefrak EA, ed. *Cardiac Valve Prosthesis*. New York, NY: Appleton-Centory-Crofts; 1979:181–96.

14. Beall AC Jr, Bloodwell RD, Liotta D, Cooley DA, DeBakey ME. Elimination of sewing ring metal seat interface in mitral valve prostheses. *Circulation*. 1968;37(Suppl 11): 184.

15. DeWall RA, Qasim N, Carr L. Evolution of mechanical heart valves. *Ann Thorac Surg*. 2000;69: 1612-1621.

16. Beall AC Jr, Morris GC Jr, Howell JF Jr, Guinn GA, Noon GP, Reul GJ Jr, et al. Clinical experience with an improved mitral valve prosthesis. *Ann Thorac Surg*. 1973;15: 601-606.

17. Topaz O, Rutherford MS, Mackey-Bojack S, Polkampally PR, Topaz A, Prinz A, et al. Beware of the B(e)all valve: mistaken valve identity, 30-year survival, and valve replacement. *Tex Heart Inst J*. 2010;37(2): 237-239.

18. Winters Jr., William L. (Methodist DeBakey Heart & Vascular Center, The Methodist Hospital, Houston, TX). Interview with: Michael Ellis DeBakey (Methodist DeBakey Heart & Vascular Center, The Methodist Hospital, Houston, TX). 2007 Dec 20.

19. Maxwell, Zella (Texas Children's Hospital History Project, Texas Children's Hospital Archives, The John P. McGovern Historical Collections and Research Center in The Texas Medical Center Library Houston, TX). Interview with: Denton A. Cooley (Texas Heart Institute, Houston, TX). 1979 Jul.

20. Minetree H. *Cooley, The Career of A Great Surgeon*. New York, NY: Harper & Row, Publishers; 1973: 148.

21. Cooley DA. A brief history of the Texas Heart Institute. *Tex Heart Inst J*. 2008;35(3): 235-239.

22. Hopper H. Hollywood Today. *Chicago Tribune* Syndicate. February 9, 1963.

23. Connolly M. Notes from Hollywood. *The Hollywood Reporter* syndicated column, April 23, 1963

24. McComb D. *Oral History Interview of Michael E. DeBakey from the Lyndon Baines Johnson Library*. Bethesda, MD: National Library of Medicine; 1969.

25. Lindberg DAB. Interview with Dr. Michael DeBakey. Profiles in Science, National Library of Medicine website. http://profiles.nlm.nih.gov/RM/G/G/A/K/_/rmggak.html. Created August 17, 1991. Accessed September 11, 2013.

26. Mary Lasker: Notable New Yorkers. Columbia University Libraries Oral History Research Office website. http://www.columbia.edu/cu/lweb/digital/collections/nny/laskerm/index.html. Created July 6, 1965. Accessed September 11, 2013.

27. Citation, the 1963 Albert Lasker Award for Clinical Research. *Bulletin of the New York Academy of Medicine*. 1963;39(11): 704-706.

28. Half-heart replacement. *Time*. November 8, 1963.

29. Plastic pump keeps heart ticking. *Associated Press*. October 28, 1963.

30. Liotta D. Early clinical application of assisted circulation. *Tex Heart Inst J*. 2002;29(3): 229-230.

31. DeBakey ME. The odyssey of the artificial heart. *Artif Organs*. 2000;24(6): 405-411.

32. C. William Hall, M.D., Biography. Society for Biomaterials website. http://www.biomaterials.org/c_william_hall_bio.cfm. Accessed September 11, 2013.

33. Cromie WJ. Substituting pumps for sick hearts. World Book Encyclopedia Science Services, *St. Petersburg Times*. February 19, 1966.

34. *U.S. Congress, Senate Subcommittee of the Committee of Appropriations for 1964, Hearings on Department of Health, Education, and Welfare Appropriations*. Washington D.C.: Government Printing Office; 1963:1402.

35. Strauss MJ. The political history of the artificial heart. *New Engl J Med*. 1984;310(5): 332-336.

36. Nosé Y. Tribute to Dr. C. William Hall, founding director of U.S. Artificial Heart Program at NIH (1922-1992). *Artif Organs*. 1993;17(2): 71-72.

37. Glick MR. The technological imperative and the battle for the hearts of America. *Perspect Biol Med*. 2007;50(2): 276-294.

38. DeBakey ME. Left ventricular bypass pump for cardiac assistance, clinical experience. *Am J Cardiol*. 1971;27: 3-11.

39. Andelman D. Dogs get rubber hearts–for humans in 1970? *Oakland Tribune*. September 11, 1968.

40. Artificial heart object of science team project. *UPI*. May 3, 1965.

41. Leading killers. *Associated Press*. September 13, 1964.

42. Woolley JT, Peters G. Lyndon B. Johnson: 211-The President's News Conference, March 7, 1964. The American Presidency Project website. http://www.presidency.ucsb.edu/ws/?pid=26101. Accessed September 11, 2013.

43. Woolley JT, Peters G. Remarks at the first Meeting of the President's Commission on heart disease, cancer, and stroke. The American Presidency Project website. http://www.presidency.ucsb.edu/ws/?pid=26163. Accessed September 11, 2013.

44. Goor DA. *The Genius of C. Walton Lillehei and The True History of Open Heart Surgery*. New York, NY: Vantage Press; 2007:273-274.

45. Garrett HE, Dennis EW, DeBakey ME. Aortocoronary bypass with saphenous vein graft, seven-year follow-up. *J Am Med Assoc*. 1973;223(7): 792-794.

46. Favaloro RG. Saphenous vein autograft replacement of severe segmental coronary artery occlusion: operative technique. *Ann Thorac Surg*. 1968;5: 334-339.

47. Fuster V, Willerson JT. In memoriam - Rene G Favaloro, MD: The passing of a pioneer. *Circulation*. 2001;103(4): 480-481.

48. Groundbreaking for Fondren and Brown buildings an inspiring occasion. *The Journal*, a publication of The Methodist Hospital, Houston. Oct-Nov. 1964:1

49. Starr P. *The Social Transformation of American Medicine: The rise of a sovereign profession and the making of a vast industry*. New York, NY: Basic Books; 1982: 370.

50. Woolley JT, Peters G. Lyndon B. Johnson: Remarks upon receiving report of the president's commission on heart disease, cancer and stroke. The American Presidency Project website. http://www.presidency.ucsb.edu/ws/?pid=26751. Accessed September 11, 2013.

Chapter 7: The Price of Fame, 1964-1970

1. Duke of Windsor faces arterial surgery. *Associated Press*. December 11, 1964.

2. DeBakey, Michael E. (The Methodist Hospital, Houston, TX). Letter to: Dr. Alton Ochsner (Tulane University School of Medicine, New Orleans, LA). 1964 Dec.

3. Duke of Windsor undergoing tests. *Associated Press*. December 13, 1964.

4. Garrett HE, Crawford ES, Beall AC Jr, Howell JF, DeBakey ME. Surgical Treament Of Aneurysm Of The Thoracoabdominal Aorta. Surg Clin North Am. 1966 Aug;46(4):913-8.

5. Crawford ES, De Bakey ME, Morris GC Jr, Garrett HE, Howell JF. Aneurysm Of The Abdominal Aorta. Surg Clin North Am. 1966 Aug;46(4):963-78.

6. Dennis EW, Kinard SA Jr, McCall BW, DeBakey ME, Howell JF, Garrett HE. Aneurysms Of The Aorta; A Consideration Of Pre- And Postoperative Medical Management. Prog Cardiovasc Dis. 1965 May;7:544-64.

7. DeBakey ME, Crawford ES, Cooley DA, Morris GC Jr, Royster TS, Abbott WP. Aneurysm Of Abdominal Aorta Analysis Of Results Of Graft Replacement Therapy One To Eleven Years After Operation. Ann Surg. 1964 Oct;160:622-39.

8. 20 hour day is usual for Dr. DeBakey. *Associated Press*. December 14, 1964.

9. Full recovery seen for duke of Windsor. *United Press International*. December 16, 1964.

10. Duke's surgery successful. *Associated Press*. December 20, 1964.

11. It's jolly Christmas for Duke. *Associated Press*. December 26, 1964.

12. Royal flowers for Duke on eve of surgery. *The Sydney Morning Herald*. December 16, 1964.

13. Repairing the royal aorta. *Time*. December 25, 1964.

14. Edward H.R.H. Windsor finds there is no job for an ex-king. *Chicago Tribune*. December 16, 1966.

15. Sibley MM. *The Methodist Hospital of Houston, Serving the World.* Austin, TX: Texas State Historical Association; 1989:5.

16. Duke of Windsor leaving hospital. *Associated Press.* December 31, 1964.

17. Duke ends his hospital stay. *Associated Press.* January 1, 1965.

18. McComb D. *Oral History Interview of Michael E. DeBakey from the Lyndon Baines Johnson Library.* Bethesda, MD: National Library of Medicine; 1969.

19. Surgery viewed around world on satellite TV. *Associated Press.* May 12, 1965.

20. Lemann N. Super medicine. *Texas Monthly.* April 1979; page 126.

21. The Texas tornado. *Time* magazine. May 28, 1965.

22. DeBakey ME. Report of president's Commission on Heart Disease, Cancer, and Stroke, editorial. *Circulation.* 1965;32: 686.

23. DeBakey ME. Concepts of the president's Commission on Heart Disease, Cancer, and Stroke. *Clin Res.* 1965;13: 146.

24. Dog lives several hours with an artificial heart. *Associated Press.* April 3, 1965.

25. Dutton DB. *Worse than the disease: pitfalls of medical progress.* Cambridge, UK: Cambridge University Press; 1988:98-99.

26. Altman LK. The doctor's world; artificial heart in turmoil. *New York Times.* May 17, 1988.

27. Fox RC, Swazey JP. *The Courage to Fail, a Social View of Organ Transplants and Dialysis.* Chicago, IL: The University of Chicago Press; 1974:157-158.

28. DeBakey ME, Hall CW. Toward the artificial heart. *New Scientist.* 1964:538-541.

29. At Texas Medical Center, specialist team varies each day. *Associated Press.* April 24, 1966.

30. Thompson T. *Hearts, Of Surgeons and Transplants, Miracles and Disasters along the Cardiac Frontier.* New York, NY: McCall Publishing Company; 1971:136.

31. Thompson T. *Hearts, Of Surgeons and Transplants, Miracles and Disasters along the Cardiac Frontier.* New York, NY: McCall Publishing Company; 1971:138.

32. Arizona Heart Institute remembers heart surgery pioneer Dr. Michael E. DeBakey. Medindia website. http://www.medindia.net/health-press-release/Arizona-Heart-Institute-Remembers-Heart-Surgery-Pioneer-Dr-Michael-E-DeBakey-26558-1.htm#ixzz0pAPkM3yw. Created July 15, 2008. Accessed September 13, 2014.

33. Herbaugh S. He pumps energy into heart surgery. *Associated Press.* July 23, 1985.

34. Porretto J. Pioneering heart doctor Michael DeBakey dead at 99. *Associated Press.* July 12, 2008.

35. Altman LK. Dr. Michael E. DeBakey, rebuilder of hearts, dies at 99. *The New York Times.* July 13, 2008.

36. Television surgery and the Duke. *Associated Press.* November 10, 1965.

37. Duke praises DeBakey. *Associated Press.* November 2, 1965.

38. Speer, James B. (The Methodist Hospital History Project, The Methodist Hospital Archives at The John P. McGovern Historical Collections and Research Center in the Texas Medical Center Library, Houston, TX). Interview with: Mrs. Margaret McElhany (The Methodist Hospital, Houston,TX). 1979 Mar.

39. Sibley MM. *The Methodist Hospital of Houston, Serving the World.* Austin, TX: Texas State Historical Association; 1989:168.

40. Winters Jr., William L (Methodist DeBakey Heart & Vascular Center, The Methodist Hospital, Houston, TX). Interview with: DeBakey, Michael Ellis (Methodist DeBakey Heart & Vascular Center, The Methodist Hospital, Houston, TX). 2007 Dec 20.

41. Fussman C. What I've learned: Michael DeBakey. *Esquire.* March 1, 2001.

42. Roberts WC. Michael Ellis DeBakey: a conversation with the editor. *Am J Cardiol.* 1997;1;79(7):929-950.

43. Manus O'Donnell, M.D., *Interview with Dr. William L. Winters Jr.,* Date unknown

44. Shearer L. Dr. Michael DeBakey, he is turning the dream of artificial arteries and artificial hearts into reality. *Parade.* May 16, 1965.

45. *The Texas Tornado. Time.* May 28, 1965.

46. SoRelle R. Lessons from the heart. *The Journal,* a magazine of The Methodist Hospital System. 1995;34(1):8-13.

Chapter 8: A New Era of Transplantation, 1966-1968

1. DeBakey ME, Hall CW. Towards the artificial heart. New Scientist 22:538-541, May 28, 1964
2. Liotta D, Hall CW, Cooley DA, DeBakey ME. Prolonged ventricular bypass with intrathoracic pumps. *Trans Am Soc Artif Intern Organs.* 1964;10:154-6.
3. Liotta D, Hall CW, Maness JH, DeBakey ME. The Implantable Intrathoracic Circulatory Pump: Surgical Technique. *Cardiovasc Res Cent Bull.* 1964 Oct-Dec;92:54-61
4. Hall CW, Akers WW, O'Bannon W, Liotta D, DeBakey ME. Intraventricular Artificial Heart. *Trans Am Soc Artif Intern Organs.* 1965;11:263-4.
5. Liotta D, Maness J, Bourland H, Rodwell D, Hall CW, DeBakey ME. Recent Modifications In The Implantable Left Ventricular Bypass. *Trans Am Soc Artif Intern Organs.* 1965;11:284-90.
6. Hall CW, Liotta D, Henly WS, Crawford ES, DeBakey ME. Development Of Artificial Intrathoracic Circulatory Pumps. *Am J Surg.* 1964 Nov;108:685-92
7. Bailey R, Kerr A. A patient's gift to the future of heart repair. *Life.* May 6, 1966.
8. 50 years marked by heart group. *The New York Times.* January 27, 1966.
9. Woolley JT, Peters G. Lyndon B. Johnson, remarks upon presenting the heart-of-the-year award to John E. Fogarty, February 3, 1966. The American Presidency Project website. http://www.presidency.ucsb.edu/ws/?pid=27892. Accessed September 14, 2013.
10. Cromie WJ. Substituting pumps for sick hearts. *World Book Encyclopedia* Science Service. February 19, 1966.
11. Human getting human heart. *Associated Press.* April 17, 1966.
12. Artificial heart put in chest of patient. *Associated Press.* April 21, 1966.
13. Doctors implant artificial heart. *Associated Press.* April 21, 1966.
14. Tomlin R. Lights . . .Camera. . .Surgery! DeBakey Museum to include innovative filming platform. *Findings.* 2007;5(1).
15. DeBakey ME. Odyssey of the artificial heart. *Artif Organs.* 2000;24(6): 406-411.
16. Glubok N. 'Heart' saved hubby, surgeon tells wife. *Chicago Daily News.* April 24, 1966.
17. Willingly risked death as a human guinea pig. *Associated Press.* April 24. 1966.
18. Surgery: a better half-heart. *Time.* April 29, 1966.
19. Implanted "heart" pumps life into doomed patient. *St. Petersburg Times.* April 22, 1966.
20. Science and publicity. *The New York Times.* April 22, 1966.
21. Schmeck HM Jr. A successful artificial heart could be a boon to mankind. *The New York Times.* April 22, 1966.
22. Nelson H. Artificial heart pioneer called 'publicity seeker.' *Los Angeles Times.* May 29, 1966.
23. Plastic heart patient dies. *Associated Press.* April 26, 1966.
24. The 'heart' may get new trial. *Associated Press.* April 27, 1966.
25. Death of a patient. *Time.* May 6, 1966.
26. Getz G. Dr. DeBakey denies he arranged publicity. *Los Angeles Times.* May 27, 1966.
27. Artificial heart by 1971 is predicted by DeBakey. *Associated Press.* May 1, 1966.
28. Bailey R, Kerr A. A patient's gift to the future of heart repair. *Life.* May 6, 1966.
29. Artificial heart put in woman. *UPI.* August 9, 1966.
30. Heart pump patient well. *Associated Press.* September 3, 1966.
31. Heart pump used again by DeBakey. *UPI.* October 29, 1966.
32. Campbell M. President top newsmaker of '66. *Associated Press.* December 27, 1966.
33. Noted heart surgeon 'a man in a hurry.' *Associated Press.* April 24, 1966.
34. Cooley DA. Growth of open heart surgery. *Medical Record and Annals.* 1967;60: 266-269.
35. Cooley DA. Early development of congenital heart surgery: open heart surgeries. *Ann Thorac Surg.* 1997 Nov; 64(5):1544-1548.
36. Sones FM, Shirey EK, Proudeft WL, Westcott RN. Cine-coronary arteriography. *Circulation.* 1959;22(4 Part 2): 773-774.
37. Fye WB. President's page: cardiology and technology: an enduring and energizing partnership. *J Am Coll Cardiol.* 2002;40(6): 1192-1195.
38. Schmeck HM Jr. 12 federal heart attack centers to seek data on basic questions. *New York Times.* February 27, 1967

39. U.S. to emphasize heart pump study. *The New York Times*. November 29, 1966.

40. Strauss MJ. The political history of the artificial heart. *New Engl J Med*. 1984;310(50: 332-336.

41. DeBakey ME, Liotta D, Hall CW. Prospects for and implications of the artificial heart and assistive devices. *J Rehabil* March-April, 1966. 32(2):106-107

42. DeBakey ME, Liotta D, Hall CW. "Left-heart bypass using an implantable blood pump" in *Mechanical Devices to Assist the Failing Heart*, National Academy of Sciences – National Research Council, Washington, D.C., 1966, Chap 19, pp. 223-239

43. Liotta D, Hall CW, DeBakey ME. "Heart Failure and implantable circulatory pumps: Physiology and clinical application" in *Heart Substitutes*, Brest, Albert N. (ed.), Springfield, Illinois, Charles C Thomas, 1966, Chap 18, pp 225-237

44. Hall CW, Liotta D, DeBakey ME. Bioengineering efforts in developing artificial hearts and assistors. Am J Surg July, 1967 114(1):24-30

45. Hall CW, Liotta D, DeBakey ME. "Artificial heart – Present and future," in *Research in the Service of Man: Biomedical Knowledge, Development and Use*. Washington, D.C., U.S. Printing Office, 1967, pp 201-216

46. South African 'feeling better' after heart transplant. *Associated Press*. December 4, 1967.

47. Surgeon confident. *AAP News*. December 23, 1967.

48. Artificial heart need is seen by specialists. *Associated Press*. January 17, 1968.

49. SoRelle R. New heart, new life/in 25 years, transplants have come of age. *Houston Chronicle*. November 29, 1992.

50. William Hines, Cure, Not Treatment, Is Surgeon's Goal, World of Science, *The Free Lance-Star*, November 9, 1968

51. Implant patients all right. *UPI*. September 2, 1968.

52. Transplant surgeons plan artificial heart. *UPI*. September 28, 1968.

Chapter 9: Schism, 1968-1970

1. First at Houston, heart transplant patient succumbs. *Associated Press*. November 24, 1968.

2. Astronauts made biggest news scene splash. *Associated Press*. December 31, 1968.

3. Thompson T. *Hearts, Of Surgeons and Transplants, Miracles and Disasters Along the Cardiac Frontier*. New York, NY: The McCall Publishing Company; 1971:31.

4. 2 paid $200,000 by Medicare. *Associated Press*. August 5, 1969.

5. DeBakey ME. Michael Ellis DeBakey: a conversation with the editor. Interview by William C. Roberts. *Am J Cardiol*. 1997;79(7): 929-950.

6. Thompson T. *Hearts, Of Surgeons and Transplants, Miracles and Disasters Along the Cardiac Frontier*. New York, NY: The McCall Publishing Company; 1971:5.

7. George P. Noon (The Methodist Hospital, Houston, Texas). Fax correspondence to: William L. Winters, Jr. (The Methodist Hospital, Houston, Texas). 2013 Apr.

8. Garrett HE, Dennis EW, DeBakey ME. Aortocoronary bypass with saphenous vein graft: seven-year follow-up. *J Am Med Assoc*. 1973;223(7): 792-794.

9. Garrett H, Dennis EW, DeBakey ME. Aortocoronary Bypass With Saphenous Vein Graft: Seven-Year Follow-Up. *J Am Med Assoc*. 1996;276(18):1517-1520.

10. Favaloro RG, Effler DB, Groves LK, Sones FM Jr, Fergusson DJG. Myocardial revascularization by internal mammary artery implant procedures: clinical experience. *J Thorac Cardiovasc Surg*. 1967;54: 359-370.

11. Morris GC Jr, Howell JF, Crawford ES, et al. The distal coronary bypass. *Ann Surg*. 1970;172(4): 652-662.

12. Schmeck HM Jr. Heart transplant formula: skill and a little sugar. *The New York Times*. September 29, 1968.

13. Cooley DA. A brief history of the Texas Heart Institute. *Tex Heart Inst J*. 2008;35(3): 235-239.

14. Angelle D. An American pioneer. *Leading Health*. 2003;2(3): 11-15.

15. Thompson T. *Hearts, Of Surgeons and Transplants, Miracles and Disasters Along the Cardiac Frontier*. New York, NY: The McCall Publishing Company; 1971:14.

16. Mason JT. Mary Lasker: Notable New Yorkers. Columbia University Libraries Oral History Research Office website. http://www.columbia.edu/cu/lweb/digital/collections/nny/laskerm/index.html. Created July 6, 1965. Accessed September 15, 2013.

17. Texas Baptists to consider freeing Baylor Med College. *Baptist Press*. October 9, 1968.

18. A proposal for the development of medical education in Texas, 1969-1980. Adopted December 3, 1968. Education Resources Information Center website. http://www.eric.ed.gov. Created December 1968. Accessed September 15, 2013.

19. Church and state: government money for Baptists. *Time*. December 13, 1968.

20. Texas Baptists to vote on releasing Baylor Med. *Baptist Press*. October 23, 1968.

21. Baylor medical elects two. *The New York Times*. January 24, 1969.

22. Benson D. Baylor College of Medicine, 65 years of excellence. *Solutions Magazine*. Winter 2008;4(3).

23. Distinguished Americans are honored. *UPI*. January 22, 1969.

24. Father of Frank Sinatra in Houston hospital. *UPI*. January 20, 1969.

25. 3 of 4 survive heart surgery. *UPI*. January 6, 1969.

26. Heart donor lag upsets surgeon. *The New York Times*. February 28, 1969.

27. Brody JE. Heart transplant death rate linked to rejection. *The New York Times*. March 1, 1969.

28. Heart surgery foes 'too faint hearted.' *Associated Press*. March 2, 1969.

29. Surgery team signs as donors. *Associated Press*. February 13, 1969.

30. Stephenson LW. History of cardiac surgery. In: Cohn LH, ed. *Cardiac Surgery in the Adult*. 3rd ed. New York, NY: The McGraw Hill Companies, Inc.; 2008;23.

31. Quinn J. Strange case of the artificial heart. *New York Daily News*, News Syndicate Co. Inc. September 8, 1969.

32. Artificial heart's use questioned: Dr. Cooley is silent on transplant dispute. *Associated Press*. April 10, 1969.

33. Auerbach S. Two dispute making of plastic heart. *Washington Post*. April 10, 1969.

34. Electric Heart. NOVA online. PBS website. http://www.pbs.org/wgbh/nova/eheart. Created December 21, 1999. Accessed September 15, 2013.

35. Woman's heart implanted to replace artificial organ. *UPI*. April 8, 1969.

36. Were research guidelines violated in attempt to save Karp's life? *Associated Press*. April 9, 1969.

37. U.S. stir over plastic heart. *The Age*. April 11, 1969.

38. Artificial heart stirs medical controversy. *Associated Press*. April 9, 1969.

39. Transplant doctor ready for federal investigation. *Associated Press*. April 11, 1969.

40. Heart of fiber, plastic placed inside patient. *UPI*. April 5, 1969.

41. Bowsher M. Top surgeons' feud over artificial heart boils on in Houston. *Wall Street Journal*. July 17, 1969.

42. DeBakey ME, Hall CW, Hellums JD, et al. Orthotopic cardiac prosthesis: preliminary experiments in animals with biventricular artificial heart. *Cardiovasc Res Cent Bull*. 1969;7(4): 127-142.

43. Plastic heart doctor fired for violation. *UPI*. May 17, 1969.

44. Fox RC, Swazey JP. *The Courage to Fail, A Social View of Organ Transplants and Dialysis*. Chicago and London: The University of Chicago Press; 1974:177.

45. Cooley acted without 'clearance.' *Associated Press*. May 16, 1969.

46. Fox RC, Swazey JP. *The Courage to Fail, A Social View of Organ Transplants and Dialysis*. Chicago and London: The University of Chicago Press; 1974:178.

47. Dr. Cooley Will Continue to Use the Artificial Heart; Baylor Seeks Limitation, United Press International, May 18, 1969.

48. Cooley, associate quit Baylor. *Associated Press*. June 25, 1969.

49. Thompson T. The Texas Tornado vs. Dr. Wonderful. *Life*. April 10, 1970.

50. DeBakey, Cooley controversy: artificial heart 'stolen.' *UPI*. October 21, 1970.

51. Fox RC, Swazey JP. *The Courage to Fail, A Social View of Organ Transplants and Dialysis*. Chicago and London: The University of Chicago Press; 1974.

52. Fox RC, Swazey JP. *The Courage to Fail, A Social View of Organ Transplants and Dialysis*. Chicago and London: The University of Chicago Press; 1974:185

53. Fox RC, Swazey JP. *The Courage to Fail, A Social View of Organ Transplants and Dialysis*. Chicago and London: The University of Chicago Press; 1974:211

54. Thompson T. *Hearts, Of Surgeons and Transplants, Miracles and Disasters Along the Cardiac Frontier*. New York, NY: The McCall Publishing Company; 1971:119.

Chapter 10: The Pilgrimage, 1960-1970

1. Thompson T. *Hearts; of surgeons and transplants, miracles and disasters along the cardiac frontier*. New York, NY: McCall Publishing Company; 1971:121.

2. Wertenbaker L. *To Mend the Heart: The Dramatic Surgery and Its Pioneers*. New York, NY: The Viking Press; 1980:196.

3. She finds no help after making trip. *Associated Press*. March 12, 1973.

4. Parish, Betsy (writer). Interview with: Dr. Manus O'Donnell (The Methodist Hospital, Houston, Texas). 2009 Aug.

5. Roberts WC. John Flake Anderson, MD: a conversation with the editor. *BUMC Proceedings*. 2003;16:439-453.

6. Roberts WC. George Kennedy ("Ken") Hempel Jr., MD: a conversation with the editor. *BUMC Proceedings*. 2007;20(4):369-380.

7. Roberts WC. John Webster Kirklin. MD: a conversation with the editor. *BUMC Proceedings*. 1998;81:1027-1044.

8. Diethrich EB. Developing the DeBakey team – 15 years of faculty members: 1950-1965. Presented at: Michael E. DeBakey International Surgical Society XVth Congress; May 16, 2004; Houston, Texas.

9. Chapman DW. *Heart, Helicopters, and Houston; Fifty Golden Years of Heart Disease as seen by an Insider*. Austin, TX: Nortex Press, a division of Sunbelt Media, Inc.; 1996:150.

10. Roberts WC. Michael Ellis DeBakey: a conversation with the editor. *Am J Cardiol*. 1979;79: 929-950.

11. Chapman DW. *Heart, Helicopters, and Houston; Fifty Golden Years of Heart Disease as seen by an Insider*. Austin, TX: Nortex Press, a division of Sunbelt Media, Inc.; 1996:78.

12. Sullivan ME. A view from the millennium: the practice of cardiology circa 1950 and thereafter. *J Am Coll Cardiol*. 1999;33(5): 1141-1151.

13. Braunwald E. The rise of cardiovascular medicine. *Eur Heart J*. 2012 Apr;33(7):838-845.

14. White PD. *Heart Disease*. 4th ed. New York, NY: Macmillan; 1951:561-562.

15. Chapman DW. *Heart, Helicopters, and Houston; Fifty Golden Years of Heart Disease as seen by an Insider*. Austin, TX: Nortex Press, a division of Sunbelt Media, Inc.; 1996:51.

16. Winters, William L Jr. (Methodist DeBakey Heart & Vascular Center, The Methodist Hospital, Houston, Texas). Interview with: Dr. Manus O'Donnell (The Methodist Hospital, Houston, Texas). 2004 Aug.

17. Seldinger SI. Catheter replacement of the needle in percutaneous arteriography: a new technique. *ACTA Radiologic*. 1953;39(5): 368-376.

18. McCollum CH, Garcia-Rinaldi R, Graham JM, Noon GP, DeBakey ME. Percutaneous needle arteriography. *World J Surg*. 1980;4(1): 105-112.

19. Beall AC Jr, Henly WS, Morris GC Jr, Crawford ES, Cooley DA, DeBakey ME. Translumbar aortography: a simple, safe technic. *Ann Surg*. 1963;157(6): 882-891.

20. Winters, William L Jr. (Methodist DeBakey Heart & Vascular Center, The Methodist Hospital, Houston, Texas). Interview with: Dr. John O. Roehm (The Methodist Hospital, Houston, Texas). 2006 Dec.

21. Vineberg AA. Surgery of coronary artery disease. *Prog Cardiovasc Dis*. 1962;4: 391-418.

22. Vineberg AA. Results of 14 years experience in the surgical treatment of human coronary artery insufficiency. *Can Med Assoc J*. 1965;92: 325-332.

23. Edler I, Hertz CH. The use of ultrasonic reflectoscope for continuous recording of the movements of the heart walls. *Clin Physiol Funct Imaging.* 2004:24: 118-136.

24. Edler I. The use of ultrasound as a diagnostic aid, and its effects on biological tissues. Continuous recording of the movements of various heart-structures using an ultrasound echo-method. *Acta Med Scand Suppl.* 1961;370: 7-65.

25. Joyner CR, Reid JM, Bond JP. Reflected ultrasound in the assessment of mitral valve disease. *Circulation.* 1963;27: 503-511.

26. Lawrie GM, Morris GC, Earle N. Long-term results of coronary bypass surgery. *Ann Surg.* 1991;213: 377-385.

27. Morris GC Jr, Reul GJ, Howell JF, et al. Follow-up results of distal coronary artery bypass for ischemic heart disease. *Am J Cardiol.* 1972;29(2): 180-5.

28. Winters WL Jr. Early days of echocardiography. Echocardiography: a review of cardiovascular ultrasound. *Echo.*1984;1(2): 115-149.

29. Williamson MV. (The Methodist Hospital Archives, The Methodist Hospital, Houston,TX). *It's The Way It Was, Part Two – The Methodist Years,* September 20, 2005

Chapter 11: The Academic Building Blocks, 1969-1979

1.   DeBakey ME. The centers of excellence concept. *Methodist DeBakey Cardiovasc J.* 2004;1(1): 1.

2.   Merrill JM. *"As it was" and is: A Memoir.* Lincoln, NE: iUniverse, Inc.; 2003:58.

3.   Lynch EC. *Education in Internal Medicine: The Baylor Experience.* Houston, TX: Baylor College of Medicine; 2002:46.

4.   Sibley MM. *The Methodist Hospital of Houston, Serving the World.* Austin, TX: Texas State Historical Association; 1989:177.

5.   Speer, James B. (The Methodist Hospital History Project, The Methodist Hospital Archives at The John P. McGovern Historical Collections and Research Center in the Texas Medical Center Library, Houston, TX). Interview with: Dr. Hatch W. Cummings Jr. (The Methodist Hospital, Houston, TX). 1975 Nov.

6.   Sibley MM. *The Methodist Hospital of Houston, Serving the World.* Austin, TX: Texas State Historical Association; 1989:179.

7.   Henry D. McIntosh, M.D., joins staff. *The Journal,* the magazine of The Methodist Hospital, Houston. 1970:3.

8.   Maldonado MM. Presentation of Henry McIntosh, M.D. 1984 Founders Medal of the Southern Society for Clinical Investigation. *Am J Med Sci.* 1984;288(3): 101-103.

9.   Merrill JM. *"As it was" and is: A Memoir.* Lincoln, NE: iUniverse, Inc.; 2003:71.

10. Winters, William L. Jr. (The Methodist Hospital, Houston, TX). Interview with: Dr. Manus O'Donnell (The Methodist Hospital, Houston, TX). 2004 Aug.

11. Transplants discussed. *Associated Press.* November 10, 1972.

12. Methodist Hospital uses new noninvasive diagnostic techniques for heart problems. *The Texas Methodist.* 1973;119(4): 10.

13. Winters, William L. Jr. (The Methodist Hospital, Houston, TX). Interview with: Dr. Mark L. Entman (The Methodist Hospital, Houston, TX). 2009 May.

14. Merrill JM. *"As it was" and is: A Memoir.* Lincoln, NE: iUniverse, Inc.; 2003:82.

15. Morris, James P. (The Methodist Hospital History Project, The Methodist Hospital Archives at The John P. McGovern Historical Collections and Research Center in the Texas Medical Center Library, Houston, TX). Interview with: Dr. Antonio M. Gotto Jr. (The Methodist Hospital, Houston, TX). 1981 Mar.

16. Merrill JM. *"As it was" and is: A Memoir.* Lincoln, NE: iUniverse, Inc.; 2003:79.

17. Gotto AM Jr. Mr. Ted Bowen and the Cardiovascular Center of The Methodist Hospital. *The Journal,* the magazine of The Methodist Hospital, Houston. 1979 May.

18. Lynch EC. *Education in Internal Medicine: The Baylor Experience.* Houston, TX: Baylor College of Medicine; 2002:49.

19. Dedication of national center marked at March ceremonies. *Inside Baylor.* 1975;VI(4).

20. Lynch EC. *Education in Internal Medicine: The Baylor Experience.* Houston, TX: Baylor College of Medicine; 2002:50.

21. Winters, William L. Jr. (The Methodist Hospital, Houston, TX). Interview with: Dr. Manus O'Donnell (The Methodist Hospital, Houston, TX). 2004 Aug.

22. Winters, William L. Jr. (The Methodist Hospital, Houston, TX). Interview with: Dr. Albert E. Raizner (The Methodist Hospital, Houston, TX). 2004 Oct.

23. Winters, William L. Jr. (The Methodist Hospital, Houston, TX). Interview with: Dr. William Spencer (The Methodist Hospital, Houston, TX). 2004 Jun.

24. Jeffrey K, Parsonnet V. Cardiac pacing, 1960-1985; a quarter century of medical and industrial innovation. *Circulation.* 1998;97: 1978-1991.

25. Spencer WH 3rd, Zhu DW, Markowitz T, Badruddin SM, Zoghbi WA. Atrial septal pacing: a method for pacing both atria simultaneously. *Pacing Clin Electrophysiol.* 1997;20(11): 2739-2745.

26. Spencer WH 3rd, Zhu DW, Kirkpatrick C, Killip D, Durand JB. Subclavian venogram as a guide to lead implantation. *Pacing Clin Electrophysiol.* 1998;21(3): 499-502.

27. Spencer WH 3rd, Markowitz T, Alagona P. Rate augmentation and atrial arrhythmias in DDDR pacing. *Pacing Clin Electrophysiol.* 1990;13(12 Pt 2): 1847-1851.

28. Wright KE Jr, McIntosh HD. Artificial pacemakers: indications and management. *Circulation.* 1973;47: 1108-1118.

29. Pacemaker evaluation lab established at The Methodist Hospital. *The Journal,* the magazine of The Methodist Hospital, Houston. 1974:7-8.

30. Parsonnet V, Bernstein AD. Cardiac Pacing in the 1980s: treatments and techniques in transition. *J Am Coll Cardiol.* 1983;1(1): 339-354.

31. Lynch EC. *Education in Internal Medicine: The Baylor Experience.* Houston, TX: Baylor College of Medicine; 2002:60.

32. Fowler NO, Hultgren HN, McIntosh HD. Training programs in cardiovascular disease. *Am J Cardiol.* 1974;34: 429-438.

33. Lynch EC. *Education in Internal Medicine: The Baylor Experience.* Houston, TX: Baylor College of Medicine; 2002:61.

34. Williamson MV. (The Methodist Hospital Archives, The Methodist Hospital, Houston, TX). *It's The Way It Was, Part Two – The Methodist Years,* September 20, 2005.

35. Baylor med official to resign post. *The Houston Post.* October 15, 1976;4A.

36. Medical quarrel: coronary bypass surgery debated. *Associated Press.* September 10, 1976.

37. Brody JE. Doctors query bypass surgery as aid to heart. *The New York Times.* November 22, 1976;front page.

38. McIntosh HD. Founder's Award speech. *Am J Med Sci.* 1984;288(3): 103.

39. McIntosh HD, Garcia JA. The first decade of aortacoronary bypass grafting, 1967-1977. *Circulation.* 1978;57(3): 405.

40. McIntosh HD. Indications for coronary arteriography. *Circulation.* 1977;56(1): 1.

Chapter 12: Beyond the Stethoscope, 1970-1980

1. Transplants out, says heart man. *The Age,* Sydney Australia. July 17, 1973.

2. Greene JA. Prescribing by numbers: drugs and the definition of disease. *JHU Press.* 2007:264.

3. From bench to bedside: Mary Lasker and the drive for "payoff" from medical research. The Mary Lasker Papers; Profiles in Science, National Library of Medicine website. http://profiles.nlm.nih.gov/ps/retrieve/Narrative/TL/p-nid/202. Accessed September 18. 2013.

4. Landers A. Keep a check on hypertension. *St. Petersburg Times.* October 18, 1977.

5. Oparil S, Weber MA. *Hypertension: a Companion of Brenner and Rector's the Kidney.* Philadelphia, PA: Elsevier Saunders, Inc.; 2005:7.

6. DeBakey ME, Gotto AM Jr. *The Living Heart.* New York, NY: David McKay; 1977.

7. DeBakey ME. A conversation with the editor, Interview with William C. Roberts. *Am J Cardiol.* 1997;79(7): 929-950.

8. Dr. Gotto assumes leadership of Bob and Vivian Smith Department of Medicine. *The Journal*, the magazine of The Methodist Hospital, Houston. 1977: 3.

9. Lynch EC. *Education in Internal Medicine: The Baylor Experience*. Houston, TX: Baylor College of Medicine; 2002:64.

10. Parish, Betsy (writer). Interview with: Dr. Miguel A. Quiñones (The Methodist Hospital, Houston, Texas). 2011 Apr.

11. Parish, Betsy (writer). Interview with: Dr. Manus O'Donnell (The Methodist Hospital, Houston, Texas). 2009 Aug.

12. Gotto AM. Remembering Dr. Michael DeBakey. *Weill Cornell Medicine*. 2008: 3.

13. Veterans Administration Cooperative Study of Surgery for Coronary Arterial Occlusive Disease. III. Methods and baseline characteristics, including experience with medical treatment. By the Veterans Administration Cooperative Group for the Study of Surgery for Coronary Arterial Occlusive Disease. *Am J Cardiol*. 1977;40(2): 212-225.

14. DeBakey ME, Lawrie GM. Aortocoronary-artery bypass: assessment after 13 years. *J Am Med Assoc*. 1978;239(9) 937-939.

15. DeBakey: Awareness of heart disease causes cuts deaths. *UPI*. February 1, 1978.

16. Beck J. Heart disease: don't wait for a beta-blocker–beat it yourself. *The Evening Independent*. August 25, 1977.

17. Joan Beck, Heart Disease: Don't Wait for a Beta-Blocker–Beat It Yourself, The Evening Independent, August 25, 1977

18. DeBakey ME. Elimination of heart disease within reach. *Lakeland Ledger*. February 14, 1978.

19. Beta-Blocker Heart Attack Trial (BHAT). ClinicalTrials.gov website. http://clinicaltrials.gov/ct2/show/NCT00000492. Accessed September 18, 2013.

20. Craig M. Platt, M.D., joins NewCardio's Scientific Advisory Board. *Reuters*. March 26, 2008.

21. Executive Profile Craig M. Pratt, M.D., Newcardio, Inc. Blumberg Business Week website. http://investing.businessweek.com/research/stocks/people/person.asp?personId=9513009&ticker=NWCI&previousCapId=98509&previousTitle=ACTELION%20LTD-REG. Accessed September 18, 2013.

22. Winters, William L. Jr. (Methodist DeBakey Heart & Vascular Center, The Methodist Hospital, Houston, Texas). Interview with: Dr. W. Richard Cashion (The Methodist Hospital, Houston, Texas). 2009 Nov.

23. Director of nuclear cardiology named. *The Journal*, the magazine of The Methodist Hospital, Houston. 1979.

24. Verani MS. Cardiac scanning: an important advance in the evaluation of cardiac patients. *The Journal*, the magazine of The Methodist Hospital, Houston. 1978.

25. Verani MS. Thallium-201 myocardial scintigraphy, an overview. *Clin Nucl Med*. 1983;8(6): 276-287.

26. Cashion WR Jr. Cardiac scanning. *The Journal*, the magazine of The Methodist Hospital, Houston. 1978.

27. Winters, William L. Jr. (Methodist DeBakey Heart & Vascular Center, The Methodist Hospital, Houston, Texas). Interview with: Dr. Albert E. Raizner (The Methodist Hospital, Houston, Texas). 2004 Oct.

28. Winters, William L. Jr. (Methodist DeBakey Heart & Vascular Center, The Methodist Hospital, Houston, Texas). Interview with: Dr. Miguel A. Quiñones (The Methodist Hospital, Houston, Texas). 2008 Feb.

29. Quiñones MA. Pulsed Doppler echocardiography: application to clinical cardiology. *The Journal*, the magazine of The Methodist Hospital, Houston. 1978.

30. DeBakey ME. Research related to surgical treatment of aortic and peripheral vascular disease. *Circulation*. 1979;60(7): 1619.

31. Nathan DA, Center S, Wu C, Keller W. An implantable synchronous pacemaker for the long term correction of complete heart block. *Am J Cardiol*. 1963;II(3): 362-367.

32. Levine JH, Mellits ED, Baumgardner RA, et al. Predictors of first discharge and subsequent survival in patients with automatic implantable cardioverter-defibrillators. *Circulation*. 1991;84: 558-566.

33. Denes P, Rosen KM. The man and his science. *PACE*. 1983;6(Part II): 994.

34. Cardiac catheterization used to assess heart disease. *The Journal*, the magazine of The Methodist Hospital, Houston. 1980.

35. Winters, William L. Jr. (Methodist DeBakey Heart & Vascular Center, The Methodist Hospital, Houston, Texas). Interview with: Dr. William Spencer (The Methodist Hospital, Houston, Texas). 2004 Jun.

36. Naoer WK. Has the golden age of cardiology passed? *Am J Cardiol*. 1994;73: 724-725.

Chapter 13: New Programs, 1978-1984

1. Lemann N. Super medicine. *Texas Monthly*. April, 1979.

2. Zinman D. Michael DeBakey, doctor speaks from the heart. *Los Angeles Times* – Washington Post News Service. February 12, 1979.

3. DeBakey ME, Creech O Jr, Cooley DA. Arterial homografts for peripheral arteriosclerotic occlusive disease. *Circulation*. 1957;15: 21-30.

4. Weisse AB. *Heart to Heart: the Twentieth Century Battle Against Cardiac Disease: An Oral History*. New Brunswick, NJ: Rutgers University Press; 2002:177-178.

5. Schier MJ. Program, dinner Friday at Baylor. *The Houston Post*. February 13, 1976.

6. Altman LK. The Doctor's World: Dr. DeBakey at 90: stringent standards and a steady hand. *The New York Times*. September 1, 1998.

7. Doctor cites fat foods evils. *The Victoria Advocate*. April 24, 1982.

8. DeBakey ME, Gotto AM Jr. *The Living Heart*. New York, NY: David McKay; 1977.

9. DeBakey ME, Gotto AM Jr, Scott LW, Foreyt JP. *The Living Heart Diet*. New York, NY: Simon & Schuster; 1984.

10. Williamson MV. It's the way it was, part two – The Methodist years. The Methodist Hospital Archives, Houston, Texas. September 20, 2005.

11. Altman LK. DeBakey to remove the Shah's spleen. *The New York Times*. March 13, 1980.

12. Altman LK. The Shah's health: a political gamble. *The New York Times*. May 17, 1981.

13. Kraft J. Sadat: rare qualities of leadership. *The Milwaukee Sentinel*. April 10, 1980.

14. Howell JD. The changing face of twentieth-century American cardiology. *Ann Intern Med*. 1986;105(5): 772-782.

15. DeBakey ME, Lawrie GM. Aortocoronary-artery bypass: assessment after 13 years. *J Am Med Assoc*. 1978;239(9): 937-939.

16. Buccino RA, McIntosh HD. Aortocoronary bypass grafting in the management of patients with coronary artery disease. *Am J Med*. 1979;66: 651-666.

17. Conn R. Heart bypass debate continues. Knight Ridder Inc. November 2, 1979.

18. Engel TR, Meister SG. Coronary percutaneous transluminal angioplasty. *Ann Intern Med*. 1979;90(2): 268-269.

19. Monagan D, Williams DO. *Journey into the Heart: A Tale of Pioneering Doctors and Their Race to Transform Cardiovascular Medicine*. New York, NY: Gotham Books; 1970:149.

20. Monagan D, Williams DO. *Journey into the Heart: A Tale of Pioneering Doctors and Their Race to Transform Cardiovascular Medicine*. New York, NY: Gotham Books; 1970:140.

21. Krone RJ. Thirty years of coronary angioplasty. *Cardiology Journal*. 2008;15(2): 201-202.

22. Cohen B. Interview with Heliane Canepa. Angioplasty.Org website. http://www.ptca.org/nv/interviews.html. Accessed September 20, 2013.

23. Levy RI, Jesse MJ, Mock MB. NHLBI position on percutaneous transluminal coronary angioplasty (PTCA). *Am J Cardiol*. 1979;53: 867.

24. Mullin SM, Passamani ER, Mock MB. Historical background of the National Heart, Lung, and Blood Institute Registry for Percutaneous Transluminal Coronary Angioplasty. *Am J Cardiol*. 1984;53: 3C-6C.

25. Medicine: blowup in the arteries. *Time*. July 3, 1978.

26. Dehmer GJ, Douglas JS Jr, Abizaid A, et al. SCAI/ACCF/HRS/ESC/SOLACI/APSIC statement on the use of live case demonstrations at cardiology meetings assessments of the past and standards for the future. *Heart Rhythm*. 2010;7(10): 1522-1535.

27. Cohen B. Interview with Spencer B. King, III, M.D., Part III. Angioplasty.Org website. http://www.ptca.org/nv/interviews.html. Accessed September 20, 2013.

28. Winters, William L. Jr. (Methodist DeBakey Heart & Vascular Center, The Methodist Hospital, Houston, Texas). Interview with: Dr. Albert E. Raizner (The Methodist Hospital, Houston, Texas). 2004 Oct.

29. Raizner AE, Lewis J, Winters WL, et al. A new form of treatment of coronary artery disease. *The Journal*, the magazine of The Methodist Hospital, Houston. March 1981/

30. Zoler ML. Chez Eddy: elegant food that's easy on the heart. *The New York Times*. June 22, 1988.

31. Getting your just desserts. *Texas Monthly*/ August 1981: 19.

32. Parish, Betsy (writer). Interview with: Dr. Miguel A. Quiñones (The Methodist Hospital, Houston, Texas). 2011 Apr.

33. Roberts WC. Robert Roberts, MD: a conversation with the editor. *Am J Cardiol*. 1999;83: 1458-1475.

34. Winters, William L. Jr (Methodist DeBakey Heart & Vascular Center, The Methodist Hospital, Houston, Texas). Interview with: Dr. Robert Roberts (The Methodist Hospital, Houston, Texas). 2004.

35. Roberts R. The molecular cardiology laboratory at Baylor College of Medicine. *Cardiology*. 2002;98: 210-213.

36. Winters, William L. Jr. (Methodist DeBakey Heart & Vascular Center, The Methodist Hospital, Houston, Texas). Interview with: Dr. Miguel A. Quiñones (The Methodist Hospital, Houston, Texas). 2008 Feb.

37. Winters, William L. Jr. (Methodist DeBakey Heart & Vascular Center, The Methodist Hospital, Houston, Texas). Interview with: Patty Chesnick, RN (The Methodist Hospital, Houston, Texas). 2011 Jan.

38. Winters, William L. Jr. (Methodist DeBakey Heart & Vascular Center, The Methodist Hospital, Houston, Texas). Interview with: Dr. William Gaston (The Methodist Hospital, Houston, Texas). 2009 Jun.

39. James B. Young, M.D., helped advance subspecialty of cardiac transplantation. *Cardiology Today*. 2009 Feb. Available at: http://www.healio.com/cardiology/hf-transplantation/news/print/cardiology-today/%7Bbf688dc8-bf7d-4608-a94f-dbdfdf84a5aa%7D/james-b-young-md-helped-advance-subspecialty-of-cardiac-transplantation. Accessed September 20, 2013.

40. King W. DeBakey resumes heart transplant surgery. *The New York Times*. February 22, 1984.

Chapter 14: Opening New Channels, 1984-1989

1. Winters, William L. Jr. (Methodist DeBakey Heart & Vascular Center, The Methodist Hospital, Houston, Texas). Interview with: Dr. Mark L. Entman (Methodist DeBakey Heart & Vascular Center, The Methodist Hospital, Houston, Texas). 2009 May.

2. Parish, Betsy (writer). Interview with: Dr. Mark L. Entman (Methodist DeBakey Heart & Vascular Center, The Methodist Hospital, Houston, Texas). 2011 May.

3. History of the National Heart and Blood Vessel Research and Demonstration Center, National Heart and Blood Vessel Research and Demonstration Center Archives at the John P. McGovern Historical Collections and Research Center in the Texas Medical Center Library.

4. Private funds sought for research on heart. *Houston Chronicle*. March 1, 1985.

5. Sibley MM. *The Methodist Hospital of Houston, Serving the World*. Austin, TX: Texas State Historical Association; 1989:209.

6. Man receives new heart, lung. *Associated Press*. April 5, 1985.

7. Gotto AM Jr, DeBakey ME. Profiles in cardiology. *Clinical Cardiology*. 1991;14: 1007-1010.

8. Parish, Betsy (writer). Interview with: Dr. Albert E. Raizner (Methodist DeBakey Heart & Vascular Center, The Methodist Hospital, Houston, Texas). 2011 August.

9. Winters, William L. Jr. (Methodist DeBakey Heart & Vascular Center, The Methodist Hospital, Houston, Texas). Interview with: Dr. Robert Roberts (Methodist DeBakey Heart & Vascular Center, The Methodist Hospital, Houston, Texas). 2004.

10. Morgan HE, Paul SR. American Heart Association–Bugher Foundation Centers for Molecular Biology in the Cardiovascular System. *Circulation*. 1995;91: 487-493.

11. Roberts R. The Molecular Cardiology Laboratory at Baylor College of Medicine. *Cardiology*. 2002;98: 210-213.

12. Schneider MD. Training Grant in Molecular Cardiology, Grant 5T32HL007706-13 from the National Heart, Lung, and Blood Institute IRG:ZHLI. enGrant Scientific website. Accessed September 25, 2013. http://search.engrant.com/project/yP6zRq/training_grant_in_molecular_cardiology

13. Lynch EC. *Education in Internal Medicine: The Baylor Experience*. Houston, TX: Baylor College of Medicine; 2002:76.

14. Parish, Betsy (writer). Interview with: Dr. William A. Zoghbi (Methodist DeBakey Heart & Vascular Center, The Methodist Hospital, Houston, Texas). 2011 July.

15. Lynch EC. *Education in Internal Medicine: The Baylor Experience*. Houston, TX: Baylor College of Medicine; 2002:77.

16. Winters, William L. Jr. (Methodist DeBakey Heart & Vascular Center, The Methodist Hospital, Houston, Texas). Interview with: Dr. William Gaston (Methodist DeBakey Heart & Vascular Center, The Methodist Hospital, Houston, Texas). 2009 June.

17. Lynch EC. *Education in Internal Medicine: The Baylor Experience*. Houston, TX: Baylor College of Medicine; 2002:78.

18. King SB III. Percutaneous transluminal coronary angioplasty. *Am J Cardiol*. 1988;62: 2k-6k.

19. Hollman J. The limited impact of percutaneous coronary artery angioplasty on bypass surgery. *Intern J Cardiol*. 1988;20: 193-200.

20. By-pass effective against heart disease, surgeon says. *Lakeland Ledger*. May 10, 1982.

21. Moore TJ, York M. Hospitals review heart surgery death rates. *Knight-Ridder Newspapers*. December 22, 1986.

22. York M, Moore TJ. DeBakey: U.S. should limit bypass deaths by denying payments. *Knight-Ridder Newspapers*. September 23, 1986.

23. Voas S. DeBakey defends coronary bypass. *Pittsburgh Post-Gazette*. June 29, 1989.

24. Sibley MM. *The Methodist Hospital of Houston, Serving the World*. Austin, TX: Texas State Historical Association; 1989:205.

25. DeBakey ME, Lawrie GM, Glaeser DH. Patterns of atherosclerosis and their surgical significance. *Annals of Surgery*. 1985;201: 115.

26. Hurst JW. The value of coronary bypass surgery compared with medical therapy. *J Am Med Assoc*. 1989;261(14): 2118.

27. Winters, William L. Jr. (Methodist DeBakey Heart & Vascular Center, The Methodist Hospital, Houston, Texas). Interview with: Dr. Jack Roehm (Methodist DeBakey Heart & Vascular Center, The Methodist Hospital, Houston, Texas). 2006 Dec.

28. Winters, William L. Jr. (Methodist DeBakey Heart & Vascular Center, The Methodist Hospital, Houston, Texas). Interview with: Patty Chesnik, R.N. (Methodist DeBakey Heart & Vascular Center, The Methodist Hospital, Houston, Texas). 2011 Jan.

29. Winters WL Jr, Lawrie G. The pursuit of excellence: Michael E. DeBakey as mentor, colleague, and friend. *Methodist DeBakey Cardiovasc J*. 2008;4(2): 8-10.

30. Lawrie GM, Wyndham CRC, Krafchek J, Luck JC, Roberts R, DeBakey ME. Progress in the surgical treatment of cardiac arrhythmias. *J Am Med Assoc*. 1985;254(11): 1464-8.

31. Pacifico A, Bardy GH, Borggrefe M, et al., eds. *Implantable defibrillator therapy: a clinical guide*. New York, NY: Springer U.S.; 2002.

32. Chesebro JH, Knatterud G, Roberts R, et al. Thrombolysis in myocardial infarction (TIMI) trial, phase 1: a comparison between intravenous tissue plasminogen activator and intravenous streptokinase, clinical findings through hospital discharge. *Circulation*. 1987;76: 142-145.

33. Roberts R, Pratt CM. Value of intravenous streptokinase in acute myocardial infarction. *Int J Cardiol*. 1984;5: 637-741.

34. Relman AS. Intravenous thrombolysis in acute myocardial infarction. *New Engl J Med.* 1985;312(14): 915-916.

35. Winters, William L. Jr. (Methodist DeBakey Heart & Vascular Center, The Methodist Hospital, Houston, Texas). Interview with: Dr. William Spencer (Methodist DeBakey Heart & Vascular Center, The Methodist Hospital, Houston, Texas). 2004 Jun.

36. Roberts G, Ruplinger J, Spencer W, et al. Helicopter transport of patients with acute myocardial infarction. *Texas Medicine.* 1988;84(10): 35-37.

37. Fromm RE Jr, Hoskins E, Cronin L, Pratt CM, Spencer WH 3rd, Roberts R. Bleeding complications following initiation of thrombolytic therapy for acute myocardial infarction: a comparison of helicopter-transported and nontransported patients. *Ann Emerg Med.* 1991;20(8): 892-895.

38. Winters, William L. Jr. (Methodist DeBakey Heart & Vascular Center, The Methodist Hospital, Houston, Texas). Interview with: Dr. Albert E. Raizner (Methodist DeBakey Heart & Vascular Center, The Methodist Hospital, Houston, Texas). 2004 Oct.

39. Roehm JO Jr, Gianturco C, Barth MH, Wright KC. Percutaneous transcatheter filter for the inferior vena cava. A new device for treatment of patients with pulmonary embolism. *Radiology.* 1984;150(1): 255-257.

40. Roehm JO Jr. The bird's nest filter: a new percutaneous transcatheter inferior vena cava filter. *J Vasc Surg.* 1984;1(3): 498-501.

41. Roehm JO Jr, Johnsrude IS, Barth MH, Gianturco C. The bird's nest inferior vena cava filter: progress report. *Radiology.* 1988;168(3): 745-749.

42. Rodgers GP, Minor ST, Robinson K, et al. Adjuvant therapy for intracoronary stents. Investigations in atherosclerotic swine. *Circulation.* 1990;82(2): 560-569.

43. Rodgers GP, Minor ST, Robinson K, et al. The coronary artery response to implantation of a balloon-expandable flexible stent in the aspirin- and non-aspirin-treated swine model. *Am Heart J.* 1991;122(3 Pt 1): 640-647.

44. George BS, Voorhees WD 3rd, Roubin GS, et al. Multicenter investigation of coronary stenting to treat acute or threatened closure after percutaneous transluminal coronary angioplasty: clinical and angiographic outcomes. *J Am Coll Cardiol.* 1993;22(1): 135-143.

45. Sutton JM, Ellis SG, Roubin GS, et al. Major clinical events after coronary stenting. The multicenter registry of acute and elective Gianturco-Roubin stent placement. The Gianturco-Roubin Intracoronary Stent Investigator Group. *Circulation.* 1994;89(3): 1126-1137.

46. Winters, William L. Jr. (Methodist DeBakey Heart & Vascular Center, The Methodist Hospital, Houston, Texas). Interview with: Dr. Nadim M. Zacca (Methodist DeBakey Heart & Vascular Center, The Methodist Hospital, Houston, Texas). 2004.

47. Zacca NM, Raizner AE, Noon GP, et al. Treatment of symptomatic peripheral atherosclerotic disease with a rotational atherectomy device. *Am J Cardiol.* 1989;63: 77-80.

48. Raizner AE, Kaluza GL. Hula, pet rocks and intravascular brachytherapy. *Methodist DeBakey Cardiovasc J.* 2005;1(4): 7.

49. Kleiman NS, Raizner AE, Roberts R. Percutaneous transluminal coronary angioplasty: is what we see what we get? *J Am Coll Cardiol.* 1990;16(33): 576-577.

50. The Cardiology Working Group. Cardiology and the quality of medical practice. *J Am Med Assoc.* 1991;265: 482-485.

51. Hartzler GO. PTCA or aortocoronary bypass surgery: Perspectives. *Z. Kariol.* 1985;74(Sup 6): 111-115.

52. Fye WB. *American Cardiology, The History of a Specialty and Its College.* Baltimore and London: The Johns Hopkins University Press; 1996:305.

53. The TIMI Study Group. Comparison of invasive and conservative strategies after treatment with intravenous tissue plasminogen activator in acute myocardial infarction. *New Engl J Med.* 1989:320: 618-627.

54. Parish, Betsy (writer). Interview with: Dr. Miguel Quiñones (Methodist DeBakey Heart & Vascular Center, The Methodist Hospital, Houston, Texas). 2011 Apr.

Chapter 15: Prevention and Controversy, 1987-1988

1. Breo DL. Renowned surgery pioneer DeBakey still operating at 79. *Chicago Sun-Times.* September 11, 1988.
2. Scientists receive medals from Reagan. *The New York Times.* June 26, 1987.
3. DeBakey ME, Teitel ER. Device Profile: Use of the MicroMed® DeBakey VAD® for the treatment of end-stage heart failure. *Expert Rev Med Devices.* 2005;2(2): 137-140.
4. Electric Heart. NOVA online. PBS website. http://www.pbs.org/wgbh/nova/eheart. Created December 21, 1999. Accessed September 22, 2013.
5. Noon GP, Morley D, Irwin S, Benkowski R. Development and clinical application of the MicroMed DeBakey VAD. *Curr Opin Cardiol.* 2000;15: 166-171.
6. Braunwald E. On future directions for cardiology. The Paul D. White Lecture. *Circulation.* 1988;77(1): 13-32.
7. Breier LC. Heart to heart: Dr. DeBakey discusses effect of diet, stress and exercise on coronary health. *Chicago Sun-Times.* November 1, 1987.
8. Melnick JL, Dreesman GR, McCollum CH, Petrie BL, Burek J, DeBakey ME. Cytomegalovirus antigen within human arterial smooth muscle cells. *Lancet.* 1983;2: 644-647.
9. Gotto AM. Profiles in cardiology: Michael E. DeBakey. *Clin Cardiol.* 1991;14: 1007-1010.
10. Brody JE. Federal Heart Panel asks public to eat fewer fats. *The New York Times.* December 16, 1970.
11. Cohn V. Study is 'first conclusive proof' cutting cholesterol helps. *The Telegraph.* May 22, 1984.
12. Gotto AM Jr, Bierman EL, Connor WE, et al. Recommendations for treatment of hyperlipidemia in adults, A joint statement of the Nutrition Committee and the Council on Arteriosclerosis. *Circulation.* 1984;69(5): 1065A-1090A.
13. Lowering blood cholesterol to prevent heart diseases. NIH Consensus Development Conference Statement. *Nutr Rev.* 1985:43(9): 283-291.
14. National Cholesterol Education Program. National Heart Lung and Blood Institute website. http://www.nhlbi.nih.gov/about/ncep/ncep_pd.htm. Accessed September 22, 2013.
15. Mass cholesterol testing needed, says heart expert. *Associated Press.* March 16, 1985.
16. Greene JA. *Prescribing by Numbers: Drugs and the Definition of Disease.* Baltimore, MD: Johns Hopkins University Press; 2007:176.
17. DeBakey ME, Gotto AM Jr, Scott LW, Foreyt JP. *The Living Heart Diet.* New York, NY: Simon & Schuster; 1984.
18. Squires S. 'Living Heart Diet' satisfies the palate. *The Washington Post* news service, *Eugene Register-Guard.* March 20, 1985.
19. Research expects new center to give city major economic lift. *Houston Chronicle.* January 24, 1987.
20. Doctors call for cholesterol screen for the masses. *UPI; The Bryan Times.* May 23, 1987.
21. Results of a year-long study have far-reaching implications for the millions of Americans who don't know their cholesterol level. *PR Newswire.* May 20, 1987.
22. Steinberg D. An interpretive history of the cholesterol controversy: part 1. *J Lipid Res.* 2004;45: 1583-1593.
23. Moore TJ. The cholesterol myth. *The Atlantic.* September 1, 1989; cover.
24. Blakeslee S. Surgeon questions cholesterol role. *The New York Times.* April 9, 1987.
25. Zoler ML. Chez Eddy: elegant food that's easy on the heart. *The New York Times.* June 22, 1988.
26. Steinberg D. An interpretive history of the cholesterol controversy, part IV: The 1984 Coronary Primary Prevention Trial ends it–almost. *J Lipid Res.* 2006;47: 1-14.
27. Gotto AM Jr. The future of statins. *Dean's Bulletin,* Weill Cornel Medical College. January 28, 2008.
28. *Cholesterol Education Program: hearing before the Subcommittee on Health and the Enfironment of the Committee on Energy and Commerce, House of Representatives, One Hundred First Congress, first session, December 7, 1989.* Washington, D.C.: U.S. G.P.O.: 1990.
29. Corday E, Ryden L. Why some physicians have concerns about the cholesterol awareness program. *J Am Coll Cardiol.* 1989;13(2): 497-502.

30. Winters WL Jr. President's Page: the private practitioner and the college. *J Am Coll Cardiol.* 1990;16(1): 244-246.
31. Cholesterol drugs shown to cut healthy group's risk. *Associated Press.* November 13, 1997.
32. Downs JR, Beere PA, Whitney E, et al. Design & rationale of the Air Force/Texas Coronary Atherosclerosis Prevention Study (AFCAPS/TexCAPS). *Am J Cardiol.* 1997;80(3): 287-293.
33. Downs JR, Clearfield M, Weis S, et al. Primary prevention of acute coronary events with lovastatin in men and women with average cholesterol levels: results of AFCAPS/TexCAPS. Air Force/Texas Coronary Atherosclerosis Prevention Study. *J Am Med Assoc.* 1998;279(20): 1615-1622.
34. Kjekshus J, Pedersen TR, Reducing the risk of coronary events: evidence from the Scandinavian Simvastatin Survival Study (4S). *Am J Cardiol.* 1995;76(9): 64C-68C.
35. Steinberg D. An interpretive history of the cholesterol controversy, part V: The discovery of the statins and the end of the controversy. *J Lipid Res.* 2006;47: 1339-1351.
36. Winters WL Jr. President's Page: Inauguration Address. *J Am Coll Cardiol.* 1990; 15(5): 1193-1195.
37. Winters, William L. Jr. (Methodist DeBakey Heart & Vascular Center, The Methodist Hospital, Houston, Texas). Interview with: Dr. Miguel A. Quiñones (Methodist DeBakey Heart & Vascular Center, The Methodist Hospital, Houston, Texas). 2008 Feb.
38. Parish, Betsy (writer). Interview with: Dr. William A. Zoghbi (Methodist DeBakey Heart & Vascular Center, The Methodist Hospital, Houston, Texas). 2011 Jul.
39. Social Security Amendments, Section 1801, Title XVIII, Health Insurance for the aged and disabled, 42 USCS 1395:6811. Our Documents initiative Website: http://www.ourdocuments. gov/doc.php?flash=true&doc=99. Accessed September 25, 2013
40. Rich S. AMA assails Medicare payment scale. *The Washington Post.* June 11, 1991.
41. Frye RL. A visit to the physician payment review commission. *J Am Coll Cardiol.* 1992;19(5): 1114-1115.
42. Winters WL Jr. President's Page: RBRVS in review. *J Am Coll Cardiol.* 1991;17(4) 997-998.
43. Winters WL Jr. President's Page: ACC testimony of the increased demand for cardiovascular services. *J Am Coll Cardiol.* 1990;16(4): 1057-1059.
44. Freudenheim M. Government aims at heart test to trim expenses. *The New York Times.* November 25, 1990.
45. Winters, William L. Jr. (Methodist DeBakey Heart & Vascular Center, The Methodist Hospital, Houston, Texas). Interview with: Mr. Larry Mathis (D. **Peterson** & Associates, Houston, Texas). 2006 Apr.
46. Fye WB. *American Cardiology, The History of a Specialty and Its College.* Baltimore and London: Johns Hopkins University Press; 1996:325-326.
47. Culbertson RA, Lee PR. Medicare and physician autonomy. *Health Care Financ Rev.* 1996;18(2): 115-130.

Chapter 16: Adapting to the Evolution of Health Care, 1990s

1. Fye WB. *American Cardiology, The History of a Specialty and Its College.* Baltimore and London: The Johns Hopkins University Press; 1996:327.
2. Fox PD, Kongstvedt PR. The Origins of Managed Care. In: Kongstvedt PR, ed. *The Essentials of Managed Health Care.* 5th edition. Sudbury, MA: Jones & Bartlett; 2007:10.
3. Michael E. DeBakey, M.D., look who's talking health care reform now. *The New York Times.* October 8, 1995.
4. Thomas C. Health care: whom do you trust? *Los Angeles Times* Syndicate. February 24, 1994.
5. Dr. Michael E. DeBakey and Dr. William G. Anlyan, mismanaged health care editorial. *The Deseret News.* June 25, 1995.
6. Special Committee on Aging. *Hearing before the Special Committee on Aging, United States Senate, Ninety-Eighth Congress, Second Session.* Washington, D. C.: U.S. Government Printing Office; 1984.

7.   Rovner S. Medicare: cost of cost-cutting often life, death issue. *The Washington Post*. January 21, 1986.

8.   DeBakey ME. A surgical perspective. *Ann Surg*. 1991;213: 499-531.

9.   Myerson AR. It's a business. No, it's a religion. *The New York Times*. February 13, 1994.

10. Gratzer D. What ails health care. *The Public Interest*. March 22, 2005.

11. Mintz B. Methodist's CEO stepping down/Mathis to head hospital until successor found. *Houston Chronicle*. September 26, 1996.

12. Edmonds C, Hallman GL. CardioVascular Care Providers: a pioneer in bundled services, shared risk, and single payment. *Tex Heart Inst J*. 1995:22(1): 72-76.

13. Freudenheim M. Costs of bypass surgery studied. *The New York Times* News Service, *The Tuscaloosa News*. June 16, 1985.

14. Cooley DA. *100,000 Hearts, a Surgeon's Memoir*. Austin, TX: Dolph Briscoe Center for American History, The University of Texas at Austin; 2012:170.

15. Beachy D. Top doctors no longer charging top dollar/It's another breakthrough for Cooley. *Houston Chronicle*. July 29, 1990.

16. Cooley DA. *100,000 Hearts, a Surgeon's Memoir*. Austin, TX: Dolph Briscoe Center for American History, The University of Texas at Austin; 2012:169.

17. Herzlinger RE, ed. *Consumer-Driven Health Care: Implications for Providers, Payers, and Policymakers*. San Francisco, CA: John Wiley & Sons, Inc.; 2004:143.

18. Roberts WC. Michael Ellis DeBakey: a conversation with the editor. *Am J Cardiol*. 1997;79: 929-950.

19. Winters, William L. Jr. (Methodist DeBakey Heart & Vascular Center, The Methodist Hospital, Houston, Texas). Interview with: Dr. Jimmy F. Howell (Methodist DeBakey Heart & Vascular Center, The Methodist Hospital, Houston, Texas). 2006 Jan.

20. Eagle KA, Guyton RA, Davidoff R, et al. ACC/AHA Guidelines for Coronary Artery Bypass Graft Surgery: Executive Summary and Recommendations: A Report of the American College of Cardiology/American Heart Association Task Force on Practice Guidelines, (Committee to Revise the 1991 Guidelines for Coronary Artery Bypass Graft Surgery). *Circulation*. 1999;100: 1464-1480.

21. Winters, William L. Jr. (Methodist DeBakey Heart & Vascular Center, The Methodist Hospital, Houston, Texas). Interview with: Dr. Charles H. McCollum (Methodist DeBakey Heart & Vascular Center, The Methodist Hospital, Houston, Texas). 2005 Nov.

22. The legacy of leadership: Arthur C. Beall Jr., M.D. Baylor College of Medicine, Michael E. DeBakey Department of Surgery website. http://www.bcm.edu/surgery/index.cfm?pmid=15104. Accessed September 25, 2013.

23. Henly WS, Fitzgerald JB. Private practice of cardiac surgery at The Methodist Hospital. *Methodist DeBakey Cardiovasc J*. 2011;8(1): 19-20.

24. Nichols B. Renowned surgeon DeBakey nears 85, scorns retirement as he keeps hectic pace. *The Dallas Morning News*. September 5, 1993.

25. Lawrie GM. Patient in the spotlight: the rewards and challenges of treating VIP patients. Texas Surgical Associates website. http://www.texassurgical.com/media.html. Created March 1998. Accessed September 26, 2013.

26. Dinis da Gama A. A simplified open surgical technique for the management of thoracoabdominal aortic aneurysms. Presented at: the 38th Annual Symposium on Vascular and Endovascular Issues, Techniques, and Horizons. New York, NY; 2011 Nov 16-20.

27. Crawford ES, Crawford JL. *Diseases of the Aorta: Including an Atlas of Angiographic Pathology and Surgical Treatment*. Baltimore, MD: Lippincott Williams & Wilkins; 1984.

28. Pearce W. Diseases of the aorta: an atlas of angiographic pathology and surgical technique. *Arch Surg*. 1986;121(7): 856.

29. Hoover B. Renowned heart doc to speak at two events. *Lubbock Avalanche-Journal*. March 22, 2012.

30. Yao JST, Pearce WH, eds. *Aneurysms: New Findings and Treatments*. Norwalk, CT: Appleton & Lange; 1994:19.

31. Ernst CB. In Memoriam: E. Stanley Crawford, MD, 1922-1992. *J Vasc Surg*. 1993; 17(2): 618-619.

32. Safi HJ. In Tribute: Ernest Stanley Crawford, M.D. *Methodist DeBakey Cardiovasc J*. 2011;7(1): 53-54.

33. Cooley DA. In Memoriam: George Cooper Morris Jr. *Tex Heart Inst J*. 1996;23(4): 255-256.

34. Lawrie G, Winters WL Jr. The pursuit of excellence: Michael E. DeBakey as mentor, colleague, and friend. *Methodist DeBakey Cardiovasc J*. 2008;4(2): 8-10.

35. Winters, William L. Jr. (Methodist DeBakey Heart & Vascular Center, The Methodist Hospital, Houston, Texas). Interview with: Dr. George Noon (Methodist DeBakey Heart & Vascular Center, The Methodist Hospital, Houston, Texas). 2008 Jul.

36. Fackelmann K. Measuring a teacher's reach by his students' stature. *USA Today*. November 2, 1998.

37. McCollum CH. The distinguished service award medal for the Society of Vascular Surgery, 1999: Michael Ellis DeBakey. *J Vasc Surg*. 2000;31(2): 406-409.

38. SoRelle R. DeBakey will relinquish surgery helm at Baylor. *Houston Chronicle*. January 1, 1993.

39. Mears WR. Clinton's conference goes into overtime. *Associated Press*. December 21, 1992.

40. Beachy D. Health of the nation/Some will reap windfall, some will suffer loss/Smaller firms will feel pinch of health plan. *Houston Chronicle*. September 19, 1993.

41. Beachy D. Two Houston hospitals plan big job cuts/Health care reform. *Houston Chronicle*. September 5, 1993.

42. Zoler ML. Chez Eddy: elegant food that's easy on the heart. *The New York Times*. June 22, 1988.

43. Gotto AM Jr, Roe H, Fraser B. Manger and the staff of Chez Eddy Restaurant of the Methodist Hospital System. In: Gotto AM, ed. *The Chez Eddy Living Heart Cookbook*. Upper Saddle River, NJ: Prentice Hall, Inc.; 1991:Foreword.

44. Criswell A. The best recipes of '93. *Houston Chronicle*. January 12, 1994.

45. Beachy D. Under the knife/Doctors, hospitals and patients feel sting as managed health care plans cut costs by cutting choices. *Houston Chronicle*. February 28, 1993.

46. Montgomery J. '95 Review/The Year's Top Stories/Houston thrived in some economic sectors, but many companies continued cutbacks. *Houston Chronicle*. December 31, 1995.

47. Parish, Betsy (writer). Interview with: Dr. William L. Winters Jr. (Methodist DeBakey Heart & Vascular Center, The Methodist Hospital, Houston, Texas). 2012 Apr.

48. Thurston JM. *Death of Compassion: The endangered doctor-patient relationship*. Waco, TX: WRS Publishing; 1996:11.

49. Gillum RF. Trends in acute myocardial infarction and coronary heart disease death in the United States. *J Am Coll Cardiol*. 1994;23(6): 1273-1277.

50. Ryan TJ, Bauman WB, Kennedy JW, et al. ACC/AHA Task Force Report: guidelines for percutaneous transluminal coronary angioplasty. *J Am Coll Cardiol*. 1993;22(7): 2033-2054.

51. Beachy D. Admissions to hospitals show decline/outpatient surgery, shorter stays cited. *Houston Chronicle*. April 6, 1993.

52. Winters, William L. Jr. (Methodist DeBakey Heart & Vascular Center, The Methodist Hospital, Houston, Texas). Interview with: Dr. William Spencer (Methodist DeBakey Heart & Vascular Center, The Methodist Hospital, Houston, Texas). 2008 Jun.

Chapter 17: Changing of the Guard, 1994-1996

1. Speech by Henry Kissinger, Fourteenth Annual Ashbrook Memorial Dinner, John M. Ashbrook Center for Public Affairs, Ashland University. September 11, 1997. http://archive.is/qwju. Accessed September 25. 2013.

2. Sibley MM. *The Methodist Hospital of Houston, Serving the World*. Austin, TX: Texas State Historical Association; 1989:178.

3. Parish, Betsy (writer). Interview with: Dr. Albert E. Raizner (Methodist DeBakey Heart & Vascular Center, The Methodist Hospital, Houston, Texas). 2012 Feb.

4. Flatow I. Remembering heart surgeon Michael DeBakey; Talk of the Nation transcript, *National Public Radio*. July 18, 2008.
5. Reeves P. 'Cardiovascular Tolstoy' who is Boris's best hope. *The Independent*. November 4, 1996.
6. Yeltsin to leave hospital in days. *Associated Press*, Moscow. November 11, 1996.
7. Deener B. 9 Texas hospitals make list of best. *Dallas Morning News*. July 11, 1994.
8. Estill J. Revise Medicare heart surgery program: report. *Associated Press*. August 18, 1987.
9. Hallman GL, Emonds C. Integrated cardiac care. *Ann Thorac Surg*. 1995;60: 1486-1489.
10. Winters, William L. Jr. (Methodist DeBakey Heart & Vascular Center, The Methodist Hospital, Houston, Texas). Interview with: Dr. William Spencer (Methodist DeBakey Heart & Vascular Center, The Methodist Hospital, Houston, Texas). 2004 Jun.
11. Winters, William L. Jr. (Methodist DeBakey Heart & Vascular Center, The Methodist Hospital, Houston, Texas). Interview with: Dr. William Gaston (Methodist DeBakey Heart & Vascular Center, The Methodist Hospital, Houston, Texas). 2009 June.
12. Payne C. Methodist makes plans for medical transplant; city's largest hospital purses long-term goal to become diversified health care delivery system. *Houston Business Journal*. June 10, 1994.
13. Baird J, Vara R. Methodist-St. Luke's deal on hold/Merger hits snag in negotiations. *Houston Chronicle*. February 3, 1995.
14. Baird J. Hospitals preparing for new era/More mergers lie ahead in Houston. *Houston Chronicle*. September 30, 1994.
15. Medical chancellor to step down. *Austin American Statesman*. December 20, 1995.
16. Mintz B. Methodist to create network/Hospital targets suburbs for community health care centers. *Houston Chronicle*. June 7, 1996.
17. Mintz B. Methodist CEO's stepping down/Mathis to lead hospital until successor found. *Houston Chronicle*. September 26, 1996.
18. Darwin J. Methodist, Baylor create joint management council. *Houston Business Journal*. October 6, 1996.
19. DeMaria AN, Lee TH, Leon DF, et al. Effect of managed care on cardiovascular specialists: involvement, attitudes and practice adaptations. *J Am Coll Cardiol*. 1996:28(7): 1884-1895.
20. Winters, William L. Jr. (Methodist DeBakey Heart & Vascular Center, The Methodist Hospital, Houston, Texas). Interview with: Dr. Antonio M. Gotto (The Methodist Hospital, Houston, Texas).
21. Altman LK. In Moscow in 1996, a doctor's visit changed history. *The New York Times*. May 1, 2007.
22. Gotto AM Jr. Remembering Dr. Michael DeBakey. *WeillCornellMedicine*, the magazine of Weill Cornell Graduate School of Medical Sciences. 2008 Fall: 3.

Chapter 18: A Coming Together, 1994-2001

1. Kleinke JD. Medicine's industrial revolution. *The Wall Street Journal*. August 21, 1995.
2. Mathis LL. *The Mathis Maxims: Lessons in Leadership*. Houston, TX: Leadership Press; 2001:174.
3. Fox PD, Wasserman J. Academic medical centers and managed care: uneasy partners. *Health Affairs*. 1993;12(1): 85-93.
4. Mathis LL. *The Mathis Maxims: Lessons in Leadership*. Houston, TX: Leadership Press; 2001:175.
5. DeBakey ME, Anlyan WG. Mismanaged health care, editorial. *The Deseret News*. June 25, 1995.
6. Grover FL. The bright future of cardiothoracic surgery in the era of changing healthcare delivery. *Ann Thorac Surg*. 1996;61: 499-510.
7. Mintz B. Methodist Hospital will affiliate with primary physicians. *Houston Chronicle*. April 26, 1996.
8. Leading C.V. surgeons form group practice to expand programs throughout community. Texas Surgical Associates Press Release. November 18, 1997.
9. Mintz B. Surgeons transplant practice to suburbs/DeBakey heart team members leave Baylor. *Houston Chronicle*. July 12, 1997.

10. Becker ER, Morris DC, Culler SD, et al. The changing healthcare market and how it has influenced the treatment of cardiovascular disease, part I. *Am J Manag Care*. 1999; 5(9): 1119-1124.

11. Noon GP. Michael Ellis DeBakey, M.D., September 7, 1908 – July 11, 2008. *Methodist DeBakey Cardiovasc J*. 2008;4(4): 22-24.

12. Altman LK. The doctor's world; Dr. DeBakey at 90: stringent standards and a steady hand. *The New York Times*. September 1, 1998.

13. Nichols B. Reports of DeBakey retirement. *Albany Times Union*. November 29, 1998.

14. DeBakey M. Rx for the health care system. *The Wall Street Journal*. October 8, 1998.

15. Brooks K. Kindest heart cut? `Minimal invasion'. *Albany Times Union*; Knight Ridder News Service. August 4, 1998.

16. AHA Statistical Update: Heart Disease and Stroke Statistics—2012 Update: A Report From the American Heart Association. Circulation website. http://circ.ahajournals.org/content/125/1/e2. Created December 15, 2011. Accessed September 25, 2013

17. Noon GP. Evolution of surgical treatment of coronary artery occlusive disease. *J Am Med Assoc*. 2009;301(9): 970-971.

18. Cohn WE, de La Torre R, Liddicoat JR. Is the future of cardiac surgery in the hands of the interventional cardiologist? *Heart Surg Forum*. 2001;4(4): 297-300.

19. Winters, William L. Jr. (Methodist DeBakey Heart & Vascular Center, The Methodist Hospital, Houston, Texas). Interview with: Dr. William H. Spencer III (Methodist DeBakey Heart & Vascular Center, The Methodist Hospital, Houston, Texas). 2004 Jun.

20. Lakkis NM, Nagueh SF, Kleiman NS, et al. Echocardiography-guided ethanol septal reduction for hypertrophic obstructive cardiomyopathy. *Circulation*. 1998;98: 1750-1755.

21. Cardiac treatment inducing small heart attack can be helpful, doctors say. *Chicago Tribune*. November 18, 1996.

22. Harvin S. Dr. William Spencer, heart doctor brings innovative procedure–and caring–to MUSC. *The Post and Courier*. November 3, 2001.

23. Fernandes VL, Nielsen C, Nagueh SF, et al. Follow-up of alcohol septal ablation for symptomatic hypertrophic obstructive cardiomyopathy: The Baylor and Medical University of South Carolina Experience 1996 to 2007. *J Am Coll Cardiol Intv*. 2008;1(5): 561-570.

24. Preslon TA. Medicine: marketing an operation. *Atlantic Monthly*. 1984 Dec:32-40.

25. *Coronary artery bypass graft (CABG) surgery, assuring quality while controlling Medicare costs*. Office of Inspector General. U.S. Department of Health and Human Services website. http://oig.hhs. gov/oei/reports/oai-09-86-00076.pdf. Accessed September 25, 2013.

26. Cromwell J, Dayhoff DA, McCall NT, et al. *Medicare Participating Heart Bypass Center Demonstration, Extramural Report*. Health Care Finance Administration; Centers for Medicare & Medicaid Services website. http://www.cms.gov/Research-Statistics-Data-and-Systems/Statistics-Trends-and-Reports/Reports/downloads/oregon2_1998_3.pdf. Accessed September 2013.

27. *Bundled Payment: An AHA Research Synthesis Report*. Chicago, IL: American Hospital Association Committee on Research; 2010.

28. Parish, Betsy (writer). Interview with: Drs. Albert E. Raizner and William L. Winters Jr. (Methodist DeBakey Heart & Vascular Center, The Methodist Hospital, Houston, Texas). 2012 Feb.

29. Whitelaw NA, Warden GL. Reexamining the delivery system as part of Medicare reform. *Health Affairs*. 1999;18(1): 132-143.

30. Paone G, Higgins RSD, Spencer T, Silverman NA. Enrollment in the Health Alliance Plan HMO is not an independent risk factor for coronary artery bypass graft surgery. *Circulation*. 1995;92(9): 69-72.

31. Parish, Betsy (writer). Interview with: Mr. Ron Girotto (former CEO of The Methodist Health Care System, Houston, Texas). 2012 Aug.

32. Porter ME, Olmsted Teisberg E. How physicians can change the future of health care. *J Am Med Assoc*. 2007;297(10): 1103-1111.

33. Parish, Betsy (writer). Interview with: Mrs. Debra Feigin Sukin (St. Luke's Episcopal Health System, Houston, Texas). 2011 Nov.

34. Wittrup RD. On picking a doctor. Health Care Anew Blog. http://healthcareanew.blogspot.com/search?q=methodist+health+care. Created December 04, 2007. Accessed September 25, 2013.
35. Parish, Betsy (writer). Interview with: Dr. Albert E. Raizner (Methodist DeBakey Heart & Vascular Center, The Methodist Hospital, Houston, Texas). 2011 Aug.
36. Parish, Betsy (writer) Interview with: Mrs. Lynn M. Schroth (former executive vice president for The Methodist Hospital, Houston, Texas). 2012 Aug.
37. Wendler R. Another DeBakey milestone. *Texas Medical Center News*. March 15, 2001.

Chapter 19: A Parting of the Way, 2004

1. Tropical Storm Allison Overview. Harris County Flood Control District website. http://www.hcfcd.org/F_tsa_overview.html. Accessed September 27, 2013.
2. Dr. Feigin reports on flood damage and recovery. The Portal. 2001;2(3): 2.
3. Turner A. Allison's Legacy / The figures are numbing: 22 deaths, $5 billion in area damage. One year ago, the nation's worst tropical storm left its mark but didn't dampen Houston's spirit. Houston Chronicle. June 2, 2002.
4. All Methodist buildings flooded by storm reopen. Houston Chronicle. July 17, 2001.
5. Lezon D. Patients and patience / Power failures force hospitals to scramble staff. Houston Chronicle. June 11, 2001.
6. Rother K. Surviving the flood: Texas Medical Center's unsinkable spirit. Heartwire. July 30, 2001.
7. Williams S. Be prepared, unpredictability of mother nature - and human nature - prompts more hospitals to examine and upgrade their emergency response systems. Nurse Week News. January 30, 2003.
8. Parish, Betsy (writer). Interview with: Dr. Mark Entman (DeBakey Heart Center, The Methodist Hospital, Houston, Texas). 2011 Oct.
9. Of Note: Methodist upgrading its cardiac cath labs. Houston Chronicle. January 23, 2001.
10. Parish, Betsy (writer). Interview with: Drs. Albert E. Raizner and William L. Winters Jr. (Methodist DeBakey Heart & Vascular Center, The Methodist Hospital, Houston, Texas). 2012 Feb.
11. The Methodist DeBakey Heart Center Market Plan. Houston, TX: The Methodist Hospital; 2001.
12. Parish, Betsy (writer). Interview with: Dr. Lynn M. Schroth (former executive vice president for The Methodist Hospital, Houston, Texas). 2012 Aug.
13. Christian C. Threat to medicine's lifeblood / Methodist Hospital will end year in red /U.S. funding cutbacks cited as reason. Houston Chronicle. October 24, 1999.
14. Darwin J. Budget act keeps hospitals off balance. Houston Business Journal. October 17, 1999.
15. Wollam A. Methodist sells long-struggling HMO to national, publicly traded health insurer. Houston Business Journal. February 3, 2002.
16. Asin S. Change in leadership [press release]. Houston, TX: The Methodist Hospital; September 28, 2001.
17. Kreimer S. Methodist hospital, CEO part ways out of the blue. Houston Chronicle. September 29, 2001.
18. Lezon D. Woman, 57, resting after rare surgery. Houston Chronicle. November 16, 2000.
19. Carreau M. DeBakey is still trailblazing. Houston Chronicle. June 29, 2002.
20. Fairchild E. The Methodist Hospital is ranked among the country's top centers in 10 specialties [press release]. Houston, TX: The Methodist Hospital; July 17, 2003.
21. Parish, Betsy (writer). Interview with: Mr. Ron Girotto (former CEO of The Methodist Health Care System, Houston, Texas). 2012 Aug.
22. Schlegel D. To the leading edge' / Methodist expects huge expansion to propel hospital. Houston Chronicle. February 11, 2004.
23. Wendler R. New research institute slated to open in 2009. Texas Medical Center News. February 15, 2007.

24. Swartz M. Till death do us part. Texas Monthly. March 2005.
25. Ackerman T. Behind the split / Uncertainty, hope as giants part ways / Baylor's choice for a new partner put plenty at stake. Houston Chronicle. February 22, 2005.
26. Schlegel D, Ackerman T. Baylor, Methodist in historic split / St. Luke's picked as medical affiliate. Houston Chronicle. April 22, 2004.
27. Parish, Betsy (writer). Interview with: Dr. Miguel Quiñones (Methodist DeBakey Heart & Vascular Center, The Methodist Hospital, Houston, Texas). 2011 Apr.
28. Baylor College of Medicine, St. Luke's sign new affiliation agreement [press release]. Houston, TX: Baylor College of Medicine; April 22, 2004. http://www.bcm.edu/pa/affiliationagreement.htm
29. Ackerman T. Methodist Hospital pairing with Cornell / New partners say distance not a problem. Houston Chronicle. June 24, 2004.
30. Manners M, Narvaez F. Weill-CU and NewYork-Presbyterian ally with large Houston hospital. Cornell Chronicle. July 1, 2004.
31. Ackerman T. Baylor, Methodist battle to employ doctors, Longtime partners face new era as medical rivals. Houston Chronicle. June 14, 2004.
32. Ackerman T. Baylor's pathology chief takes Methodist offer/Doctor will lead hospital's new research institute. Houston Chronicle. July 13, 2004.

Chapter 20: The Fork in the Road, 2004-2008

1. Nissimov R. Letter warned of 'crisis' if Baylor, hospital split. Houston Chronicle. April 30, 2004.
2. Parish, Betsy (writer). Interview with: Dr. William L. Winters Jr. (Methodist DeBakey Heart & Vascular Center, The Methodist Hospital, Houston, Texas). 2012 Aug.
3. Parish, Betsy (writer). Interview with: Dr. Miguel A. Quiñones (Methodist DeBakey Heart & Vascular Center, The Methodist Hospital, Houston, Texas). 2011 Apr.
4. Ackerman T. Baylor president says faculty lured / New Methodist Hospital partner Cornell denies recruiting claims. Houston Chronicle. January 15, 2005.
5. Winters WL Jr. Attitudes are contagious. Methodist DeBakey Cardiovasc J. 2005;1(3): 1.
6. DeBakey ME. The centers of excellence concept. Journal Methodist DeBakey Cardiovasc J. 2005;1(1): 1.
7. Berger E, Ackerman T. Behind the split / Methodist taps talent from Baylor / School worries as hospital lures some staff from its former partner to research institute. Houston Chronicle. March 20, 2005.
8. Ackerman T. It's a good first step / Baylor and Methodist agree to a training contract after an impasse. Houston Chronicle. December 11, 2004.
9. Winters, William L. Jr. (Methodist DeBakey Heart & Vascular Center, The Methodist Hospital, Houston, Texas). Interview with: Dr. Miguel A. Quiñones (Methodist DeBakey Heart & Vascular Center, The Methodist Hospital, Houston, Texas). 2008 Feb.
10. Winters WL Jr. Portrait of a chairman. Methodist DeBakey Cardiovasc J. 2006;2(1): 15.
11. ACGME program requirements for graduate medical education in cardiovascular disease (internal medicine). ACGME website. http://www.acgme.org/acgmeweb/Portals/0/PFAssets/2013-PR-FAQ-PIF/141_cardiovascular_disease_int_med_07132013.pdf. Accessed September 29, 2013.
12. Wendler R. DeBakey recovering, library and museum named in his honor. Texas Medical Center News. November 1, 2006.
13. Altman LK. The doctor's world / The man on the table devised the surgery. The New York Times. December 25, 2006.
14. Winters WL Jr. In memory of Dr. Don W. Chapman. Methodist DeBakey Cardiovasc J. 2007;3(2): 1.
15. Winters, William L. Jr. (Methodist DeBakey Heart & Vascular Center, The Methodist Hospital, Houston, Texas). Interview with Dr. Michael E. DeBakey (Methodist DeBakey Heart & Vascular Center, The Methodist Hospital, Houston, Texas). 2007 Dec.

16. Roberts WC. Michael Ellis DeBakey: A conversation with the editor. Am J Cardiol. 1997;79: 929-950.

17. Sorrel AL. Heart surgeon pioneer wins highest civilian honor, A Congressional Gold Medal has been awarded to Michael E. DeBakey, MD, whose medical career spans 60 years. American Medical News. May 19, 2008.

18. Angelle D. An American pioneer. Leading Medicine. 2003;2(3): 11-17.

19. American correction used to repair a mitral valve. News-Medical.Net website. http://www.news-medical.net/news/2007/08/17/28861.aspx. Created August 17, 2007. Accessed September 29, 2013.

20. Dunkin BJ Methodist Institute for Technology, Innovation, and Education – MITIE – an educational home for health care professionals. Methodist DeBakey Cardiovasc J. 2009;5(2): 10-12.

21. Robotic heart repair. NewsChannel 5 WTVF-TV, Nashville, TN. January 25, 2008.

22. Ackerman T. DeBakey approaches 100 with renewed vigor. Houston Chronicle. March 9, 2008.

23. Coleman AP. DeBakey VAD beat goes on at international clinical trials. Houston Business Journal. January 22, 1999.

24. History of MicroMed and the DeBakey VAD®. MicroMed Cardiovascular Inc. website. http://www.micromedcv.com/eu/index.php/Media/technology-history.html. Accessed September 28, 2013.

25. $2.8 Million grant renewed for development of "pulse-less" total artificial heart. Business Wire. August 6, 2009.

26. Frazier OH. Michael E. DeBakey, 1908 to 2008. J Thorac Cardiovasc Surg. 2008:136(4): 809-811.

27. Williams L. Congressional Gold Medal for DeBakey heads to President Bush [press release]. Houston, TX: Baylor College of Medicine; October 2, 2007.

28. Powell SM. Houston's DeBakey gets congressional medal in D.C., Famed surgeon calls for lawmakers to use VA system as a model for health care reform. Houston Chronicle. April 23, 2008.

29. DeBakey ME. Dr. DeBakey's Comments [press release]. Houston, TX: Baylor College of Medicine; April 23, 2008.

30. Ackerman T. Legendary heart surgeons DeBakey, Cooley mend rift, Top heart surgeons Cooley and DeBakey put their decades-old feud to rest. Houston Chronicle. November 6, 2007.

31. Ackerman T. DeBakey inducts Cooley into his surgical society / putting the past to rest bond between top surgeons grows. Houston Chronicle. May 3, 2008.

32. DeBakey ME, Gotto AM. The Living Heart in the 21st Century. Amherst, NY: Prometheus Books; 2012:1.

33. Hassan A. Colleagues, officials salute legendary Dr. DeBakey. Houston Chronicle. July 12, 2008.

34. Ackerman T, Feibel C. Remembering Dr. Michael DeBakey / `His patients felt his concern' / Public viewing at City Hall draws diverse mourners. Houston Chronicle. July 16, 2008.

35. DeBakey S, DeBakey L. Michael E. DeBakey, M.D., and the collegial family triad. CV Network. 2008;7(3): 6-9.

36. Mattox KL. Michael E. DeBakey: the consummate leader. Methodist DeBakey Cardiovasc J. 2009:5(2): 32.

37. DeBakey L, DeBakey S. Michael E. DeBakey, M.D.: beloved brother, master mentor, compatible colleague, professional paragon. Methodist DeBakey Cardiovasc J. 2009:5(3): 49-56

INDEX

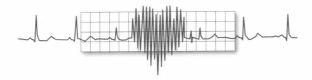

ACKNOWLEDGEMENTS

William L. Winters Jr., MD, MACC

The inspiration for this chronicle came to me one day several years ago when Dr. Don W. Chapman and I were philosophizing about the extraordinary changes that had taken place in the practice of medicine, and in particular the advances in cardiovascular medicine over the past 60 years, most all of which we had each experienced or participated in personally.

Acutely aware that many other physicians on The Methodist Hospital medical staff also were active participants in this exceptional history, we knew a story was there to be told. It was then I began to conduct video interviews with long-standing members of the medical staff. Starting with Dr. Chapman and ultimately including Drs. DeBakey and Cooley, among more than 70 others, it was an effort to chronicle some of that story for our medical archives to prevent it being lost from memory.

It was about that time that Betsy Parish, a longtime friend as well as a patient of mine, finished writing her book, *Legacy, 50 Years of Loving Care at Texas Children's Hospital 1954 – 2004*. After its publication in 2006, I suggested to her that we might collaborate on this project – A History of Cardiovascular Surgery and Medicine at The Methodist Hospital in Houston. She was receptive, and so we began.

Our reference sources were many, including some of the 70-plus video interviews that I have conducted with The Methodist Hospital medical staff over the past seven years, the scientific medical literature, the lay press, my personal experience and, most importantly, Betsy Parish's interviews with selected individuals and her unique ability to plumb the internet and the archives at the John P. McGovern Historical Collections and Research Center at the Houston Academy of Medicine – Texas Medical Center Library for pertinent information. She has my lasting appreciation for her literary skills and gratitude for persistence and patience in the face of inevitable and unavoidable delay and changing winds. Her indomitable spirit overcame all.

We wish to acknowledge with special appreciation the financial support of the John S. Dunn Sr. Endowment for Cardiovascular Research and Education, the Houston Methodist Foundation, and Houston Methodist Hospital.

For their assistance in reviewing sections of this work as it developed, we wish to thank Drs. George P. Noon, Mark Entman, Richard Cashion, Miguel Quiñones, Albert Raizner, Daniel Jackson, Jimmy F. Howell, Robert Roberts, James B. Young, Roy Sessions, and William H. Spencer III. We also are indebted to the input provided by John Bookout, Susan Coulter, Ron Girotto, Larry Mathis, and Lynn Schroth. Our gratitude goes to Dr. William C. Roberts for writing the Foreword and to Drs. Antonio M. Gotto Jr. and George P. Noon for contributing their thoughts for the "Reflections of Two Principals."

I am personally indebted to the following for their solicited reviews of the completed manuscript: Drs. Catherine DeAngelis, Bruce Fye, James B. Young, Robert Roberts, Roy Sessions, Richard Wainerdi, PhD and Ron Girotto and Larry Mathis.

We also wish to thank JoAnne Pospisil, Archives Director at Baylor College of Medicine, Houston Methodist Hospital librarian Linné Girouard, Jean Nelson, and Denny Angelle of the Houston Methodist Hospital Foundatiion for their much-needed assistance in photograph research.

I am indebted to Lois DeBakey for her reading a pre-publication draft of this book. It was delivered to her at a late stage of development for a variety of reasons. But I did not think it appropriate to send it to publication without her having seen it. She did kindly read and review it, without putting her imprimatur upon it, citing differences of style and substance throughout—some of which we reconciled and some of which we did not. Ultimately, we agreed to disagree. I admit to this with some trepidation because of potential fallout from our readers who may recognize her as "the conscience of American medical letters,"[1] or to those who subscribe to the philosophy of Dr. Robert Moser, former editor of the Journal of the American Medical Association, "To put it simply, Dr. Lois DeBakey has done more to bring literacy to medical writing than any other person in the country. If you write well and are an honest person, she rewards you; but if not, she can come down on you like a ton of bricks."[2] Well, there are bricks on the ground. Perhaps there will be some future author(s) who, in different times, will enlarge upon the enormous influence of Dr. Michael E. DeBakey's sisters on his life and career as well as the extraordinary careers they have fashioned for themselves in the literacy world of medical communication.

And there will be future authors in years to come who will likely review part or all of *Houston Hearts* from a different point of view, especially the account of the historic dissolution of the Baylor College of Medicine/The Methodist Hospital fifty-year collaboration and its consequences.

Remember as you read *Houston Hearts*, there is a bias rule that says every source is biased in some way. Historians are not free from bias, though usually not intentional, but may be accused of selective retelling of the facts. The authors have striven to minimize personal bias and the bias of others, and to respect the sentiments of those still living who were involved. Some aspects of more recent events await a future telling of the story.

Our appreciation goes to James Shanahan, photographer, who voluntarily contributed many hours to the taping of more than 70 video interviews since 2004, and to the many physicians from the cardiology and CV medical staff who participated. Linné Girouard, Houston Methodist Hospital librarian, kept us safe from interruptions in the Ory Room during the interviews.

A special thank you to Anne Robbins, archivist at Houston Methodist Hospital, who, alone and in her spare time, spent endless hours transcribing the interviews for all posterity to read. The DVDs with the recorded interviews and transcriptions are in safe keeping in The Methodist Hospital Library for all who care to view or read them.

The one who deserves the most praise is my priceless secretary, Kathleen Kindel, who, without a single complaint, ever, has typed and retyped endless versions of my myriad recollections, references, and rhyming rhetoric for Betsy Parish to incorporate into the final manuscript.

Responsibility and kudos for the final edit of the manuscript goes to Shelley Norden Barnes, longtime editor of the Methodist DeBakey Cardiovascular Journal.

Last, but certainly not least, I wish to thank my very loving wife of 60 years, Barbara, for her patience in looking endlessly at my back during the last few years as I worked on this monumental project at my desk at home.

---

1. Manning, PR, DeBakey, L., *Medicine, Preserving the Passion in the 21st Century*, Springer-Verlag. NY. 1987.

2. Wendler, R. DeBakey Sisters Teach Logic and Language of Medicine, *Texas Medical Center News*. May 2008

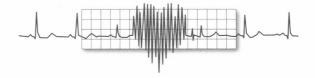

ABOUT THE AUTHORS

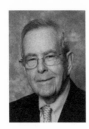

William L. Winters Jr., MD, BS, MS, MACC

Dr. Winters has been a member of the Methodist DeBakey Heart & Vascular Center since 1968, 33 years before its formal, 2001 inception. Board-certified in Internal Medicine with specialty certification in cardiovascular diseases, he is a senior attending staff member in the Department of Cardiology at The Methodist Hospital and holds the John S. Dunn Foundation Chair for Clinical Cardiovascular Research and Education. He serves as Editor in Chief of *The Methodist DeBakey Cardiovascular Journal*, and Director of The Methodist Hospital Education Institute. Dr. Winters attended Princeton University and then Northwestern University where he received his Bachelor of Science and medical degree, earning membership in Alpha Omega Alpha for top scholastic honors. He completed a medical residency and cardiology fellowship at Temple Medical School in Philadelphia. At the invitation of Dr. Don W. Chapman, Dr. Winters relocated to Houston in 1968 and joined "The Chapman Group" in their cardiovascular medicine practice. With him he brought to Houston his knowledge of echocardiography, a "then-new" diagnostic test to determine heart structure and function. In 1980, in conjunction with Drs. Albert Raizner and John Lewis, he was among the first to perform angioplasties in Houston. Dr. Winters holds a number of prestigious academic titles including Master of the American College of Cardiology, President of the American College of Cardiology (1990-91), and President of The Methodist Hospital Medical Staff. A past

President of the American Heart Association, Texas Affiliate, he has been consistently named among the "Best Doctors in America" and recognized by H Texas Magazine as one of Houston's Top Doctors. Dr. Winters has been the recipient of many awards, including the John W. Overstreet Award from The Methodist Hospital Medical Staff, and the first George P. Noon, MD, Award, presented in 2011. *Houston Hearts* is his first book.

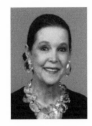

Betsy Parish

Betsy Parish is a former newspaper columnist who also had a lengthy career as a marketing and public relations executive in the retail and hospitality industries. She is a fifth generation descendent of one of the pioneering families who settled Houston in 1838. Her grandfather, Dr. E. Freeman Robbins, was a 1911 alumnus of Baylor University College of Medicine in Dallas who became the first intern at Houston's Baptist Sanitarium and Hospital and practiced in Houston for more than six decades. The author of *Legacy: Fifty Years of Loving Care, Texas Children's Hospital, 1954-2004*, published in 2008, Ms. Parish is a past President of the Friends of the Texas Medical Center Library and continues to serve on its board of directors. She is an advocate of all efforts to document and preserve the history of Houston health care.